Michael Chapman · Gedis Grudzinskas
Tim Chard (Eds.)

THE EMBRYO

Normal and Abnormal Development and Growth

With 91 Figures

Springer-Verlag
London Berlin Heidelberg New York
Paris Tokyo Hong Kong

M.G. Chapman, MBBS, MRCOG
Department of Obstetrics and Gynaecology,
Guy's Hospital,
London SE1 9RT, UK

J.G. Grudzinskas, MD, MRCOG, FRACOG
Academic Unit of Obstetrics and Gynaecology,
The London Hospital, Whitechapel,
London E1 1BB, UK

T. Chard, MD, FRCOG
Academic Unit of Reproductive Physiology,
St Bartholomew's Hospital Medical College,
London EC1A 7BE, UK

ISBN 3-540-19630-7 Springer-Verlag Berlin Heidelberg New York
ISBN 0-387-19630-7 Springer-Verlag New York Berlin Heidelberg

British Library Cataloguing in Publication Data
The Embryo.
1. Man. Embryos
I. Chapman, Michael *1949–*
612.64
ISBN 3-540-19630-7 W. Germany

Library of Congress Cataloging-in-Publication Data
The Embryo: normal and abnormal development and growth/Michael Chapman . . . (eds.)
p. cm. Includes index.
ISBN 0-387-19360-7 – ISBN 3-540-19630-7
1. Prenatal diagnosis. 2. Human embryo. I. Chapman, Michael, 1949–
[DNLM: 1. Fetal Development. 2. Fetal Diseases—diagnosis. WQ 211 E53]
RG628.E45 1990
618.3'2075—dc20
DNLM/DLC
for Library of Congress

Typeset by Nuts and Muttons Typesetting Ltd, Linton, Cambridgeshire
Printed by Henry Ling Ltd, The Dorset Press, Dorchester, UK
2128/3916-543210 Printed on acid-free paper

Preface

Recent years have seen the introduction of a variety of new techniques which promise to revolutionize the clinical management of early pregnancy, particularly with respect to the diagnosis and possible avoidance of congenital abnormalities. The present book brings together papers from a number of leading international research workers in this field.

The techniques of assisted reproduction have made available, for the first time, living embryonic material which can be used both for research and clinical management. For example, study of the early embryo in the test-tube has provided new information which reflects on the problem of early pregnancy loss as a potential cause of infertility. Of even greater potential importance is the fact that the embryo is now available for diagnosis. Single cells can be removed without affecting the viability of the remainder. These cells can be subjected to the sophisticated techniques of molecular biology, and allow selection of embryos prior to replacement in the uterus.

Another area of advance is in the diagnosis of major congenital abnormalities in late first trimester and midtrimester. Chorion villus biopsy provides fetal tissue for diagnosis at a much earlier stage than that which has hitherto been possible with amniocentesis. Ultrasound imaging permits the identification of congenital malformations in utero with an accuracy almost equivalent to that which can be achieved in the neonate. A spectrum of simple biochemical tests performed on maternal blood can greatly enhance the ascertainment of Down's syndrome and other chromosome defects.

All of these techniques were devised during the 1980s and many will come into routine clinical use in the 1990s. This book provides a full description of the state-of-the-art in this exciting and fast moving topic.

London
1990

Michael Chapman
Gedis Grudzinskas
Tim Chard

Contents

Contributors

V.N. Bolton, MA, PhD
Assisted Conception Unit, Department of Obstetrics and Gynaecology, King's College Hospital, London, UK

B. Brambati, MD
First Institute of Obstetrics and Gynaecology, Perinatal Unit, University of Milan, Milan, Italy

P. Braude, BSc, MB, PhD, MRCOG
Embryo and Gamete Research Group, Department of Obstetrics and Gynaecology, University of Cambridge, UK

T. Chard, MD, FRCOG
Academic Unit of Reproductive Physiology, St Bartholomew's Hospital Medical College, London, UK

A.J. Copp, MBBS, MA, DPhil
Imperial Cancer Research Fund, Developmental Biology Unit, Department of Zoology, University of Oxford, Oxford, UK

H. Cuckle, BA, MSc, DPhil
Department of Environmental and Preventive Medicine, The Medical College of St Bartholomew's Hospital, London, UK

C.M. Gosden, FRCPath
Medical Research Council, Western General Hospital, Edinburgh, UK

J.G. Grudzinskas, MD, MRCOG, FRACOG
Academic Unit of Obstetrics and Gynaecology, The London Hospital, London, UK

J.K. Gupta, MBChB
Department of Obstetrics and Gynaecology, St James' University Hospital, Leeds, UK

A. Handyside, MA, PhD
Royal Postgraduate Medical School, Institute of Obstetrics and Gynaecology, Hammersmith Hospital, London, UK

J.C. Hobbins, MD
Division of Maternal-Fetal Medicine, Department of Obstetrics and Gynecology, Yale University School of Medicine, New Haven, Connecticut, USA

H. Irving, DMRD, FRCR
Department of Radiology, St James' University Hospital, Leeds, UK

M. Johnson, MA, PhD
Embryo and Gamete Research Group, Department of Obstetrics and Gynaecology, and Anatomy, University of Cambridge, UK

M. Julkunen, MD
Department of Obstetrics and Gynaecology, Helsinki University Central Hospital, Helsinki, Finland

R. Koistinen, PhD
Department of Obstetrics and Gynaecology, Helsinki University Central Hospital, Helsinki, Finland

A. Lanzani, MD
First Institute of Obstetrics and Gynaecology, Perinatal Unit, University of Milan, Milan, Italy

R.J. Lilford, PhD, MRCOG, MRCP
Department of Obstetrics and Gynaecology, St James' University Hospital, Leeds, UK

G. Linton, MLSO
Department of Obstetrics and Gynaecology, St James' University Hospital, Leeds, UK

K.H. Nicolaides, BSc, MRCOG
Harris Birthright Research Centre for Fetal Medicine, King's College School of Medicine and Dentistry, London, UK

B. Nørgaard-Pedersen, MSc
Hormone Department, Statens Seruminstitut, Copenhagen, Denmark

P. O'Donovan, MRCOG
Department of Obstetrics and Gynaecology, St James' University Hospital, Leeds, UK

S. Pickering, BSc
Embryo and Gamete Research Group, Department of Obstetrics and Gynaecology, University of Cambridge, UK

E.A. Reece, MD
Division of Maternal-Fetal Medicine, Department of Obstetrics and Gynecology, Yale University School of Medicine, New Haven, Connecticut, USA

L. Riittinen, MSc
Department of Obstetrics and Gynaecology, Helsinki University Central Hospital, Helsinki, Finland

M. Seppälä, MD, FRCOG
Department of Obstetrics and Gynaecology, Helsinki University Central Hospital, Helsinki, Finland

J.L. Simpson, MD
Department of Obstetrics and Gynecology, University of Tennessee, Memphis, Tennessee, USA

R.J.M. Snijders, BSc
Harris Birthright Research Centre for Fetal Medicine, King's College School of Medicine and Dentistry, London, UK

I. Stabile, MRCOG, PhD
Center for Environmental Toxicology, University of Florida, Gainesville, Florida, USA

A.M. Suikkari, MD
Department of Obstetrics and Gynaecology, Helsinki University Central Hospital, Helsinki, Finland

L. Tului, PhD
Italian Association for the Study of Malformations (A.S.M.), Milan, Italy

C. Vincent, PhD
Embryo and Gamete Research Group, Department of Obstetrics and Gynaecology, University of Cambridge, UK

N. Wald, DSc (Med), FRCP, FFCM
Department of Environmental and Preventive Medicine, The Medical College of St Bartholomew's Hospital, London, UK

J.D. West, BSc, PhD
Department of Obstetrics and Gynaecology, University of Edinburgh, Centre for Reproductive Biology, Edinburgh, UK

J.L. Yovich, MBBS, MD, FRCOG, FRACOG, MAIBiol
Pivet Medical Centre and Department of Obstetrics and Gynaecology, University of Western Australia, Perth, Western Australia, Australia

1. Mechanisms of Early Embryonic Loss In Vivo and In Vitro

P. Braude, M. Johnson, S. Pickering and C. Vincent

Introduction

Much of our knowledge about the earliest stages of human development derives from observations on oocytes and preimplantation embryos in vitro during gamete intrafallopian transfer (GIFT) and in vitro fertilization (IVF) procedures (Edwards 1984; Edwards et al. 1981). Although patients' expectations of pregnancy following these newer methods of assisted conception are high, overall success rates in terms of live births per attempted cycle are low (10% per treatment cycle) (VLA 1989; Wagner and St Clair 1989). Even when pregnancies are established, many fail within the first few weeks after diagnosis. However, it is often forgotten that major losses occur also in spontaneous cycles (Vessey et al. 1978). In this chapter we compare losses for natural cycles with those in assisted conception cycles and examine mechanisms which may explain some of these failures.

Outcome of Spontaneous Ovulatory Cycles

Although cumulative conception tables suggest a clinical pregnancy rate of between 12% and 20% per cycle (Cooke et al. 1981), between 12% and 16% of these pregnancies are likely to end in overt spontaneous abortion (Huisjes 1984). However, these estimates of the incidence of spontaneous abortion are average figures, obtained largely from retrospective studies of hospital-based populations where early losses in particular may be missed. Thus they may not be a true reflection of the incidence of spontaneous loss in the population. More recently a prospective study has suggested that the incidence of spontaneous abortion depends to some extent on previous pregnancy outcome. Thus spontaneous loss seems to be lower in primigravidae (about 5%) and those who have had successful pregnancies, than in those who have experienced a pregnancy failure previously (19%) (Regan et al. 1989). Although the reasons for this discrepancy are not known, simply basing estimates of recurrence on average figures, or on gravidity tables, is likely to be inaccurate and thus inadequate for clinical prognosis.

Besides overt losses, the use of sensitive assays for hCG has demonstrated the occurrence of substantial subclinical losses. Wilcox et al. (1988) showed that 22% of conceptions detectable by elevated hCG levels during the late luteal phase failed to survive to the stage of being recognized clinically (6% of cycles). Based on these figures we can estimate that at least 70% of ovarian cycles do not result in a detectable pregnancy, those failures being accounted for by anovulation, failure of fertilization, or preimplantation losses. What data are there for estimating the contribution of each of these factors?

During their classic 16-year study of women undergoing hysterectomy in cycles in the absence of contraception, Hertig and Rock were able to detect "ova" (i.e. either oocytes, preimplantation cleavage stages or implantation sites) in only 34% of the 107 women in whom they considered conception to be likely from recent coital history (Hertig et al. 1959). Recent confirmation of this poor conception rate has come from studies of "ova" obtained from women who had been inseminated at the time of ovulation and then subjected to uterine lavage 5 days later for the purposes of recovering blastocysts for donation (Buster et al. 1985; Formigli et al. 1987). Only 41% of the cycles yielded oocytes or preimplantation cleavage stages. Thus even allowing for the fact that 10% of the oocytes or pre-embryos may not have been found due to errors or inefficiency of the flushing apparatus (Sauer et al. 1988), these figures suggest that at least 50% of cycles do not yield ova or cleavage stage embryos. Furthermore in Buster's study, only 24% of the preimplantation stages that were obtained were found to be blastocysts and thus at the appropriate stage for implantation. Similar results were found by Bolton et al. (1988), who reported that less than 20% of oocytes fertilized in vitro formed cavitating or expanded blastocysts, most failing in development at, or shortly after the four to eight cell stages, and Hardy et al. (1989) reported a blastocyst rate on day 5 or 6 of culture in vitro of 42%. Taken together, these data suggest that only around 10% of cycles will produce a continuing pregnancy (Vessey et al. 1978) (Table 1.1).

Table 1.1. Outcome of an ovulatory cycle

	Cumulative % pregnancy
Women initiating cycle	100
Proportion achieving fertilization	50
30% of these produce embryos capable of implanting	15
22% lost subclinically	12
12% overt spontaneous abortion	11 = ongoing pregnancy rate

What May Account for this Prodigious Loss?

Although our knowledge of early human development is scant, a number of mechanisms can be suggested to explain this early loss.

Failure of Gene Activation

Several lines of evidence suggest that a major burst of transcriptional activity occurs between the four and eight cell stages of preimplantation development. At this stage ribosomal particles mature into a functional morphological form (Tesarik et al. 1988), uptake and incorporation of uridine into ribosomes increases (Tesarik et al. 1986), and development is blocked for the first time by transcriptional inhibitors (Braude et al. 1988; Tesarik 1989). This activity is accompanied by changes in the type of proteins that are synthesized by the conceptus (Fig. 1.1). If activation of the genome is blocked experimentally, development continues up to the time of activation and then ceases (Braude et al. 1988).

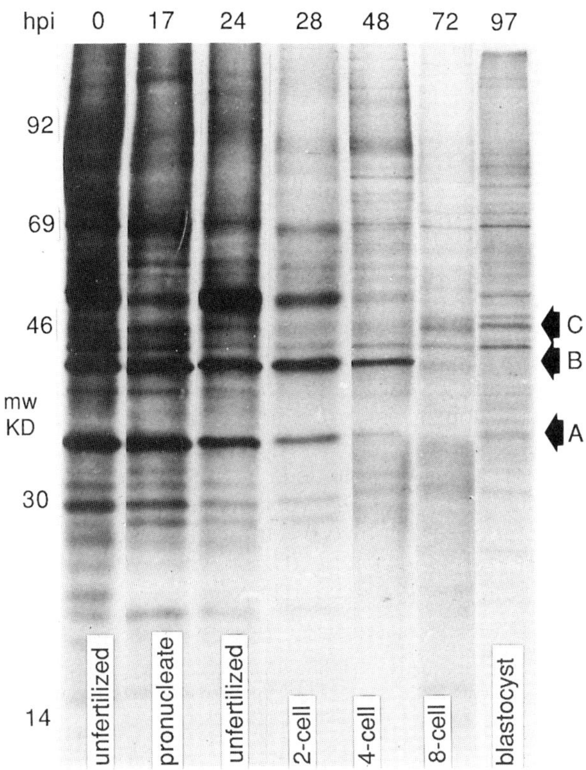

Fig. 1.1. Composite autoradiograph of proteins synthesized by oocytes, zygotes, and cleavage stage pre-embryos up to the blastocyst stage separated in one dimension by polyacylamide gel electrophoresis. Each track shows ^{35}S-methionine labelled polypeptides synthesized by a single oocyte or pre-embryo at the state indicated. Synthesis of certain polypeptides (examples A and B) decrease after the 4-cell stage, whereas others (shown by C) increase following the 4- or 8-cell stage. Synthesis of these latter polypeptides is prevented by transcriptional inhibition. (Details of methods in Braude et al. 1988.)

Although most oocytes fertilized in vitro are able to cleave to four cells, there is an increasing likelihood of cleavage arrest after these stages, with ony 20%–40% forming fully expanded blastocysts (Bolton et al. 1988; Handyside et al.

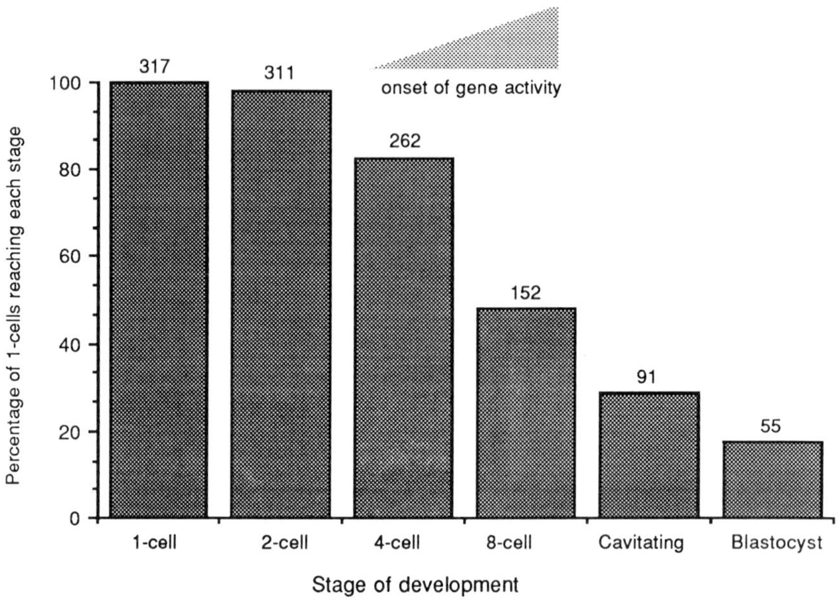

Fig. 1.2. Development of 317 fertilized oocytes, surplus to a therapeutic IVF programme, cultured in vitro for 5 days. The number of the original zygotes reaching each stage is shown above each bar. (Adapted from Bolton et al. 1988.)

1989). Thus the maximum likelihood of failure follows the period of gene activity (Fig. 1.2). It is therefore tempting to speculate that the failure of development may be a result of failure of genomic expression. However, preliminary evidence from arrested human 6- and 8-cell stages suggests that those new proteins synthesized after gene activation are nonetheless synthesized by the arrested conceptuses (Braude and Artley; unpublished data). Furthermore, the arrest seen in vitro in other species at around the time of gene activation (the 2-cell stage in the mouse (Goddard and Pratt 1983), the 8-cell stage in the sheep (Crosby et al. 1988)) are likewise not accompanied by a failure to produce proteins whose synthesis is dependent on embryonic gene activity. However, it cannot be precluded that more subtle expressions of new genomic activity are disturbed. Additionally it may well be that the change from total dependence on maternally derived information to increased dependence on newly synthesized zygotic information coincides with other developmental transitions that show an increased sensitivity to environmental factors in vivo or to culture conditions in vitro (Nasr-Esfahani et al. 1990).

Chromosomal Abnormalities

Karyotypic analysis of spontaneous pregnancy losses suggest aneuploidy rates of between 60% and 84% (Boue et al. 1975; Brambati 1989). Most of these are either trisomies or polyploidies, the deficiency of monosomies being ascribed to an earlier loss at pre- or peri-implantation stages. Although trisomies may arise as a result of non-disjunction during meiosis or mitosis during oogenesis, polyploidies could arise as a result of polyspermy, fertilization by diploid sperm, or by failure of extrusion of the polar body during meiosis.

It is now known that between 20% and 30% of human pre-embryos karyotyped after fertilization and culture in vitro are aneuploid (Angell et al. 1983; Plachot et al. 1988). However, it is unclear whether this level of aneuploidy is representative of the frequency of chromosomal abnormality in human cycles in vivo, or only of pre-embryos resulting from fertilization in vitro. These data have been obtained from pre-implantation stages which have developed from oocytes collected in superovulated cycles and which are usually surplus to therapeutic regimes after the pre-embryos with "best" morphology have been transferred to the uterus of the recipient. The superovulation procedures (Wramsby et al. 1987) and the egg retrieval processes themselves could affect the quality of the oocytes and the resulting conceptuses. Experiments in our laboratories have suggested that the in vitro handling of oocytes can produce chromosomal aberrations at alarmingly high frequencies.

(a) Temperature. The preovulatory oocyte in humans is arrested in metaphase of the second meiotic division. The chromosomes are aligned in a compact array on the metaphase plate of a spindle of microtubules, which has no asters or centrioles and is oriented perpendicular to the cell membrane (Pickering et al. 1988). Following the fusion of the spermatozoon with the cell membrane, meiosis is reactivated and the second polar body is shed. It is clear from experiments in sheep (Moor and Crosby 1985), and mice (Magistrini and Szollosi 1980; Pickering and Johnson 1987), that the spindle structure is exquisitely sensitive to a reduction from body temperature towards room temperature. Microtubules depolymerize to free tubulin under these conditions causing the spindle to dismantle with dispersion of the chromosomes. If mouse oocytes cooled to 4°C are then restored to 37°C, some do not regroup their chromosomes on the metaphase plate, but have abnormal spindles with detached clusters of chromosomes. The human oocyte seems even more sensitive to cooling and less able to repair damage on return to body temperature. Thus, freshly recovered oocytes exposed to room temperature for periods of 10 or 30 min show abnormalities of spindle organization, and even after restoration to 37°C for 1 or 4 hours, almost three-quarters remain abnormal (Pickering et al. 1989). It is not unlikely that transient cooling of oocytes towards room temperature does occur during egg retrieval and during the replacement procedure at GIFT. It is therefore not inconceivable that cooling-induced defects could account for a significant fraction of the high levels of aneuploidy which are seen in cytogenetic studies of surplus human pre-embryos, and may also contribute to the high pregnancy loss rates seen in some clinics following GIFT or IVF procedures. The contribution of such effects to the subclinical loss rate is not determined.

(b) Therapeutic Manipulations. In addition to temperature-induced chromosomal abnormalities, it is clear that the application of new techniques for enhancing fertilization with poor quality spermatozoa may also generate problems. For example, the exposure of human and murine oocytes to acidic conditions, as can occur during zona drilling (Gordon and Talansky 1986) is associated with an increased rate of parthenogenetic activation (Johnson et al. 1990). It is known that mouse parthenogenotes will develop through cleavage to post-implantation stages before failing (Barton et al. 1984). Attempts to cryopreserve human oocytes have met with little success (Chen 1986), and likewise, the oocytes of other species are difficult to freeze. It is now clear that cyroprotectants can have profound effects on the organization of the spindle in the mouse and rabbit oocytes (Johnson and Pickering 1987; Van der Elst et al.

1988; Vincent et al. 1989) and also have deleterious effects on the organization of the microfilament system (Vincent et al. 1989, 1990a) which can lead to problems with polar body extrusion and the block to polyspermy (Johnson 1989; Vincent et al. 1990b). Thus, the preparation of oocytes for freezing and their recovery after thawing may lead to chromosomal damage which, even if fertilization occurs, will preclude successful development of the resulting conceptus.

(c) Ageing. If mouse oocytes are not fertilized within a few hours of ovulation, their ability to be fertilized is reduced (Thibault 1970) and the level of aneuploidy in the zygotes that do form increases. This deleterious effect of ageing is observed whether eggs are maintained in vitro or in vivo. Our studies on the cytoskeletal organization of mouse oocytes aged in vitro or in vivo have revealed that the spindle develops characteristic patterns of disorganization. As a result, when activated to develop, abnormalities of chromosomal number result (Webb et al. 1986). Human oocytes aged in vitro for 24 hours also seem to show an increased incidence of abnormalities of cytoskeletal organization (Pickering et al. 1988). Although these studies are not as comprehensive as those for the mouse, and although as yet the impact that these changes in the oocyte might have on the chromosomal organization of the human zygote have not been assessed fully, it seems likely that the deleterious effects of ageing may be an important cause of early pregnancy loss in vivo and even in vitro. Whereas in most species coitus is restricted by female behaviour to the fertile period, thereby, assuring the presence of spermatozoa in the oviduct at the time of ovulation, in the human no such coital restriction operates. Thus the chance of freshly ovulated oocytes immediately encountering a spermatozoon will be reduced. It will be important to determine the relationship in the human between oocyte ageing, cytoskeletal disorganization and fertilizability.

Even in vitro, oocytes are inseminated conventionally some hours after retrieval (Harrison et al. 1988; Trounson et al. 1982), and some clinics, reinseminate oocytes with a fresh spermatozoal preparation 24 hours or more after the initial failed attempt (Trounson and Webb 1984). The use of these delayed insemination regimes might result in fertilization being initiated 24 hours or more after ovulation might have occurred, with potentially deleterious consequences for zygote survival.

Errors of Cytokinesis and Karyokinesis

As mentioned previously, the formation of expanded blastocysts in the human in vitro and in vivo is low. However, the simple observation that a blastocyst has formed does not necessarily imply that even this minority have normal developmental potential. Thus although little is known about the cell biology of the human blastocyst, it is clear that in mice important rearrangements of cellular organization occur during the compaction stages (around 8-cell stage)(Pratt et al. 1982; Johnson et al. 1986; Fleming and Johnson 1988). These changes influence decisively the contribution to the two tissues of the blastocyst, namely the inner cell mass (from which the embryo proper will eventually develop) and the trophectoderm, which will form part of the extraembryonic membranes (Johnson 1986). It is not yet clear when or whether compaction occurs in the human and how the primary cell lineages are established. Nevertheless, the

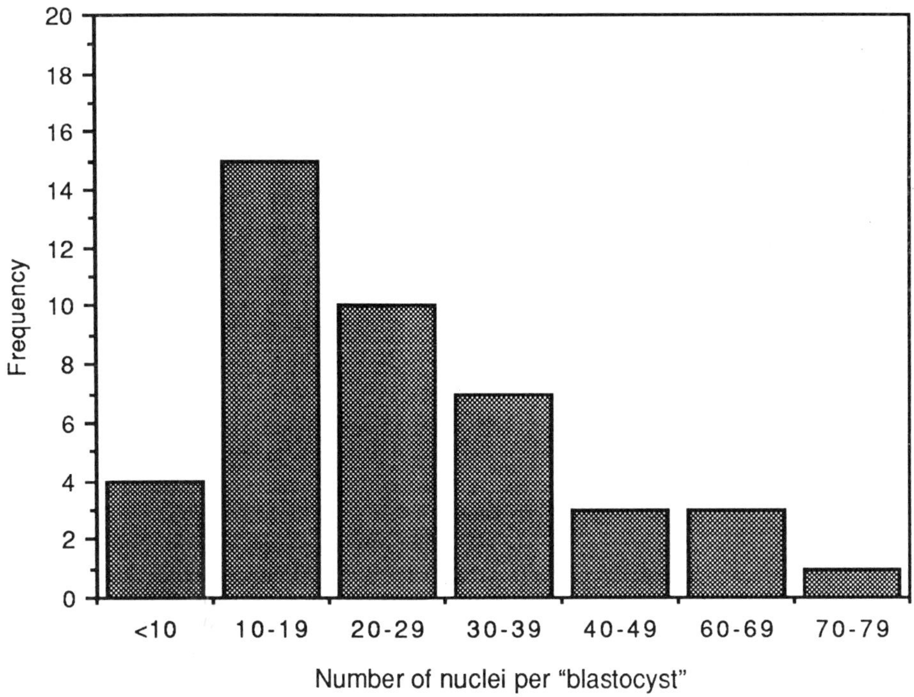

Fig. 1.3. Distribution of cell number in 43 blastocysts on day 5 of culture. Fertilized eggs surplus to therapeutic requirements were cultured in vitro to between 130 and 140 hours after insemination. Those zygotes which had formed blastocysts were stained with a fluorecent dye (DAPI) and the number of nuclei in each counted.

results of experiments in mice and other species reveal that a critical cell number is necessary for normal-sized inner cell mass formation and thus for the emergence of an embryo (Smith and McLaren 1977). However, expansion of the cleaving pre-embryo to form a blastocyst-like structure with a very reduced inner cell mass can nonetheless occur even when as few as two cells are present. In these cases a trophoblastic vesicle forms which, although it cannot generate embryonic cells, can appear grossly to be remarkably normal in appearance and is capable of outgrowing in vitro to give rise to trophoblast cells (Braude et al. 1983), of implanting (Gardner and Johnson 1972), and of secreting trophoblast marker proteins (Summers et al. 1987). If, as seems likely, this model is also appropriate for human pre-embryos, it provides a mechanism for the generation of an anembryonic pregnancy which would manifest as a transient rise in hCG and the appearance of an empty sac on ultrasound scan.

Our preliminary examination of day 5 cavitating pre-embryos developing in vitro (124–134 hours after insemination) has revealed that the number of nuclei present in the majority of blastocysts is far less than one would predict from a series of cleavage divisions based over the first three days of development. Although at least 60 cells might be expected to be present by day 5, in our study of 43 blastocysts, only 3 had number of cells in that order, with an average of only 25 nuclei per "blastocyst" (Fig. 1.3). Thus most "blastocysts" developing in vitro, even if appearing to be grossly normal when assessed in their culture drops under a dissecting microscope, may simply be slowed or arrested cleavage stages which accumulate fluid or cavitate at the appropiate time. It thus seems that the programme of "differentiation", as manifested by cell properties, has become uncoupled from the programme of cell division as assessed by cell numbers. This rather disturbing finding may explain the poor pregnancy rates following transfer of blastocysts to the uteri of patients on day 5 after insemination (Dawson et al. 1988; V.N. Bolton, in preparation). This absence of developmental potential may reflect inherent defects in the embryo which are only manifested after the onset of gene activation, but could also reflect suboptimal culture conditions in vitro. The use of more refined analytical criteria of blastocyst normality may provide us with a method for assessing the quality of different culture conditions, and replace the use of mouse embryos which have been shown repeatedly to be suboptimal (Fleming et al. 1987; George et al. 1989).

The study of oocytes and zygotic development in vitro has provided some pointers which may help our understanding of preclinical losses both natural and following therapeutic intervention. Although losses occur in both types of pregnancy their origins may be different. Thus some may be specific to assisted conception procedures such as IVF and GIFT and reflect suboptimal handling procedures. In these cases, the knowledge that has been gained from research on pre-embryos in vitro should enable appropriate precautionary measures to be taken. Losses in natural cycles which are independent of assisted conception techniques, and which occur at much higher frequencies that those observed in domestic and wild animal species, should also be susceptible to analysis by the study of early development in vitro. This may enable us to understand the underlying causes and to propose preventive measures to improve outcome (Braude and Johnson 1989).

References

Angell RR, Aitken RJ, Van Look PFA, Lumsden MA, Templeton AA (1983) Chromosome abnormalities in human embryos after in vitro fertilization. Nature 303: 336–338

Barton SC, Surani MAH, Norris ML (1984) Role of paternal and maternal genomes in mouse development. Nature 3: 374–376

Bolton VN, Hawes SM, Taylor CT, Parsons JH (1988) Development of spare human preimplantation embryos in vitro: An analysis of the correlations among gross morphology, cleavage rates and development to the blastocyst. J In Vitro Fertil Embryo Transfer 6: 30–35

Boue J, Boue A, Lazar P (1975) Retrospective and prospective epidemiological studies of 1500 karyotyped spontaneous human abortions. Teratology 12: 11–26

Brambati B (1989) Fate of human pregnancies. Patrick Steptoe Memorial Symposium, Cambridge

Braude PR, Bolton VN, Moore S (1988) Human gene expression first occurs between the four- and eight-cell stages of preimplantation development. Nature 332: 459–461

Braude PR, Johnson MH (1989) Embryo Research – yes or no? Br Med J 229: 1349–1351

Braude P, Johnson M, Bolton V, Pratt H (1983) Cleavage and differentiation of the early embryo. In: Cosignani PG, Rubin BL (eds) In Vitro fertilization and embryo transfer. Academic Press, London, pp 212–228

Buster JC, Bustillo M, Rodi IA, et al. (1985) Biologic and morphologic description of donated human ova recovered by non-surgical uterine lavage. Am J Obstet Gynecol 153: 211–217

Chen C (1986) Pregnancy after human oocyte cryopreservation. Lancet i: 884–886

Cooke ID, Sulaiman RA, Lenton EA, Parsons RJ (1981) Fertility and infertility statistics: their importance and application. Clin Obstet Gynaecol 8: 531–48

Crosby IM, Gandolfi F, Moor RM (1988) Control of protein synthesis during early cleavage of sheep embryos. J Reprod Fertil 82: 769–775

Dawson KJ, Rutherford AJ, Winston NJ, Subak-Sharpe R, Winston RML (1988) Human blastocyst transfer, is it a feasible proposition? Hum Reprod Suppl: 44

Edwards RG (1984) Human conception in vitro: new opportunities in medicine and research. In: Trounson AO, Wood C (eds) In Vitro fertilization and embryo transfer. Churchill Livingstone, Edinburgh, pp 217–250

Edwards RG, Purdy JM, Steptoe PC, Walters DE (1981) The growth of human preimplantation embryos in vitro. Am J Obstet Gynaecol 141: 408–416

Fleming TP, Johnson MH (1988) From egg to epithelium. Ann Rev Cell Biol 4: 459–485

Fleming TP, Pratt HMP, Braude PR (1987) The use of mouse preimplantation embryos for quality control of culture reagents in human in vitro fertilization programs: a cautionary note. Fertil Steril 47: 858–860

Formigli L, Formigli G, Roccia C (1987) Donation of fertilized uterine ova to infertile women. Fertil Steril 47: 162–165

Gardner RL, Johnson MH (1972) An investigation of inner cell mass and trophoblast tissues following isolation from the mouse blastocyst. J Embryol EVXP Morphol 28: 279–312

George MA, Braude PR, Johnson MH, Sweetnam DG (1989) Quality control in the IVF laboratory: in vitro and in vivo development of mouse embryos is unaffected by the quality of water used in culture media. Hum Reprod 4: 826–831

Goddard MJ, Pratt H (1983) Control of events during early cleavage of the mouse embryo: an analysis of the "2-cell block". J Embryol Exp Morphol 73: 111–133

Gordon JW, Talansky BE (1986) Assisted fertilization by zona drilling; a mouse model for correction of oligospermia. J Exp Zool 239: 247–354

Handyside AH, Pattinson JK, Penketh RJA, Delhanty JDA, Winston RML, Tuddenham EGD (1989) Biopsy of human pre-embryos and sexing by DNA amplification. Lancet i: 347–349

Hardy K, Handyside AH, Winston RML (1989) The human blastocyst: cell number, death and allocation during late preimplantation development in vitro. Development 107: 597–604

Harrison KL, Wilson LM, Breen TM, Pope AK, Cummins JM, Hennessey JF (1988) Fertilization of human oocytes in relation to varying delay before insemination. Fertil Steril 50(2): 294–297

Hertig AT, Rock J, Adams EC (1959) Thirty-four fertilized human ova, good, bad and indifferent, recovered from 210 women of known fertility. Pediatrics 23: 202–211

Huisjes HJ (1984) Spontaneous abortion. Churchill Livingstone, Edinburgh

Johnson M (1986) Manipulation of early mammalian development. What does it tell us about cell lineages? In: Gwatkin RBL (ed) Development biology. Plenum Press, New York, pp 279–296

Johnson MH (1989) The effect on fertilization of exposure of mouse oocytes to dimethylsulphoxide: an optimal protocol. J In Vitro Fertil Embryo Transfer 6:168–175

Johnson MH, Pickering SJ (1987) The effect of dimethylsulphoxide on the microtubular system of the mouse oocyte. Development 100: 313–324

Johnson MH, Chisholm JC, Fleming TP, Houliston E (1986) A role for cytoplasmic determinants in the development of the mouse early embryo? J Embryol Exp Morphol 97 (suppl): 97–121

Johnson MH, Pickering SJ, Braude PR, Vincent C, Cant A, Currie J (1990) Analysis of factors causing parthenogenic activation of human oocytes Fertil Steril 53: 266–270

Magistrini M, Szollosi D (1980) Effects of cold and isopropyl-N-phenylcarbamate on the second meiotic spindle of mouse oocytes. Eur J Cell Biol 22: 699–707

Moor RM, Crosby IM (1985) Temperature-induced abnormalities in sheep oocytes during maturation. J Reprod Fertil 75: 467–473

Nasr-Esfahani MH, Aitken JR, Johnson MH (1990) Hydrogen peroxide levels in oocytes and early cleavage stage embryos from blocking and non-blocking strains of mice. Development 109: 501–507

Pickering SJ, Johnson MH (1987) The influence of cooling on the organization of the meiotic spindle of the mouse oocyte. Hum Reprod 2: 207–216

Pickering SJ, Johnson MH, Braude PR (1988) Cytoskeletal organization in fresh, aged and spontaneously activated human oocytes. Hum Reprod 3: 978–979

Pickering SJ, Braude PR, Johnson MH, Cant A, Currie J (1990) Transient cooling to room temperature can cause irreversible disruption of the meiotic spindle in the human oocyte. Fertil Steril (in press)

Plachot M, Veiga A, Montagut J, et al. (1988) Are clinical and IVF parameters correlated with chromosomal disorders in early life: a multicentric study. Hum Reprod 3: 627–635

Pratt H, Ziomek C, Reeve W, Johnson M (1982) Compaction of the mouse embryo: an analysis of its components. J Embryol Exp Morphol 70: 113–132

Regan L, Braude PR, Trembath PL (1989) Influence of past reproductive performance on risk of spontaneous abortion. Br Med J 299: 541–545

Sauer MV, Bustillo M, Cohen SW, et al. (1988) An instrument for the recovery of preimplantation ova. Obstet Gynaecol 71: 804–806

Smith R, McLaren A (1977) Factors affecting the time of formation of the mouse blastocoele. J Embryol Exp Morphol 41: 79–92

Summers PM, Taylor CT, Hearn JP (1987) Characteristics of trophoblast tissue derived from in vitro culture of preimplantation embryos of the common marmoset monkey. Placenta 8: 411–422

Tesarik J (1989) Involvement of oocyte-coded message in cell differentiation control of early human embryos. Development 105: 317–322

Tesarik J, Kopecny V, Plachot M, Mandelbaum J (1988) Early morphological signs of embryonic genome expression in human preimplantation development as revealed by quantitative electron microscopy. Dev Biol 128: 15–20

Tesarik J, Kopecny V, Plachot M, Mandelbaum J, DeLage C, Flechon J (1986) Nucleogenesis in the human embryo developing in vitro: Ultrastructural and autoradiographic analysis. Dev Biol 115: 193–203

Thibault C (1970) Normal and abnormal fertilization in mammals. In: Raspe G (ed) Advances in the biosciences. Pergamon Press, Oxford, pp 63–85.

Trounson AO, Mohr LR, Wood C, Leeton JF (1982) Effect of delayed insemination on in vitro fertilization, culture and transfer of human embryos. J Reprod Fertil 64: 285–294

Trounson AO, Webb J (1984) Fertilization of human oocytes following reinsemination in vitro. Fertil Steril 41: 816–819

Van der Elst J, Van den Abbeel E, Jacobs R, Wisse E, Van Stierteghem AC (1988) Effect of 1,2-propanediol and dimethyl sulphoxide on the meiotic spindle of the mouse oocyte. Hum Reprod 3: 960–967

Vessey MP, Wright NH, McPherson K, Wiggins P (1978) Fertility after stopping different methods of contraception. Br Med J i: 265–267

Vincent C, Garnier V, Heyman H, Renard JP (1989) Solvent effects on cytoskeletal organization and in vivo survival after freezing of rabbit oocytes. J Reprod Fertil 87: 809–820

Vincent C, Pickering SJ, Johnson MH, Quick SJ (1990a) Dimethylsulfoxide affects the organization of microfilaments in the mouse oocyte. Mol Reprod Dev 26: 227–235

Vincent C, Pickering SJ, Johnson MH (1990b) The zona hardening effect of dimethylsulphoxide requires the presence of an oocyte and is associated with a reduction in the number of cortical granules present. J Reprod Fertil 89: 253–259

VLA (1989). Voluntary Licensing Authority for Human Fertilization and Embryology: Fourth Report. Medical Research Council, 20 Park Crescent, London W1N 4AL

Wagner MG, St Clair PA (1989) Are in vitro fertilisation and embryo transfer of benefit to all? Lancet ii: 1027–1029

Webb M, Howlett S, Maro B (1986) Parthenogenesis and cytoskeletal organization in ageing mouse eggs. J Embryol Exp Morphol 95: 131–145

Wilcox AJ, Weinberg CR, O'Connor JF, et al. (1988) Incidence of early loss of pregnancy. N Engl J Med 319: 189–194

Wramsby H, Fredga K, Leidholm P (1987) Chromosome analysis of human oocytes recovered from preovulatory follicles in stimulated cycles. N Engl J Med 316: 121–124

2. Aetiology of Pregnancy Failure

J.L. Simpson

Introduction

Pregnancy failure in humans is a common event. Utilizing beta-hCG assays to detect preclinical pregnancies shows that about 30%–40% of such pregnancies do not survive, two-thirds being lost prior to clinical recognition (Wilcox et al. 1988). That the rate-limiting step in IVF is embryo transfer further suggests that many conceptuses are lost prior to implantation, as indeed shown by the morphologic studies of Hertig and Rock (1973). Once recognized, the frequency of loss is 12%–15% (Simpson and Mills, 1985). Most of these losses occur before 8 weeks gestation (6 embryonic weeks). After 8 weeks only 3% of viable pregnancies are lost (Simpson et al. 1987) and after 16 weeks only about 1% (Tabor et al. 1986). If bleeding occurs in the first trimester, however, the associated loss rate is much higher (approximately 50%) (Stabile et al. 1987).

The aetiology of pregnancy loss is not the same throughout gestation. Genetic factors are far more likely to be responsible for early losses, whereas maternal illness is more likely to be responsible for third trimester losses. In this communication we systematically consider the aetiology of pregnancy loss, emphasizing factors responsible for early clinical losses. Elsewhere the author has discussed in more detail the timing of losses throughout gestation (Simpson 1990) and recurrence risks following repeated losses (Simpson and Carson 1991); Carson and Simpson 1990). This review inevitably reflects not only those but other reviews on the topic (Simpson 1991; Simpson and Golbus 1991).

Numerical Chromosomal Abnormalities (Aneuploidy and Polyploidy)

Preclinical Losses

There are several potential explanations for the general phenomenon of preclinical losses, but the one unequivocal explanation is morphologic abnormalities in early embryos. In turn, the most likely explanation for morphologic abnormalities is genetic factors. Over many years Hertig and Rock (Hertig et al. 1956, 1959; Hertig and Rock 1973) recovered 8 preimplantation embryos (less than 6 days from conception). Four of these embryos were morphologically abnormal. These embryos presumably would not have implanted or would not have survived long thereafter. Similarly, 9 of 26 implanted embryos (6–14 embryonic days) were morphologically abnormal, also unlikely to develop further.

There are now several cytogenetic studies of early human embryos fertilized in vitro. Chromosomal abnormalities are observed in approximately 20% of in vitro fertilized embryos (Angell et al. 1983; Rudak et al. 1985; Zenzes et al. 1985; Michelman et al. 1986; Plachot et al. 1987) In the study of Plachot et al. (1987), 69 human embryos were recovered at the 2- to 8-cell stages. Three of 68 showed only a single pronucleus, presumably being haploid; 1 of the 3 was also monosomic for a C group chromosome. Of 15 embryos showing 3 or more pronuclei, 7 were grossly triploid, 3 triploid-diploid mosaics, 2 polypoid and only 3 grossy diploid. However, none of the 3 diploid embryos each showed 2 pronuclei and would be considered normal; 37 of these 50 could not be karyotyped. However, of the 13 that could be karyotyped, only 5 were cytogenetically normal. Thus chromosomal abnormalities are not only frequent, but could be responsible for many of the early morphological abnormalities documented by Hertig and Rock.

Consistent with this conclusion are the animal studies of Gropp (1973, 1975). Mice heterozygous for various Robertsonian translocations were mated to produce various monosomies and trisomies. By selective mating and sacrifice of pregnant females, both survivability and phenotypic characteristics of the aberrant complements could be determined. In mice, as in man, autosomal monosomy was non-viable. Monosomes usually aborted within 4–5 days of conception (i.e. around implantation). Trisomies were lost later, with only a few (Nos. 12 and 19) surviving until live birth.

First Trimester

Cytogenetic abnormalities are by far the most frequent explanation for the 12%–15% of clinically recognized pregancy losses. Approximately 50% of such losses show chromosomal abnormalities. The relatively minor differences in frequencies among various studies are readily attributable to differences in maternal age or gestational stage.

Autosomal *trisomies* comprise the largest single class of abnormal chromosomal complements in spontaneous abortions. Of all abnormal complements 48.6%

are trisomic; thus, approximately 25% of all abortuses are trisomic (Table 2.1). Trisomy for every chromosome except No. 1 has been reported, and trisomy for that chromosome has been observed in an 8-cell embryo (Watt et al. 1987).

Table 2.1. Chromosomal complements in spontaneous abortions: recognized clinically in the first trimester

Complement		Frequency	(%)
Normal			
46,XX or 46,XY			54.1
Triploidy			7.7
69,XXX		2.7	
69,XYX		0.2	
69,XXY		4.0	
Other		0.8	
Tetraploidy			2.6
92,XXXX		1.5	
92,XXYY		0.55	
Not Stated		0.55	
Monosomy X			8.6
Structural abnormalities			1.5
Sex chromosomal polysomy			0.2
47,XXX		0.05	
47,XXY		0.15	
Autosomal monosomy (G)			0.1
Autosomal trisomy	Chromosome		22.3
	No. 1	0	
	No. 2	1.11	
	No. 3	0.25	
	No. 4	0.64	
	No. 5	0.04	
	No. 6	0.14	
	No. 7	0.89	
	No. 8	0.79	
	No. 9	0.72	
	No. 10	0.36	
	No. 11	0.04	
	No. 12	0.18	
	No. 13	1.07	
	No. 14	0.82	
	No. 15	1.68	
	No. 16	7.27	
	No. 17	0.18	
	No. 18	1.15	
	No. 19	0.01	
	No. 20	0.61	
	No. 21	2.11	
	No. 22	2.26	
Double trisomy			0.7
Mosaic trisomy			1.3
Other abnormalities or not specified			0.9
			100.0

Pooled data from several series, referenced elsewhere (Simpson JL, Bombard AT (1987) Chromosomal abnormalities in spontaneous abortions: frequency, pathology and genetic counselling. In: Edmonds K, Bennet MJ (eds) Spontaneous abortion. Blackwell, London).

Boué et al. (1976) observed that most trisomic conceptuses fail to progress beyond the stage expected for 8 gestational weeks or less. This is consistent with observations that even most *clinically* recognized losses occur before 8 weeks, albeit many are not manifest until several weeks after fetal demise (missed abortion) (Simpson et al. 1987).

Autosomal trisomy has a cytological counterpart – autosomal *monosomy*. The latter is rarely, if ever, observed in humans. Data in humans are thus comparable to those in the mouse, a species in which Gropp (1973, 1975) observed that murine monosomies fail to survive implantation.

Polyploidy is the presence of more than two haploid chromosome sets. Triploidy (3n = 60) and tetraploidy (4n = 92) occur frequently in abortuses (Table 2.1). The mean duration of survival for triploid conceptuses is about 5 weeks (7 weeks gestation) (Boué et al. 1976). Triploid abortuses are usually 69,XXY or 69,XXX, resulting from dispermy (Jacobs et al. 1978).

Tetraploid conceptuses are uncommon, rarely progressing beyond 2 to 3 weeks (4–5 weeks gestation).

Monosomy X is the single most common chromosomal abnormality in spontaneous abortions. Monosomy X occurs in 8.6% of all conceptions (approximately 20% of chromosomally abnormal abortions). In fetuses surviving until later in gestation, anomalies charactertistic of Turner's syndrome (Simpson 1976) may be seen: horseshoe kidney, cystic hygromas, and generalized oedema. Monosomy X occurs as result of paternal sex chromosome loss (Chandley 1981). This observation is consistent with, but does not explain, the inverse maternal age effect characteristic of 45,X.

Although the frequencies of various chromosomal abnormalities are well accepted there are some caveats. One is the impossibility of determining the status of abortuses that fail to grow in culture. Could failures be disproportionately represented by chromosomal abnormalities? Indeed, this is not an illogical hypothesis, since growth retardation is characteristic of 45,X and possibly autosomal trisomy (Simpson and LeBeau 1981). On the other hand, cytogenetically normal abortuses might preferentially fail to grow because of infection.

Guerneri et al. (1987) found a very high (77%) frequency of chromosomal abnormalities in women studied immediately after ultrasound diagnosis of fetal demise. Tissue for analysis was obtained by chorionic villus sampling, rather than relying upon later recovery of spontaneously expelled products. A very high proportion of specimens proved informative. The gestational age in the sample of Guerneri et al. (1987) may also have been earlier than in other studies (Boué et al. 1975).

Another difficulty is determining whether the material (villi or membrane) truly reflects embryonic status. In chorionic villus sampling (CVS), the frequency of cytogenetic abnormalities in villi that are not confirmed in the embryo is about 1% (Ledbetter et al. 1990). In particular, there is growing recognition that 45,X cells and certain lethal trisomies (e.g. trisomy 16) in villi need not necessarily indicate an abnormal embryo (Tharapel et al. 1989).

Second and Third Trimester

It would be of great interest to know the prevalence of chromosomal abnormalities in losses occurring in pregnancies known to have been viable at

8 weeks gestation. However, the high frequency of unrecognized missed abortion in the first trimester invalidates earlier reports that attempted to correlate precisely the frequency of chromosomal abnormalities with gestational interval. However, the frequency of chromosomal errors in losses recognized between 16 and 28 week is almost certainly less than that observed in losses *recognized* earlier (Ruzicska and Cziezel 1971; Warburton et al. 1980). In the second trimester, observed chromosomal abnormalities are similar to those observed in liveborn infants: trisomies 13, 18 and 21; monosomy X; sex chromosomal polysomies. Moreoever, anatomical findings in such abortuses are reminiscent of those present in aneuploid liveborns.

Genes Causing Aneuploidy

Numerical chromosomal abnormalities (aneuploidy) may be responsible for both sporadic losses and recurrent losses. This is based on observations that the complements of successive abortuses in a given family are more likely to be either consistently normal or consistently abnormal (Table 2.2). In other words, abortuses in a given family show non-random distribution with respect to chromosomal complements. If the complement of the first abortus is abnormal, the likelihood is 80% that the complement of the second abortus will also be abnormal (Hassold, 1980). The recurrent abnormality is usually trisomy, but it may also be monosomy or polyploidy. These data suggest that certain couples are predisposed towards chromosomally abnormal conceptions, most of which naturally result in spontaneous abortion. Presumably the mechanism involves mutant genes. Indeed, in humans consanguinity increases the risk of aneuploidy (Alfi 1981). In rodents, frequency of aneuploidy varies by strain. A variety of mechanisms by which genes could cause non-disjunction can be postulated. Warburton et al. (1987) interpret these data as indicating that corrections for maternal age render the phenomenon of recurrent aneuploidy statistically non-significant; this author docs not agree with that interpretation.

The issue is clinically relevant. If a couple were predisposed to recurrent aneuploidy, they would be at increased risk of aneuploid liveborns. The autosome trisomic in a subsequent pregnancy might not be lethal (e.g. trisomy 16), but rather might be compatible with life (e.g. trisomy 21). Available data do not

Table 2.2. The relationship between karyotypes of successive abortuses. Tabulated from Warburton et al. (1987)

Complement of first abortion	Complement of second abortion					
	Normal	Trisomy	Monosomy	Triploidy	Tetraploidy	De novo rearrangement
Normal	142	18	5	7	3	2
Trisomy	31	30	1	4	3	1
Monosomy C	7	5	3	3	0	0
Triploidy	7	4	1	4	0	0
Tetraploidy	3	1	0	2	0	0
De novo rearrangement	1	3	0	0	0	0

reveal whether liveborn aneuploidy is increased following liveborn aneuploid abortions. However, several studies suggest that the risk of liveborn trisomy 21 following a trisomic abortus is about 1% (Alberman 1981).

Chromosomal Translocations

Structural chromosomal abnormalities are a well-accepted explanation for repetitive abortions and a less common explanation for losses in general.

The most common structural rearrangement is a translocation. Individuals with balanced translocations are phenotypically normal, but abortuses or abnormal liveborns may show duplications or deficiencies as result of normal meiotic segregation. About 60% of the translocations are reciprocal, and 40% are Robertsonian.

If cytogenetic studies are routinely performed on all couples experiencing recurrent fetal losses, the frequency of translocations is about 2% of individuals (Simpson et al. 1989). By contrast, investigations restricted to couples experiencing both abortions and stillborn infants or anomalous liveborn infants will yield relatively more translocations (Table 2.3). It has long been recognized that females are about twice as likely as males to show a balanced translocation (Simpson et al. 1981), but certain questions are still unanswered: (1) Are prevalence rates influenced by numbers of previous losses? (2) Does occurrence of both first- and second-trimester losses affect prevalence rates?

If a balanced translocation is detected, antenatal cytogenetic studies should obviously be offered in subsequent pregnancies. However, the frequency of unbalanced fetuses at 16 weeks (amniocentesis) is far lower if the balanced translocation is ascertained through repetitive abortions (perhaps 3%) than if ascertained through an anomalous liveborn (approximately 12%) (Daniels et al. 1989).

Chromosomal Inversions

Another parental chromosomal rearrangement causing fetal loss is an inversion. In this intrachromosomal rearrangement the order of genes is reversed. This

Table 2.3. Balanced translocations in couples experiencing repeated abortions

Repeated spontaneous abortions with or without normal liveborn		Repeated spontaneous abortions with stillborn or abnormal liveborn		Repeated spontaneous abortions with subcategorization	
Female	Male	Female	Male	Female	Male
89/3712 2.4%	57/3651 1.4%	20/432 4.6%	7/409 1.7%	100/3074 3.3%	65/3009 2.1%

Pooled data from Simpson et al. (1989.

rearrangement usually occurs when two chromosomal breaks are followed by reinsertion in reverse order of the chromosomal segment produced by the breaks. Inversions in which break points exist on opposite sides of the centromere are *pericentric*; those in which break points are on the same side of the centromere are *paracentric*.

Heterozygotes for either pericentric or paracentric inversions may be normal if genes are neither lost, gained, nor altered as a result of the breaks. However, individuals with inversions suffer abnormal reproductive consequences as a result of normal meiotic phenomena, namely crossing-over during meiosis I. In order for genes within inversions to pair, a loop must form during meiosis I. Crossing-over may or may not occur within an inversion loop, but it is likely to do so if the loop encompasses a large portion of the chromosome. If crossing-over occurs, certain gametes are unbalanced.

Inversion is an infrequent cause of fetal loss, even among repeated aborters. However, inversions are highly deleterious (Sutherland et al. 1976; Martin et al. 1983). A single crossover within a *paracentric* inversion results in both dicentric and acentric products. Both acentric and dicentric gametes contribute to fetal wastage. Both outcomes are usually lethal; thus, paracentric inversions are rarely associated with anomalous livebirths.

By contrast, *pericentric* inversions are likely to cause both abortions and anomalous livebirths. After crossing-over, we have noted that two of the four gametes represent the parental sequences (one normal, one inverted). The other two gametes represent recombinants, genes distal to one breakpoint deficient and genes distal to the other breakpoint duplicated. The prevalence of pericentric inversions among couples experiencing repetitive abortions is considerably lower than the prevalence of balanced translocations. Pooled data suggest that inversions exist in 0.1% of females and 0.1% of males experiencing repeated spontaneous abortions.

Luteal Phase (Progesterone) Deficiency (LPD)

Early pregnancy abnormalities resulting from implantation in an unsupportive endometrial environment might explain some spontaneous abortions. The term luteal phase deficiency (LPD) is used to describe an endometrium manifesting an inadequate progesterone effect. Such an abnormality could be the result of either inadequate endometrial progesterone receptor function or low progesterone production. In the latter, the corpus luteum may be unable to secrete progesterone in quantities sufficient to maintain the pregnancy until placental secretion becomes self-sustaining (5 weeks post conception or 7 weeks gestation).

LPD is believed by many to be a cause of recurrent pregnancy loss, although its frequency has never been determined. Some have estimated that it occurs in 35% of patients experiencing recurrent losses (Jones 1976); this figure is derived from patients first ascertained on the basis of prior losses and then subjected to endometrial biopsy (Daya et al. 1988). Usually such patients were treated; rarely were patients diagnosed and left untreated for a control comparison. Furthermore, subjects with no losses (controls) were not concurrently studied by endometrial biopsy to determine if the luteal phase defect existed in fertile populations. Indeed, when regularly menstruating, fertile women with no history of abortions were biopsied in up to 10 serial cycles, the frequency of luteal phase defect proved to be 51.4% in any single cycle and 26.7% in sequential cycles (Davis et al. 1989). Thus, the existence of luteal phase defect as both an entity and an explanation for repetitive abortions is doubtful.

Determining the frequency of luteal phase defect is made difficult by the lack of uniform diagnostic criteria. LPD was originally diagnosed on the basis of an endometrial biopsy lagging at least two days behind the actual postovulation date, as determined by counting backward from the next menstrual period (assuming 14 days from ovulation to menses). Minor variations in histologic dating and in the monthly cycle may account for much of the 40% occurrence of "luteal phase defect" as diagnosed in normal women by one endometrial biopsy. Even the original endometrial dating by Noyes, Hertig, and Rock showed a mean error of 1.81 days (Noyes et al. 1950). This report recommended that an endometrial biopsy be called "out of phase" only if it lags 3 or more days behind the actual postovulation date. More recently, 62 endometrial biopsies read by five different pathologists resulted in an interobserver variation that would have altered management in 22%–39% of patients (Scott et al. 1988). Reading endometrial biopsy slides a second time, the same pathologist agreed with his initial diagnosis is only 25% of samples (Li et al. 1989). Therefore, at least two "out-of-phase" biopsies are necessary to make the diagnosis of LPD. It has recently been suggested that LPD can be diagnosed by histologic endometrial dating correlated with a postovulation date calculated from the date of the LH rise, rather than by counting backwards from the succeeding menses (Li et al. 1987).

Others have suggested that the diagnosis of LPD can be based on one (Daya and Ward, 1988) or more (Wu and Minassian, 1987) progesterone concentrations in the luteal phase. Progesterone was measured in women with a history of three spontaneous abortions by Horta et al. (1977). Of 15 such women 10 had lower luteal progesterone concentrations than 15 healthy non-pregnant control women; all 10 went on to abort during the first trimester. However, in patients with two or more spontaneous abortions, low progesterone in the luteal phase had a predictive value of only 71% in respect of LPD diagnosed by an abnormal endometrial biopsy. Others have suggested that the diagnosis can be made by observing the length of basal body temperature elevation, proposing that a luteal length of 11 days or less indicates a high likelihood of LPD (Downs and Gibson, 1983). A modification of this proposal is that an LH surge–menses interval of less than 10 days can be considered as diagnostic of a luteal phase defect (Smith et al. 1984). Progesterone receptors measured in the luteal endometrium do not usually correlate with pathologic dating (McRae et al. 1984; Jacobs et al. 1987). One group found lower progesterone receptor concentrations in the endometrium of women with LPD, but a large overlap with normal women was observed (Spiritos et al. 1985). Another study showed higher progesterone receptor concentrations accompanied by low serum progesterone in patients with an out-of-phase endometrial biopsy (Saracoglu et al. 1985). However, perturbations in endometrial receptors have not been correlated with actual pregnancy loss.

With so much doubt on the diagnostic criteria for LPD, it is hardly surprising that no randomized studies exist to document the efficacy of therapy, principally progesterone. Over 100 published studies since 1965 discuss LPD, usually ascertained in infertile women; however, none of these studies were controlled with a randomized placebo group. A typical study claiming effective treatment is that of Tho et al. (1979); 23 of 100 women with repetitive spontaneous abortions had "documented" luteal phase defects on the basis of "out-of-phase" endometrial biopsies. All 23 women were treated with progesterone suppositories and 21 completed their pregnancies. The closest approximation to a control group was 37 other women who had no obvious cause for their losses. Twenty-two of these 37 were treated with "empiric" progesterone; 15 were not. Of the treated women, 73% had successful pregnancies compared to 47% of the untreated women.

Daya et al. (1988) investigated 65 patients with recurrent abortions and found 26 (40%) to have both two consecutive out-of-phase biopsies and low progesterone levels. All were treated with progesterone, after which the endometrium appeared normal. Only three (19%) of 16 subsequent pregnancies aborted. However, there was no control group. The best data suggesting that LPD is a valid entity are derived from a study of 33 infertile women whose luteal phase defect was documented by two out-of-phase biopsies (Daly et al. 1983). Although the study involved women having infertility rather than recurrent abortions, the investigators observed no abortions in the 14 women who conceived after demonstration of an in-phase endometrial biopsy following progesterone treatment. Among the 16 women whose biopsy was not corrected, there were four pregnancies, all of which ended in spontaneous abortion (Daly et al. 1983). The study suggests a role for LPD in infertility, and also hints that LPD indeed may lead to spontaneous abortion.

In conclusion, critical analysis of available data is suggestive of the efficacy of progesterone, but prospective randomized studies are needed (Daya, 1988).

Thyroid Abnormalities

Decreased conception rates occur with overt hypothyroidism or hyperthyroidsim. However, data implicating subclinical thyroid dysfunction with fetal losses are lacking (Montero et al. 1981). Studies purporting to show a relationship may be questioned on the basis of the diagnostic criteria, and the lack of proper controls.

Carbohydrate Abnormalities

It is usually thought that spontaneous abortion rates are no higher among patients with diabetes mellitus than among controls. However, the large prospective collaborative study conducted by myself and colleagues (Diabetes in Early Pregnancy Study) (Mills et al. 1988) sugggested that women whose diabetes is poorly controlled are at increased risk. In our study metabolic data were gathered from the fifth week of gestation, and data allowing a variety of confounding variables to be taken into account were collected. Overall, no significant

Table 2.4. Diabetic control and fetal losses

Initial glycosylated haemoglobin (S.D. control mean)	N	Fetal losses (%)	Mean glycosylated haemoglobin, first trimester	N	Fetal losses (%)
<2	137	9.5	<2	137	10.3
2–4	131	14.5	2–4	121	15.2
>4	112	21.4	>4	112	20.2

Relationship of diabetic control of fetal loss rates, assessed by (a) initial glycosylated haemoglobin, obtained at 6 or 7 weeks gestation, and (b) mean weekly first trimester glycosylated haemoglobin. Derived from data reported by Mills, Simpson, Driscoll, et al. (1988).

differences in loss rates existed between controls (15.6%) and women with insulin-dependent diabetes mellitus (15.9%). However, subjects whose glycosylated haemoglobin was greater than 4 S.D. above the mean showed the highest pregnancy loss rates (Table 2.4). Miodnovic and colleagues (1984; 1985; 1986) have accumulated data consistent with this, as have Greene et al. (1989) in a retrospective analysis. Thus, poorly controlled diabetes mellitus is probably a cause of early pregnancy loss. However, well-controlled and subclinical diabetes should not be considered causes.

Intrauterine Adhesions (Synechiae)

Intrauterine adhesions could interfere with implantation or early embryonic development. Adhesions may follow overzealous curettage of the uterus during the postpartum period, intrauterine surgery (e.g. myomectomy), or endometritis. Curettage accounts for most cases, with adhesions most likely to develop when the procedure is performed 3 or 4 weeks postpartum. The diagnosis is usually suggested by menstrual abnormalities, but 15%–30% show repeated abortions. If adhesions are detected in a woman experiencing repetitive losses, lysis of the adhesions under direct hysteroscopic visualization should be performed. Approximately 50% of subjects conceive after surgery, but the frequency of abortions remains high.

Incomplete Müllerian Fusion and Other Uterine Anomalies

In incomplete uterine fusion, the pregnant uterus may be unable to accommodate the growing fetus, and the placenta may implant on a poorly vascularized septum. First-trimester abortions occurring after ultrasonographic confirmation of a viable pregnancy at 8 or 9 weeks may also be attributed to uterine fusion defects. Abortions at 10 to 12 weeks gestation *without* confirmation of prior viability are more likely to represent missed abortions, fetal demise having occurred before 8 weeks gestation.

Uterine fusion defects are widely accepted as a cause of second-trimester abortions, but have not been rigorously studied. The prevalence of abortions in patients with such defects may be as high as 20%–25% (Heinonen et al. 1982). Loss rates may be higher with septate and bicornuate uteri than with unicornuate uteri or uteri didelphys; however, data are sparse.

Women experiencing second-trimester abortions and shown to have a Müllerian fusion anomaly can probably benefit from uterine reconstruction; however, careful selection is important for optimal results.

Women exposed to diethylstilbestrol in utero are also at increased risk of pregnancy loss (Herbst et al. 1989). The aetiology is considered to involve a structurally abnormal (T-shaped) uterus.

Leiomyomas

Uterine leiomyomas are an uncommon contribution to pregnancy wastage. Location is probably more important than size. Submucous leiomyomas are the most likely to cause fetal loss, acting through several mechanisms:

1. Thinning of the endometrium over the surface, leading to implantation in a poorly decidualized site.
2. Rapid growth in the hormonal milieu of pregnancy can compromise the blood supply of the leiomyoma, resulting in necrosis ("red degeneration") that in turn leads to uterine contractions and fetal expulsion.
3. Large leiomyomas may encroach upon the space required by the developing fetus, thereby leading to premature delivery through mechanisms analogous to those present in incomplete Müllerian fusion. Lack of space can also lead to fetal deformations.

Myomectomy may occasionally be warranted for women experiencing repetitive second-trimester abortions.

Incompetent Cervix

A functionally intact cervix and lower uterine cavity are obvious necessities for a successful intrauterine pregnancy. Cervical incompetence is characterized by painless dilatation and effacement, usually during the mid-second or early third trimester. Cervical incompetence frequently follows traumatic events such as surgical dilatation, cervical lacerations, cervical amputations, conization, or cauterization. A history of premature cervical dilatation during pregnancy suggests the diagnosis, which is not always easy to verify. Diagnosis may be confirmed in the non-pregnant state if a dilator (e.g. No. 8 Hegar) easily traverses the internal os. Ultrasonography can confirm that dilatation has already occurred, but is less helpful in identifying women destined to experience premature cervical dilatation.

Various operations for correcting cervical incompetence have been proposed, with success rates approximating 80% (Rock and Jones 1977). One study attempted to determine the value of cerclage in the absence of demonstrable abnormality (Edmonds 1988) but this was not obviously successful. It should also be noted that two randomized trials have failed to show a statistically significant positive effect in perinatal outcome in women undergoing cervical cerclage (Lazar and Guegen 1984; Rush et al. 1984). However, the samples were heterogeneous and included women having both first trimester losses as well as any deliveries before 37 weeks.

Infections

Infections are well-known causes of late fetal wastage, and could be responsible for early fetal loss as well. Any of several mechanisms could be responsible: (1) intrauterine fetal demise resulting from overwhelming infection; (2) microorganisms interfering with organogenesis so that differentiation can no longer proceed; (3) fever per se; and (4) teratogenic action of agents used to treat the infection. A question which is often unanswered is whether a given infectious agent actually caused the demise, or merely arose after the fetal demise.

Microorganisms claimed to be associated with spontaneous abortion include *Variola, Vaccinia, Salmonella typhi, Vibrio fetus, Malaria, Cytomegalovirus, Brucella, Toxoplasmosis, Mycoplasma hominis, Chlamydia trachomatis,* and *Ureaplasma urealyticum*. However, data showing relative risk for fetal loss are not available for any of these. Antibodies to *Chlamydia trachomatis* are not increased in women having spontaneous abortions (Quinn et al. 1987). The only solid data are for *Ureaplasma urealyticum*.

Stray-Pedersen et al. (1978) studied 46 women with histories of three or more consecutive losses of unknown aetiology. Endometrial *Ureaplasma* colonization was significantly more frequent among women with repetitive abortions (28%) than among controls (7%). Of 43 women in the former group, 13 harboured *Ureaplasma* in both cervix and endometrium. The 43 women and their husbands were then treated with doxycycline for 11 days, with subsequent cultures showing no *Ureaplasma*. Nineteen of the 43 women became pregnant after treatment. Of these 19 women, 3 experienced another spontaneous abortion and 16 had normal full-term infants. Among 18 women with *Ureaplasma* who were not treated, there were 5 more abortions and 5 full-term pregnancies.

Empiric antibiotic therapy has been claimed to be of benefit to couples experiencing repetitive spontaneous abortions, thus suggesting an infectious etiology. In one study, only 10% of patients who were treated with tetracycline for 4 weeks and who became pregnant experienced another spontaneous abortion (Toth et al. 1986). By contrast, 38% of patients who did not choose to take antibiotics and who later became pregnant had a further spontaneous abortion. However, antibiotics were given or not given in accordance with the patients wishes; thus, the validity of the "control" group is arguable.

Anti-Fetal Antibodies

It is obvious that alterations of the immune system could be responsible for fetal wastage. However, the nature of the immunological process responsible for maintaining pregnancy is complex. Both autoimmune as well as alloimmune factors have been identified as causes of pregnancy loss.,

A familiar example of an immunological mechanism causing fetal wastage is the production of maternal antibodies against the fetus on the basis of genetic dissimilarities at a given locus. Mid- or late-gestational fetal loss is well documented in Rh-negative (D negative) women having anti-D antibodies. A rare situation involves anti-P antibodies (Levine 1978). Most individulas are genotype PP or Pp. However, an occasional female is homozygous pp. If a women of genotoype pp mates with a PP or Pp male, offspring may be Pp. If the mother develops anti-P antibodies, Pp fetuses are rejected early in gestation. Plasmapheresis may be efficacious (Rock et al. 1985).

Autoimmune Disease

The association between pregnancy loss and certain autoimmune disease is generally accepted (Branch and Ward 1989). Individuals with lupus anticoagulant (LAC) antibodies and anticardiolipin antibodies have an increased likelihood of fetal wastage. These two antibodies have closely related specificities. Anticardiolipin antibody may be the more sensitive indicator of the two (Locksin et al. 1985), but may also be less specific. In vitro, LAC is an anticoagluant; in vivo it paradoxically increases the likelihood of thrombosis (Gastineau et al. 1985). Lupus anticoagulant has been associated with subplacental clotting and fetal losses in all trimesters, as well as with poor reproductive history in general (Elias and Eldor 1984; Harris 1988). Thus, the abortifacient mechanism is presumably decidual. Because only 5%–10% of patients with systemic lupus erythematosus (SLE) have LAC, individuals with antinuclear antibodies (ANA) may or may not have LAC (Exner et al. 1978). Similarly, not all patients with LAC will have SLE.

Unander et al. (1987) studied 99 women having three or more abortions, 68 with no liveborns. Increased anticardiolipin antibodies were found in 42. The proportion in "primary" and "secondary"" aborters was the same, but the highest levels of anticardiolipin antibodies were observed in the former. Unfortunately, there were no control data. Howard et al. (1987) observed LAC in 9 of 29 women having "three spontaneous miscarriages or stillbirths." Cowchock et al. (1986) observed anticardiolipin antibodies in 13.1% of 61 women with repeated abortions. The first controlled study was by Petri et al. (1987): The frequency of LAC was 9% and anticardiolipin antibodies 11%; neither was different from control subjects.

Although the significance of these antibodies in clinically asymptomatic subjects is probably limited, evaluation of repetitive pregnancy losses should include a search for both LAC (or activated thromboplastin time or platelet neutralization tests) and anticardiolipin antibodies (Harris et al. 1986; Harris

1988). Scott et al. (1987) state that the incidence of midtrimester fetal death in women with LAC or anticardiolipin antibodies is 91%. This was based on a literature survey of 242 untreated pregnancies in 65 women; 220 losses occurred. In their own experience, 83% of 162 prior pregnancies in such women were lost. There is also an increased frequency of other pregnancy complications (e.g. growth retardation, preeclampsia). Treatment with prednisone and low-dose aspirin may improve the outcome (Branch et al. 1985), but treatment should be restricted to couples with midtrimester losses. Harris (1988) seems similarly sceptical in treating women with early losses.

Evidence for a relationship between autoimmune phenomena and early losses is even more arguable than that of LAC and anticardiolipin antibodies. In the study by Cowchock et al. (1986), the frequency of other antibodies to nuclear antigens (DNA, Ro or SS-A, La, Smith, ribonucleoprotein) was somewhat higher in 61 women with unexplained fetal losses than in 21 women with explained losses (e.g. balanced translocation, uterine anomaly). However, no control subjects were studied. A later study showed a pregnancy loss of 17% in 96 pregnancies in anti-SS-A women; the loss rate was 21% in 235 pregnancies in women without anti-SS-A antibodies (Ramsey-Goldman et al. 1986). Hass et al. (1986) studied antisperm antibodies in 109 women "without an immunologic cause for their recurrent abortions." The frequencies of antibodies as assessed by tray agglutination test (TAT), sperm immobilization test (SIT), and ELISA against solubilized sperm and seminal fluid antigens were 2.7%, 8.3% and 19.3% respectively. No control group was available.

In summary, the role of autiommune factors in early pregnancy loss is controversial. Some association probably exists, given data concerning LAC and anticardiolipin antibodies in midtrimester losses. However, the extent to which autoimmune factors should be sought in otherwise healthy couples is arguable. Assays for antinuclear antibodies and either LAC or anticardiolipin antibodies are probably sufficient.

Finally, claims of increased pregnancy losses in women with endometriosis (Damewood 1989) could be explained on an autoimmune basis, if indeed such an association exists.

Alloimmune Disease (Shared Parental Histocompatibility)

Rejection of the fetal allograft is prevented by maternal blocking or suppressive factors which protect the fetus. Blocking antibodies paradoxically seem to develop or to be enhanced by paternal antigens. This is assumed to be the explanation for the fact that pregnant women develop antipaternal leukocytotoxic antibodies.

About 20% of women develop such antibodies following their first pregnancy, and about 65% of multiparous women have such antibodies (Beard et al. 1983; Gill 1983; Weksler et al. 1983). These cytotoxic antibodies may or may not be of primary importance, but rather could serve as markers. Such antibodies, recognised by inhibition of the one-way mixed lymphocyte reaction, are believed to be anti-idiotypic antibodies that interact with maternal lymphocyte antigen receptors.

It follows that maternal–fetal histo*in*compatibility should enhance pregnancy maintenance. By contrast, greater than normal sharing of histocompatibility antigens (HLA) (or, as preferred by some, trophoblast-like antigens or TLX) (McIntyre et al. 1986; Faulk et al. 1989) between mother and father could be deleterious because fetus and mother would be less likely to differ antigenically. Direct experimental support for a beneficial effect of maternal–fetal incompatability includes: (1) increased placental size in mouse fetuses that result from matings in which paternally derived histocompatibility antigens differ from maternal antigens, (2) higher implantation frequencies in histoincompatible murine zygotes, and (3) maintenance of generic polymorphisms at major histocompatibility loci despite over 70 generations of brother–sister mating in rats (Beer and Billingham 1976).

In addition to parental HLA sharing, there is other circumstantial support for the benefits of parental histoincompatibility. Only 16.6% of women with multiple abortions have antipaternal antileukocytotoxic antibodies, in contrast to 64% of multiparous women and 20% of primiparous women (Thomas et al. 1983). Similarly, 50% of women with three or more recurrent abortions show no blocking factors, as evidenced by failure to demonstrate a mixed lymphocyte reaction when their lymphocytes are exposed to their spouse's lymphocytes (Beer et al. 1987). Blocking antibodies have been observed in women having successful pregnancies, but may be lacking in those having abortuses (Rocklin et al. 1976; 1982; Stimson et al. 1979; Fitzet and Bousquet 1983).

Other interpretations are also possible. Not all investigators have observed increased HLA sharing, depressed MLR, or decreased blocking antibodies (Oksenberg et al. 1984). Some couples sharing HLA-DR antigens have shown no spontaneous abortions, despite 10 or more pregnancies (Ober et al. 1983). In addition, the critical information of whether the abortus actually inherited the paternal antigen shared by its mother and father is often lacking. Antibodies can be absent in some women with successful pregnancy. Moreover, these antibodies develop only late in pregnancy and lack of antibodies probably does not lead to an inability to become pregnant (Regan and Braude 1987). Sargent et al. (1988) showed the rarity of cytotoxic antibodies (T cell and B cell) in both successful pregnancy (only 1 of 16 cases through 17 weeks) and abortions (0 of 9 cases). Discrepancies between the various studies are difficult to reconcile. Experimental designs have varied widely, and selection biases have not been fully evaluated. One alternative hypothesis is that blocking antibodies are the *result* of livebirths, as opposed to being necessary for pregnancy maintenance.

That some but not all couples sharing HLA antigens have deleterious effects could also be explained by postulating that normal pregnancy requires maternal–fetal histocompatibility not for HLA but rather for another closely linked locus. This hypothesis is not only consistent with HLA antigens failing to be expressed on the trophoblast but is supported by direct data. Blocking antibodies said to be present in normal pregnancies but absent in women experiencing spontaneous abortion are directed against neither HLA-A, B, C nor DR (Power et al. 1983). Thus, Faulk and McIntyre believe that immune regulation is stimulated by a series of placental antigens, so-called trophoblast lymphocyte cross-reactive (TLX) antigens (Faulk and McIntyre 1981; Faulk et al. 1989). This group claims to have isolated TLX antigens. They further claim that couples experiencing repetitive spontaneous abortions are more likely to share "TLX antigens" than couples without pregnancy wastage (McIntyre et al. 1986; Faulk et al. 1989).

Although parental antigen sharing could be expected to lead to repetitive abortion, it is also possible to explain the same data on a non-immunologic basis. Closely linked to the mouse histocompatibility (H2) complex is locus T/t. Embryos homozygous for certain alleles at this locus die at various stages of embryogenesis. Whether a T/t-like complex exists in humans is arguable. If it does, and if it is linked to HLA on human chromosome 6, histocompatibility between mother and her fetus and (her spouse) for this or another locus could merely reflect homozygosity for lethal T/t alleles. In fact, evidence for such an effect has been presented by Schacter et al. (1984).

If fetal rejection occurs as a result of diminished fetal–maternal immunologic interaction, it follows that immunotherapy might be effective. Indeed, pretransplant blood transfusions have been used to decrease allograft rejection after kidney transplantation (Norman et al. 1986). This beneficial effect appears due to the lymphocyte-rich fraction ("buffy-coat"). Immunization with lymphocytes of the paternal strain increases fetal survival in donkey–horse matings from 20% to 65% (Allen et al. 1986).

These studies served as the experimental basis for human studies in which women lacking blocking antibodies but sharing HLA antigens with their spouse were immunized with either paternal leukocytes (Beer et al. 1981; Mowbray et al. 1985; Takakuwa et al. 1986) or third party leukocytes (McIntyre and Faulk, 1986; Unander et al. 1986). Trophoblast membrane transfusion has also been attempted (McIntyre and Faulk 1986; Johnson et al. 1986).

The efficacy of immunotherapy was the subject of detailed consideration at a recent symposium sponsored by the Royal College of Obstetricians and Gynaecologists (Beard and Sharp, 1988). It is apparent that only a single, large prospective randomized trial has been published (Mowbray et al. 1985). The apparent improvement in outcome in the treated group (77% livebirths) compared to the untreated group (37% livebirths) was accompanied by lower-than-expected successes in the control group [a priori 60%–70%, as reviewed by Simpson and Carson (1991) and Vlaanderen and Treffers (1987)]. Thus, there could be a selection bias. It is also uncertain whether pregnancy complications are increased in immunized pregnancies. Multicentre randomized trials are currently in progress.

Irradiation and Antineoplastic Agents

X-irradiation and antineoplastic agents are accepted abortifacients, showing that exogenous factors during embryogenesis can cause fetal loss. However, therapeutic X-rays or chemotherapeutic drugs are administered during pregnancy only to seriously ill women. In diagnostic doses, X-rays have not been proven to cause fetal demise, though it would be prudent to consider X-rays as a potential confounding variable. Even relatively low levels of antimetabolites (e.g. methotrexate) might be abortifacient (Selevan et al. 1985), as shown by the successful use of such agents in ectopic gestation.

Cigarette Smoking

Smoking during pregnancy has been positively correlated with spontaneous abortion. Kline et al. (1980) found increased abortion rates in smokers, independent of maternal age and alcohol consumption. A positive dose–response curve was observed. Alberman et al. (1976) also reported that smokers showed a higher (albeit not significantly higher) proportion of abortuses with normal karyotypes, which suggest that smoking might affect the conceptus directly.

It is possible that smoking and other toxins might exert deleterious effects only on susceptible hosts. Genetic susceptibility might exist, though most exposed pregnancies end normally. Nonetheless, smoking is a significant confounding variable in determining fetal loss rate.

Alcohol

Several studies have reported an association between fetal loss and alcohol consumption. In one study, 616 women experiencing spontaneous abortions were compared with 632 women delivering at 28 weeks or more (Kline et al. 1980). Among women whose pregnancies ended in spontaneous abortion, 17% drank at least twice per week whereas 8.1% of controls drank similar quantities. After adjusting for smoking, age, prior abortions, etc. the association between alcohol and abortion remained significant. Harlap and Shiono (1980) also found a slightly increased risk for abortion in women who drank in the first trimester. The increase failed to reach statistical signficance, but could not be explained on the basis of smoking, prior abortion, age, or other factors.

By contrast, Halmesmärki (1989) found that alcohol consumption was nearly identical in women who did and did not experience an abortion; 13% of aborters and 11% of control women drank on average 3–4 drinks per week. Alcohol consumption was also similar in their spouses.

Other Environmental Factors

A few chemical agents have been claimed to have an association with fetal loss. These chemicals include anaesthetic gases, arsenic, aniline, benzene, ethylene oxide, formaldehyde and lead (Barlow and Sullivan 1982; Figa-Talamanaca and Settimi, 1984). Although many environmental toxicologists accept these agents as proved, evidence is far from convincing for low level exposures. Of topical interest is a study which claimed an association between pregnancy loss and exposure to video display terminals of greater than 20 hours per week (Goldhaber et al. 1988). However, the consensus based on other studies is that no such association exists (Blackwell and Chang 1988). Other studies show no increased risk for either pregnant laboratory workers (Heidam 1984) or pregnant pharmaceutical industry workers (Taskinen et al. 1984).

Intrauterine Devices and Other Contraceptive Agents

Conception with an intrauterine device (IUD) in situ markedly increases the risk of fetal loss. The presumed cause is infection. However, exposure to an IUD prior to pregnancy does not increase the risk of fetal loss.

At one time it was believed that use of other contraceptives – before and during pregnancy – was associated with fetal loss. This is now known to be untrue, both for women who discontinue oral contraceptives before conception (see Simpson 1985), as well as those exposed to spermicides prior to or after conception (Mills et al. 1985).

Trauma

Women commonly attribute pregnancy loss to trauma, such as a fall or blow to the abdomen. However, the fetus is well protected from external trauma by maternal structures and amniotic fluid. The relative safety of amniocentesis and chorionic villus sampling attests to this.

Psychological Factors

Impaired psychological well-being as a cause of early fetal loss has been claimed but not proved. Neurotic or mentally ill women abort, but whether the frequency of losses is higher than that in normal women is unknown. A well-known study is that of Stray-Pedersen and colleagues (Stray-Pedersen and Stray-Pedersen 1985; 1988). This group believe there is a beneficial effect of increased attention for women having repetitive abortions ("tender-loving-care") in the absence of specific medical therapy. In their most recent study, 116 women were more likely (85%) to complete their pregnancy than were 24 women not provided such care (36%). A deficiency in the study design was that only women living "close" to the university were eligible for the increased attention. Women living further away served as "controls" and thus may have differed in unknown ways from the experimental group.

This author suspects that any beneficial effect of enhanced psychological well-being is probably either more apparent than real or is merely secondary to other factors.

Generalized Effects of Severe Maternal Illness

Almost all debilitating maternal diseases have been implicated in spontaneous abortion. Various mechanisms could be invoked, specifically endocrinologic, immunologic or infectious. Examples already cited include diabetes mellitus and lupus erythematosus.

Other maternal diseases that may be associated with fetal wastage include Wilson's disease, maternal phenylketonuria, cardiac insufficiency (e.g. cyanotic heart disease), and haematologic disorders (e.g. haemoglobinopathies or aplastic anaemia). In fact, any life-threatening disease would be expected to be associated with increased abortion rates. Seriously ill women rarely become pregnant, but in some cases the disease process may deteriorate after the onset of pregnancy. Overall, only a small fraction of all fetal losses can be attributable to severe maternal disease.

The well-known maternal age effect is highly relevant to fetal wastage. Women aged 40–44 have approximately twice the likelihood of fetal loss than that of women two decades younger. Interestingly, this risk holds for both trisomic as well as euploid abortuses (Stein et al. 1980). This is consistent with animal studies showing decreased ability of older animals to retain embryos transferred from young mothers (Biggers 1969). Possible explanations include infections, diminished luteal response, and a poorly vascularized endometrium. Any of these would be exacerbated in serious maternal illness.

References

Alberman ED (1981) The abortus as a predictor of future trisomy 21. In: De La Cruz FF, Gerald PSA (eds) Trisomy (Down's syndrome). University Park Press, Baltimore, p.69

Alberman E. Creasy M, Elliott M. Spicer C (1976) Maternal effects associated with fetal chromosomal anomalies in spontaneous abortions. Br J Obstet Gynaecol 83: 621–627

Alfi OS. Chang R, Azen SP (1981) Evidence for genetic control of nondisjunction in man. Am J Hum Genet 32: 477–483

Allen WR, Kydd JH, Antczak DF (1986) Successful application of immunotherapy to a model of pregnancy failure in equids. In: Clark DA, Croy BA (eds) Reproductive immunology. Elsevier, New York, p 253

Angell RR, Aitken JR, van-Look PFGA, et al. (1983) Chromosome abnormalities in human embryos after in vitro fertilization. Nature 303: 336–338

Barlow S, Sullivan FM (1982) Reproductive hazards of industrial chemicals: an evaluation of animal and human data. Academic Press, New York

Beard RW, Sharp F (1988) Early pregnancy loss: mechanism and treatment. Proceedings of the 18th Study Group of the Royal College of Obstetricians and Gynaecologists. Royal College of Obstetricians and Gynaecologists, London

Beard RW, Braude P, Mowbray JF, et al. (1983) Protective antibodies and spontaneous abortion. Lancet i: 1090

Beer AE, Billingham RF (1976) The immunology of mammalian reproduction. Prentice-Hall, Englewood Cliffs, NJ

Beer AE, Quebbeman JF, Ayers JW, et al. (1981) Major histocompatibility complex antigens, maternal and paternal immune responses, and chronic habitual abortions in humans. Am J Obstet Gynecol 141: 987–999

Beer AE, Quebbeman JF, Sempirini AE (1987) Immunopathological factors contributing to recurrent and spontaneous abortion in humans. In: Bennet MJ, Edmonds DK (eds) Spontaneous and recurrent abortions. Blackwell, Oxford, p 90–108

Biggers JD (1969) Problems concerning the uterine causes of embryonic death, with special reference to the effects of aging of the uterus. J Reprod Fertil (Suppl) 8: 27–43

Blackwell R, Chang A (1988) Video display terminals and pregnancy. A review. Br J Obstet Gynaecol 95: 446–453

Boué J, Boué A, Lazar P (1975) Retrospective and prospective epidemiological studies of 1500 karyotyped spontaneous human abortions. Teratology 12: 11–26

Boué J, Phillipe E, Giroud A, et al. (1976) Phenotypic expression of lethal chromosomal anomalies in human abortuses. Teratology 14: 3–19

Branch DW, Scott JR, Kochenour NK, et al. (1985) Obstetric complications associated with the lupus anticoagluant. N Engl J Med 313: 1322–1326

Branch DW, Ward K (1989) Autoimmunity and pregnancy loss. Semin Reprod Endocrinol 7: 168–179

Carson SA, Simpson JL (1990) Spontaneous abortion. In: Eden Rd, Boehm FH (eds) Fetal assessment: physiological, clinical and medico-legal principles. Appleton-Century-Crofts, Norwalk, CT, pp 559–574

Chandley AC (1981) The origin of chromosomal aberrations in man and their potential for survival and reproduction in the adult human populations. Ann Genet 24: 5–11

Cowchock S, Smith JB, Gocial B (1986) Antibodies to phospholipids and nuclear antigens in patients with repeated abortions. Am J Obstet Gynecol 155: 1002–1010

Daly DC, Walters CA, Soto-Albers CE, et al. (1983) Endometrial biopsy during treatment of luteal phase defects is predictive of therapeutic outcome. Fertil Steril 40: 305–312

Damewood MD (1989) The association of endometriosis and repetitive (early spontaneous) abortions. Semin Reprod Endocrinol 7: 155–160

Daniels A, Hook EB, Wulf G (1989) Risks of unbalanced progengy at amniocentesis to carriers of chromosome rearrangements: data from United States and Canadian laboratories. Am J Med Genet 31: 14–53

Davis OK, Berkley AS, Cholst IN, Nause GJ, Freedman KS (1989) The incidence of luteal phase defect in normal, fertile women, determined. Fertil Steril 51: 582–586

Daya S, Ward S (1988) Diagnostic test properties of serum progesterone in the evaluation of luteal phase defects. Fertil Steril 49: 168–170

Daya S, Ward S, Burrows E (1988) Progesterone profiles in luteal phase defect cycles and outcome of progesterone treatment in patients with recurrent spontaneous abortions. Am J Obstet Gynecol 158: 225–232

Downs KA, Gibson M (1983) Basal temperature graph and luteal phase defect. Fertil Steril 40: 466–468

Edmonds RF (1988) Use of cervical cerclage in patients with recurrent first trimester abortions. In: Beard RW, Sharp F (eds) Early pregnancy loss: mechanism and treatment. Proceedings of the 18th Study Group of the Royal College of Obstetricians and Gynaecologists. Royal College of Obstetricians and Gynaecologists, London, pp 411–415

Elias M. Eldor A (1984) Thromboembolism in patients with "lupus" type circulating anticoagluant. Arch Intern Med 1244: 510–515

Exner T. Richard KA, Kronenberg H (1978) A sensitive test demonstrating LAC and its behavioural patterns. Br J Haematol 40: 143–151

Faulk WP, McIntyre JA (1981) Trophoblast survival. Transplantation 32: 1–5

Faulk WO, Coulam CB, McIntyre JA (1989) The role of trophoblast antigens in repetitive spontaneous abortions. Semin Reprod Endocrinol 7: 182–187

Figa-Talamanaca I, Seltimi L (1984) Occupational factors and reproductive outcome. In: Hafez ESE (ed) Spontaneous abortion. MTP Press, Lancaster, pp 61–80

Fitzet D. Bousquet J (1983) Absence of a factor blocking cellular cytotoxicity in the serum of women with recurrent abortion. Br J Obstet Gynaecol 90: 453–456

Gastineau DA, Kazimier FJ, Nichols WL, et al. (1985) Lupus anticoagulant: an analysis of the clinical and laboratory features of 219 cases. Am J Hematol 19: 265–275

Gill TH III (1983) Immunogenetics of spontaneous abortions in humans. Transplantation 35: 1–6

Goldhaber MK, Polen MR, Hiatt RA (1988) The risk of miscarriage and birth defects among women who use visual display terminals during pregnancy. Am J Industrial Med 13: 695–706

Greene MF, Hare JW, Cloherty JP, et al. (1989) First trimester hemoglobin A1 and risk for major malformation and spontaneous abortion in diabetic pregnancy. Teratology 32: 225–231

Gropp A (1973) Fetal mortality due to aneuploidy and irregular meiotic segregation in the mouse. In: Boué A, Thibault C (eds) Les accidents chromosiques de la réproduction. INSERM, Paris, p 225

Gropp A (1975) Chromosomal animal model of human disease. Fetal trisomy and development failure. In: Berry L. Poswillo DE (eds) Teratology. Springer-Verlag, Berlin, 17–35

Guerneri S. Bettio D, Simoni G, et al. (1987) Prevalence and distribution of chromosome abnormalities in a sample of first trimester internal abortions. Hum Reprod 2: 735–739

Hass GG Jr, Kubota K, Quebbeman JF, et al. (1986) Circulating antisperm antibodies in recurrently aborting women. Fertil Steril 45: 209–215

Halmesmärki E (1989) Maternal and paternal alcohol consumption and miscarriage. Br J Obstet Gynaecol 96: 186–191

Harlap S, Shiono PH (1980) Alcohol smoking and incidence of spontaneous abortions in the first and second trimester. Lancet ii: 173

Harris EN (1988) Clinical and immunological significance of anti-phospholipid antibodies. In: Beard RW, Sharp F (eds) Early pregnancy loss: mechanism and treatment. Proceedings of the 18th Study Group of the Royal College of Obstetricians and Gynaecologists. Royal College of Obstetricians and Gynaecologists, London, pp 43–60

Harris EN, Chan JKH, Asherson RA, et al. (1986) Thrombosis, recurrent fetal loss and thrombocytopenia: predictive value of the anticardiolipin test. Arch Intern Med 146: 2153–2156

Hassold T (1980) A cytogenetic study of repeated spontaneous abortions. Am J Hum Genet 32: 723–730

Heidam LZ (1984) Spontaneous abortions among laboratory workers: a follow up study. J Epidemiol Community Health 38: 36–41

Heinonen P. Saarikoski S. Pystynen P (1982) Reproductive performance of women with uterine anomalies: an evaluation of 182 cases. Acta Obstet Gynecol Scand 61: 157–162

Herbst AL, Senekjian EK, Frey KW (1989) Abortion and pregnancy loss among diethylstilbestrol-exposed women. Semin Reprod Endocrinol 7: 124–129

Hertig AT, Rock J (1973) Searching for early human ova. Gynecol Invest 4: 121–139

Hertig AT, Rock J, Adams EC (1956) Description of human ova within the first 17 days of development. Am J Anat 98: 435–493

Hertig AT, Rock J, Adams EC, Menkin MC (1959) Thirty-four fertilized human ova, good, bad and indifferent, recovered from 210 women of known fertility. A study of biologic wastage in early human pregnancy. Pediatrics 25: 202–211

Horta JLH, Fernandez JG, DeSoto LB (1977) Direct evidence of luteal insufficiency in women with habitual abortion. Obstet Gynecol 49: 705–708

Howard MA, Firkin BG, Healy DL, Choong SC (1987) Lupus anticoagulant in women with multiple spontaneous miscarriage. Am J Hematol 26: 175–178

Jacobs MH, Balasch J, Gonzalez-Merlo JM et al. (1987) J Clin Endocrinol Metab 64: 472–475

Jacobs PA, Angell RR, Buchanan IM, et al. (1978) The origin of human triploids. Ann Hum Genet 42: 49-57

Johnson PM, Chia KV, Risk JM (1986) Immunological question marks in recurrent spontaneous abortion. In; Clark DA, Croy BA (eds) Reproductive immunology. Elsevier, New York, p 239–245

Jones GS (1976) The luteal phase defect. Fertil Steril 27: 351–356

Kline J. Shrout P, Stein ZA, et al. (1980) Drinking during pregnancy and spontaneous abortion. Lancet ii: 176–180

Lazar P. Gueguen S (1984) Multicentred controlled trial of cervical cerclage in women at moderate risk of preterm delivery. Br J Obstet Gynaecol 91: 731–735

Ledbetter DH, Gilbert F, Jackson L, et al. (1990) Cytogenetic results of chorionic villus sampling: high success rate and diagnostic accuracy in the US Collaborative Study. Am J Obstet Gynecol 162: 495–501

Levine P (1978) ABO, P and MN blood group determinants in neoplasm foreign to the host. Semin Oncol 5: 25–34

Li TC, Rogers AW, Lenton EA, Dockery P, Cooke I (1987) A comparison between 2 methods of chronological dating of human endometrial biopsies during the luteal phase and their correlation with histological dating. Fertil Steril 48: 928–932

Li TC, Dockery P, Rogers AW, Cooke ID (1989) How precise is histologic dating of endometrium using the standard dating criteria? Fertil Steril 51: 759–763

Lockshin MD, Druzin ML, Goei S, et al. (1985) Antibody to cardiolipin as a predictor of fetal distress or death in pregnant patients with systemic lupus erythematosus. N Engl J Med 313:152–156

Martin AO, Simpson JL, Deddish RB, et al. (1983) Clinical implications of chromosomal inversions. A pericentric inversion in No. 18 segregating in a family ascertained through an abnormal proband. Am J Perinatol 1: 81–88

McIntyre JA, Faulk WP (1986) Trophoblast antigens in normal and abnormal human pregnancy. Clin Obstet Gynecol 29: 976–998

McIntyre JA, Faulk WP, Nichols-Johnson VR, et al. (1986) Immunological testing and immunotherapy in recurrent spontaneous abortion. Obstet Gynecol 67: 169–172

McRae MA, Blasco L, Lyttle CR (1984) Serum homones and their receptors in women with normal and inadequate corpus luteum function. Fertil Steril 42: 58–63

Michelman HW, Bonhoff A, Mettler L (1986) Chromosome analysis in polypoid human embryos. Hum Reprod 1: 243–246

Mills JL, Reed GF, Nugent RP, et al. (1985) Are there adverse effets of periconceptional spermicide use? Fertil Steril 43: 442–446
Mills JL, Simpson JL, Driscoll SG, et al. (1988) Incidence of spontaneous abortion among normal women and insulin-dependent diabetic women whose pregnancies were identified within 21 days of conception. N Engl J Med 319: 1617–1623
Miodnovic M. Lavin JP, Knowles HC, et al. (1984) Spontaneous abortion among insulin dependent diabetic women. Am J Obstet Gynecol 150: 372–376
Miodovnic M, Skillman C. Holroyde JC, et al. (1985) Elevated maternal glycohemoglobin in early pregnancy and spontaneous abortion among insulin dependent diabetic women. Am J Obstet Gynecol 153: 439–443
Miodovnic M, Mimouni F, Tsang RL, et al. (1986) Glycemic control and spontaneous abortion in insulin dependent diabetic women. Obstet Gynecol 68: 366–369
Montero M, Collea JV, Frasier D, Mestman J (1981) Successful outcome of pregnancy in women with hypothyroidism. Ann Intern Med 94· 31–34
Mowbray JG, Gibbing C, Liddell H, et al. (1985) Controlled trial of treatment of recurrent spontaneous abortion by immunization with paternal cells. Lancet ii: 941–943.
Norman DJ, Barry JM, Fischer S (1986) The beneficial effect of pretransplant third-party blood transfusions on allograft rejection in HLA identical sibling kidney transplants. Transplantation 41: 125–126
Noyes RW, Hertig ATR, Rock J (1950) Dating the endometrial biopsy. Fertil Steril 1: 3–25
Ober CL, Martin AO, Simpson JL, et al. (1983) Shared HLA antigens and reproductive performance among Hutterites. Am J Hum Genet 35: 994–1004
Oksenberg JR, Persitz E, Amar A, et al. (1984) Maternal-paternal histocompability: lack of association with habitual abortion. Fertil Steril 42: 389–395
Petri M, Golbus M, Anderson R, et al. (1987) Antinuclear antibody, lupus anticoagulant, and anticardiolipin antibody in women with idiopathic habitual abortion. Arthritis Rheum 30: 601–606
Plachot M, Junca AM, Mandelbaum J (1987) Chromosome investigations in early life. II. Human preimplantation embryos. Hum Reprod 2: 29–35
Power DA, Mason RJ, Stewart GM, et al. (1983) The fetus as an allograft: evidence for protective antibodies to HLA-linked paternal antigens. Lancet II: 701–704
Quinn PA, Petrie M, Barking M, et al. (1987) Prevalence of antibody to *Chlamydia trachomatis* in spontaneous abortion and infertility. Am J Obstet Gynecol 156: 291–296
Ramsey-Goldman R, Hom D, Deng JS, et al. (1986) Anti-SS-A antibodies and fetal outcome in maternal systemic lupus erythematosus. Arthritis Rheum 29: 1269–1273
Regan L, Braude PR (1987) Is antipaternal cytotoxic antibody a valid marker in the management of recurrent abortion? Lancet ii: 1280
Rock J, Jones HW Jr (1977) The clinical management of the double uterus. Fertil Steril 28: 798–806
Rock JA, Shirey RS, Braine HG, et al. (1985) Plasmapheresis for the treatment of repeated early pregnancy wastage associated with anti-P. Obstet Gynecol 66: 57S–60S
Rocklin RE, Kitzmiller JL, Carpenter CB, et al. (1976) Absence of an immunologic blocking factor from the serum of women with chronic abortion. N Engl J Med 295: 1209–1213
Rocklin RE, Kitzmiller JL, Garvoy MR (1982) Further characterization of an immunologic blocking factor that develops during pregnancy. Clin Immunol Immunopathol 22: 305–315
Rudak E, Dor J, Mashiach S, et al. (1985) Chromosome analysis of human oocytes and embryos fertilized in vitro. Ann NY Acad Sci 442: 476–486
Rush RW, McPherson K, Jones L, et al. (1984) A randomized controlled trial of cervical cerclage in women at high risk of spontaneous preterm delivery. Br J Obstet Gynaecol 91: 724–730
Ruzicska P. Cziezel A (1971) Cytogenetic studies on midtrimester abortuses. Humangenetik 10: 273–297
Saracoglu OF, Aksel S, Yeoman RR, et al. (1985) Endometrial estradiol and progesterone receptors in patients with luteal phase defects and endometriosis. Fertil Steril 43: 851–855
Sargent IL, Wilkins T, Redman CWG (1988) Maternal immune responses to the fetus in early pregnancy and recurrent miscarriage. Lancet ii: 1099–1104
Schacter B, Weitkamp LR, Johnson WE (1984) Paternal HLA compatibility, fetal wastage and neural tube defects: evidence for a T/t-like locus in humans. Am J Human Genet 36: 1082–1091
Selevan SG, Lindbohm M-L, Hornung RW, Hemminki K (1985) A study of occupational exposure to antineoplastic drugs and fetal loss in nurses. N Engl J Med 313: 1173–1178
Scott JR, Rote NS, Branch DW (1987) Immunologic aspects of recurrent abortions and fetal death. Obstet Gynecol 70: 645–656
Scott RT, Synder RR, Strickland DM, et al. (1988) The effect of interobserver variation in dating endometrial history on the diagnosis of luteal phase defect. Fertil Steril 50: 888l–892

Simpson JL (1976) Disorders of sex differentiation: etiology and clinical delineation. Academic Press, New York

Simpson JL (1985) Relationship between congenital anomalies and contraception. Adv Contracept 1: 3–30

Simpson JL (1990) Incidence and timing of pregnancy losses: relevance to evaluating safety of early prenatal diagnosis. Am J Med Genet 35: 165–173

Simpson JL (1991) Fetal wastage. In: Gabbe SA, Niebyl JF, Simpson JL (eds) Obstetrics: normal and abnormal pregnancies, 2nd edn. Churchill-Livingstone, New York.

Simpson JL, Bombard AT (1987) Chromosomal abnormalities in spontaneous abortions: frequency, pathology and genetic counselling. In: Edmonds K, Bennet MJ (eds) Spontaneous abortion. Blackwell, London pp 51–76

Simpson JL, Carson SA (1991) Causes of fetal loss. In: Gray R, Leridon L, Spira F (eds) Symposium on biological and demographic determinants of human reproduction. Oxford University Press, Oxford (in press)

Simpson JL, LeBeau MM (1981) Gonadal and statural determinants on the X chromosome and their relationship to in vitro studies showing prolonged cell cycles in 45,X;46,X,del(X)(p11); 46,Xdel,(X)(q13) and q(22) fibroblasts. Am J Obstet Gynecol 141: 930–939

Simpson JL, Golbus MS (1991) Genetics in obstetrics and gynecology, 2nd edn. WB Saunders, Philadelphia (in press)

Simpson JL, Mills JL (1985) Methodologic problems in determining fetal loss rates: relevance to chorionic villus sampling. In: Fraccaro M, Simoni G, Brambati B (eds) First trimester fetal diagnosis. Springer-Verlag, Berlin, pp 321–333

Simpson JL, Elias S, Martin AO (1981) Parental chromosomal rearrangements associated with repetitive spontaneous abortions. Fertil Steril 36: 584–590

Simpson JL, Mills JL, Holmes LB, et al. (1987) Low fetal loss rates after ultrasound-proved viability in early pregnancy. JAMA 258: 2555–2557

Simpson JL, Meyers, CM, Martin AO, et al. (1989) Translocations are infrequent among couples having repeated spontaneous abortions but no other abnormal pregnancies. Fertil Steril 51: 811–814

Smith SK, Lenton EA, Landgren BM, Cooke ID (1984) The short luteal phase and infertility. Br J Obstet Gynaecol 91: 1120–1122

Spiritos NJ, Yurewicz EC, Moghissi KS, et al. (1985) Pseudocorpus luteum insufficiency: a study of cytosol progesterone receptors in human endometrium. Obstet Gynecol 65: 535–540

Stabile I, Campbell S, Grudzinskas JG (1987) Ultrasonic assessment of complications during first trimester of pregnancy. Lancet ii: 1237–1240

Stein Z, Kline J, Susser E, et al. (1980) Maternal age and spontaneous abortion. In: Porter IH, Hook EB (eds) Human embryonic and fetal death. Academic Press, New York, pp 107–127

Stimson WH, Strachnan AF, Shepard A (1979) Studies on the maternal immune response to placental antigens: absence of a blocking factor from the blood of abortion-prone women. Br J Obstet Gynaecol 86: 41–45

Stray-Pedersen B, Eng J, Reikvan TM (1978) Uterine T-mycoplasma colonization in reproductive failure. Am J Obstet Gynecol 130: 307–311

Stray-Pedersen B, Stray-Pedersen S (1984) Etiologic factors and subsequential reproductive performance in 195 couples with a prior history of habitual abortion. Am J Obstet Gynecol 148: 140–146

Stray-Pedersen B, Stray-Pedersen S (1988) Recurrent abortion: the role of psychotherapy. In: Beard RW, Sharp F (eds) Early pregnancy loss: mechanism and treatment. Proceedings of the 18th Study Group of the Royal College of Obstetricians and Gynaecologists. Royal College of Obstetricians and Gynaecologists, London, pp 433–440

Sutherland GR, Gardiner AJ, Carter RF (1976) Familial pericentric inversion of chromosome 19 inv (19) (p13q13) with a note on genetic counselling of pericentric inversion carriers. Clin Genet 10: 53–59

Tabor A, Philip J, Madsen M, et al. (1987) Randomized controlled trial of genetic amniocentesis in 4606 low-risk women. Lancet i: 1287–1293

Takakuwa K, Kanazawa K, Takeuchi S (1986) Production of blocking antibodies by vaccination with husband's lymphocytes in unexplained recurrent aborters: the role in successful pregnancy. Am J Reprod Immunol Microbiol 10: 1–9

Taskinen H, Lindbohm M-L, Hemminki K (1984) Spontaneous abortions among women working in the pharmaceutical industry. Br J Indust Med 43: 199–205

Tharapel AT, Elias S, Shulman LP, et al. (1989) Resorbed co-twin as an explanation for discrepant chorionic villus results: non-mosaic 47,XX+16 in villi (direct and culture) with normal (46,XX) amniotic fluid and neonatal blood. Prenatal Diagn 9: 467–472

Tho PT, Byrd JR, McDonough PC (1979) Etiologies and subsequent reproductive performance of 100 couples with recurrent abortions. Fertil Steril 32: 389–95

Thomas ML, Harger JH, Wegener DK, et al. (1985) HLA sharing and spontaneous abortion. Am J Obstet Gynecol 151: 1053–1058

Toth A, Lesser Ml, Brooks-Toth CW, et al. (1986) Outcome of subsequent pregnancies following antibiotic therapy after primary or multiple spontaneous abortions. Surg Gynecol Obstet 163: 243–250

Unander AM, Norberg R, Hahn L, Arfors L (1987) Anticardiolipin antibodies and complement in ninety-nine women with habitual abortion. Am J Obstet Gynecol 156: 114–119

Vlaanderen W, Treffers PE (1987) Prognosis of subsequent pregnancies after recurrent spontaneous abortion in first trimester. Br Med J 295: 92–93

Warburton D, Kline J, Stein Z, et al. (1980) Cytogenetic abnormalities in spontaneous abortion of recognized conceptions. In: Porter IH, Hatcher NH, Willey AM (eds) Perinatal genetics: diagnosis and treatment. Academic Press, Orlando, pp23–40

Warburton D, Kline, Stein Z, et al. (1987) Does the karyotype of a spontaneous abortion predict the karyotype of a subsequent abortion? Evidence from 273 women with two karyotyped spontaneous abortuses. Am J Hum Genet 41: 465–483

Watt JL, Templeton AA, Messinis I, et al. (1987) Trisomy 1 in an eight cell human pre-embryo. J Med Genet 24: 60–64

Weksler BB, Pett SB, Alsono D, et al. (1983) Differential inhibition by aspirin of vascular and platelet prostaglandin synthesis in atherosclerotic patients. N Engl J Med 308: 800–805

Wilcox AJ, Weinberg CR, O'Connor JF, et al. (1988) Incidence of early loss of pregnancy. N Engl J Med 319: 189–194

Wu CH, Minassian SS (1987) Integrated luteal progesterone: an assessment of luteal function. Fertil Steril 48: 937·940

Zenzes MT, Belkien L, Bordt J, et al. (1985) Cytologic investigation of human in vitro fertilization failures. Fertil Steril 43: 883–891

3. Anembryonic Pregnancy

I. Stabile

Introduction

Anembryonic pregnancy of blighted ovum is the most common identifiable pathology in the first trimester of pregnancy (Fukijura et al. 1966). This condition provides one of nature's experiments wherein an embryo does not develop inside a gestational sac. This is, however, difficult to prove unless the gestational sac has been followed carefully from the time of conception. In this chapter the hypothesis will be proposed that all empty gestational sacs contained an embryo at one time which subsequently was resorbed. When embryonic remnants are present within the gestational sac, this is commonly referred to as a missed abortion. Perhaps a better term for this condition is early embryonic arrest. The time interval between arrest of embryonic development and clinical presentation will determine the sonographic features upon which diagnosis is based. Throughout this chapter the term anembryonic pregnancy and blighted ovum will be used interchangeably, although the former may be more appropriate. To aid understanding of the structures visible by ultrasound, an outline of the important early embryologic changes is given.

Embryology

Soon after the blastocyst implants (days 19 to 21 from the last menstrual period), a germ disc develops from the inner cell mass consisting of the ectoderm attached to the trophoblast and the endoderm facing the cavity of the blastocyst. The embryo at this stage measures approximately 0.05 mm, while the gestational sac is 0.3 mm in diameter. By the fourth week of gestation the amniotic sac forms between the ectoderm and the adjacent trophoblast. At this time, the embryo is 0.3 mm in length and has developed a primitive streak. It lies within a 2.5 mm diameter gestational sac which should be visible using high frequency transvaginal sonography (TVS). By the start of the fifth week the gestational sac (more accurately termed the chorionic cavity) has enlarged fivefold (12 mm) and the embryo now measures 2 mm. The first somites have appeared as well as the neural folds. At this stage, the gestational sac contains the amniotic sac and the much larger extraembryonic coelom with the yolk sac within. During the sixth week, the embryo grows to 4–5 mm in length and is now within the resolution of most current abdominal ultrasound equipment. By this time the cervical and thoracic somites as well as the neural tube have developed. The gestational sac is now 2–2.5 mm in diameter (volume 1.0 ml). By the start of the seventh week, the embryo measures 7–10 mm, the limb buds have fully formed and the primordial germ cells have reached the genital ridges (Altman and Dittmer 1972).

Pathology

Previous pathological studies have identified an intact empty gestational sac in 5%–10% of abortions (Mikamo 1970). Many abortions, however, yield ruptured or incomplete sacs, such that the true frequency of anembryonic pregnancy may be difficult to assess. The rate will also vary with differing clinical management such as hospital admission policies and the timing of curettage. An 11-year pathological study of 1426 specimens revealed blighted ova in 47% of cases (Rushton 1988). In this study, the selection of material reaching the laboratory (and hence the frequency with which anembryonic pregnancy was diagnosed by pathologists as the cause of early pregnancy failure) was influenced by the local admission policy, the population served, the gestation at which abortion occurred as well as the research interests of both clinicians and pathologists. Our prospective ultrasound-based study (Stabile et al. 1989a) confirmed the pathological estimates in that anembryonic pregnancy was diagnosed in 14% of women with threatened miscarriage (TMC) but in 45% of those women whose pregnancy has already failed at the time of presentation to hospital (Table 3.1).

Table 3.1. Clinical outcome in The London Study Group (No.=466)

	No. (%)
Intrauterine pregnancy	406
Normal progress termination of pregnancy	227 (48.7)
Elective termination of pregnancy	26 (5.6)
Subsequent spontaneous miscarriage	6 (1.3)
Anembryonic pregnancy	67 (14.4)
Complete miscarriage	4 (0.9)
Incomplete miscarriage	41 (8.8)
Missed miscarriage	34 (7.3)
Hydatiform mole	1 (0.2)
Extrauterine pregnancy	60 (12.8)

The London Study Group

We have recently completed (Stabile et al. 1989a) a prospective study of 624 unselected, consecutive women with TMC, in which we assessed the diagnostic value of circulating levels of pregnancy-associated proteins and hormones in conjunction with high resolution abdominal ultrasonography. The group included 67 women with anembryonic pregnancy. This was diagnosed when an empty gestational sac was identified of volume greater than or equal to 2.5 ml. in which no fetal parts could be demonstrated by ultrasound or on subsequent histological examination (Stabile et al. 1987). If the sac volume was less that 2.5 ml, the ultrasound examination was repeated the following week.

Pregnancy was confirmed at ultrasound examination in 406 women with TMC, and a live fetus of appropriate size was identified in 259 of these women (64%), of whom 10% elected to terminate their pregnancy. The pregnancy proceeded uneventfully beyond 20 weeks in 97.4% of the remaining 233 women. The proportion of women with anembryonic pregnancy varied from 12% at 8 weeks to 37% at 10 weeks (Fig. 3.1). The clinical characteristics of this group are shown in Table 3.2 by comparison with the remaining 227 women who had a live fetus in utero and whose pregnancies progressed uneventfully beyond 20 weeks.

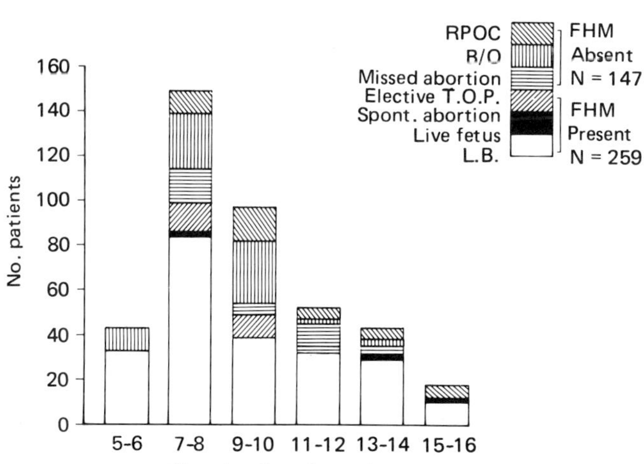

Fig. 3.1. Outcome of pregnancy in 406 women with threatened miscarriage according to gestational age.

Table 3.2. Clinical characteristics of 67 women with anembryonic pregnancy compared with 227 women with threatened miscarriage and normal outcome of their pregnancy. Mean values are shown with standard deviations in brackets

	Normal Outcome	Anembryonic pregnancy
Age	23.9 (6.2)	27.3 (7.2)
Week of first bleeding episode	6.9 (3.1)	8.5 (2.7)
Duration of first bleeding episode (days)	2.8 (1.4)	5.2 (4.7)
One or more previous pregnancies > 28 weeks	32%	47%
One or more previous spontaneous abortions	20%	43%

Anembryonic pregnancy is a common identifiable pathology in early pregnancy failure, following both spontaneous and assisted conception. Yovich and Matson (1988) identified a higher rate of anembryonic pregnancy in women conceiving after artificial insemination than after in vitro fertilization (IVF) and gamete intrafallopian transfer (GIFT).

Ultrasound Aspects

The introduction of real-time abdominal ultrasound scanning, and more recently vaginal ultrasonography, has revolutionized the clinical management of women presenting with TMC. It is now possible to confirm or exclude fetal viability after 6 weeks gestation. Traditionally, the sonographic diagnosis of anembryonic pregnancy is based on the absence of fetal or embryonic parts within a gestational sac which is large enough for such structures to be visible. When using conventional abdominal ultrasound with a sector transducer, structures as small as 5–6 mm should be visible to the experienced eye. Thus an embryo with a crown rump length of 6 mm equivalent to 6 weeks gestation (from the first day of the last menstrual period) should be identified using abdominal ultrasound. Robinson (1975) has emphasized the importance of ignoring all menstrual or clinical data in reaching the diagnosis. Other typical sonographic features include an irregular, poorly defined gestational sac situated low in the uterine cavity which is not only small for the gestational age but also fails to grow appropriately (Nyberg et al. 1986). These latter features are subjective and dependent on operator experience and the time available for examination. In our study, which was conducted as part of a busy clinical service (Stabile et al. 1989a), we were able to diagnose all cases of anembryonic pregnancy after 7 weeks or when the gestational sac volume (GSV) was greater than 3 ml. In 15 women a repeat examination was considered necessary because the GSV was less than 2.5 ml. On each occasion, the diagnosis was confirmed a week later.

It has been suggested that the use of TVS will lead to earlier diagnosis and better management of the complications of early pregnancy. While there is no doubt that high frequency vaginal sonography enables earlier visualization of the gestational sac and embryo, there is little agreement in the published literature as to the expected dimensions of the embryo and GSV at specific times during the first trimester. This may be due to biological variation and/or differences in equipment. Furthermore, precise sonographic criteria for the diagnosis of specific pregnancy complications have not as yet been established. Only one study has investigated the gestational sac size criteria for non-viable pregnancy using TVS (Levi et al. 1988). A gestational sac greater than or equal to 8 mm (mean of all three diameters; GSV 0.27 ml) without a yolk sac was noted in 10 patients, all of whom had a non-viable pregnancy. Unfortunately, the authors did not report whether the diagnosis was confirmed by histopathologic examination. In a further 5 patients a yolk sac was not seen at a gestational sac size of > 8 mm, but the pregnancy was considered normal because cardiac pulsation was identified on subsequent examination (false positives). In 3 patients an embryo was not seen in a gestational sac no greater than 16 mm (GSV 2.14 ml). All three pregnancies were defined as abnormal. There were no false positive results. In a further 3 patients the embryo was present but the pregnancy subsequently failed (at an unspecified time interval after the initial examination). Based on these small numbers of patients, the authors concluded that the criteria for the diagnosis of a non-viable pregnancy are a mean gestational sac greater than or equal to 8 mm diameter without a yolk sac and a mean gestational sac greater than or equal to 16 mm without an embryo or cardiac pulsations. It is noteworthy that the presence of a yolk sac at this stage (GSV 8 mm in diameter) did not guarantee a normal pregnancy. The authors consistently excluded a viable pregnancy if an embryo was absent at a GSV of 2.14 ml. This is not a significant improvement over the early results of Robinson (1975) who determined the GSV cut-off level of 2.5 ml and then used this to distinguish viable from non-viable pregnancies using a static B scanner. In clinical terms, it is important to ensure that the criteria of abnormality are sufficiently stringent to allow a pregnancy diagnosed as being abnormal to be terminated on sonographic evidence alone without fear of error.

Doppler studies of the maternal circulation have recently been extended to the first trimester of pregnancy. These studies have shown that a high resistance pattern with absence of the diastolic component is seen in the maternal uterine circulation up to 12 weeks gestation (Schulma et al. 1986; Stabile et al. 1988). We have previously documented the difficulties and limitations of abdominal pulsed wave examination of the uterine artery in the first trimester of normal pregnancy (Stabile et al. 1989b). More recently we have used Doppler ultrasound to study 10 women with TMC in whom a failed pregnancy was diagnosed ultrasonically (Stabile et al. 1989c). Consistent with the underlying pathology of anembryonic pregnancy (which is embryonal rather than maternal in origin), there was no apparent difference in the values for Resistance Index (RI) in the uterine circulation in four patients with anembryonic pregnancy. Fetal demise, either prior to the Doppler studies (missed abortion N=1), or one week later (N=2), was not apparently reflected in alterations in resistance to flow within the uteroplacental circulation. Three patients with a live extrauterine pregnancy also had RI values within the normal range. These results suggest that pulsed Doppler examinations of the maternal circulation does not offer the clinician additional information relating to the diagnosis of failed first trimester pregnancy. Preliminary results from another centre suggest that transvaginal Doppler assessment of *ovarian* blood flow, as early as three days post embryo transfer, may be of value in distinguishing failed from ongoing pregnancies after assisted conception techniques (McSweeney et al. 1988).

Biochemical and Endocrine Aspects

Measurement of serum or plasma levels of circulating hormones and proteins derived from the trophoblast such as human chorionic gonadotrophin (HCG), Schwangerschafts protein 1 (SP1), pregnancy-associated plasma protein A (PAPP-A), and from the corpus luteum, such as oestradiol and progesterone (Masson et al. 1983; Salem et al. 1984) have been used to predict outcome in TMC. In these studies, no attempt was made to distinguish between the various groups of pregnancy failure either using ultrasonic or histological examination. In addition, these studies included heterogeneous cohorts of women with TMC, many of whom had already aborted at time of sampling.

Chapman and his colleagues (1984) observed depressed maternal serum levels of placental products in one third of 22 women with anembryonic pregnancy. These findings are in accordance with those of Yovich and his colleagues (1986), who demonstrated depressed circulating hCG levels as early as the 4th week after the last menstrual period in 16 subfertile women with anembryonic pregnancy who conceived after ovulation induction. Aspillaga et al. (1986) compared serial hCG levels in 25 women with anembryonic pregnancy with levels in 72 normal pregnancies. Although mean hCG levels were significantly lower in the abortion group from 8 weeks onwards, these authors reported a normal pattern of change in hCG levels. Similar data were reported by Whittaker et al. (1989), who noted the remarkable attempt of the placenta to produce hCG even in the absence of a fetus.

Detailed analysis of placental protein and hormone estimations in complications of early pregnancy have been published elsewhere (Stabile et al. 1989a). Fifty-eight of 67 women (86%) with anembryonic pregnancy had a depressed hCG level (less than the 10th centile of the normal range) at the time of ultrasonography (Fig. 3.2). Similarly depressed or undetectable SP1 and PAPP-A levels were present in 40 (60%) and 59 (88%) women respectively.

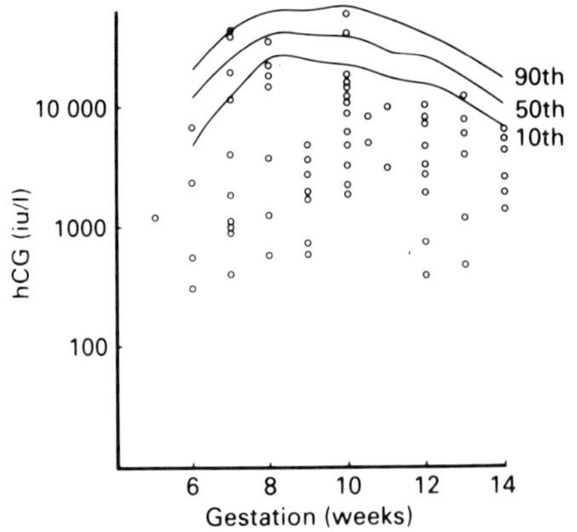

Fig. 3.2. Human chorionic gonadotrophin (hCG) measurements in 67 patients with anembryonic pregnancy at 5 to 15 weeks gestation, superimposed on the 10th, 50th and 90th centiles of the normal range.

The predictive value of an abnormal result (PV pos) was 55% for SP1, 61% or PAPP-A and 70% for hCG. A normal hCG result had 96% probability (PV neg) of excluding anembryonic pregnancy. Circulating hCG, SP1 and PAPP-A levels were not consistently depressed in women with anembryonic pregnancy suggesting that the presence of an embryo or fetus is not essential for adequate trophoblastic production of these proteins, at least in the early weeks of pregnancy.

We have recently examined the hypothesis that maternal circulating PP12 (now known as IGF-binding protein), a major product of the decidualized endometrium in the first trimester of pregnancy, is influenced by the presence or viability of the fetus (Stabile et al. 1989d). This study identified two distinct populations of women with anembryonic pregnancy (N=19). In 7 women (37%), PP12 levels were as high as twice the 90th centile of the normal range. The remaining 12 patients had normal PP12 levels. However, in four cases in which serial measurements were available PP12 levels declined. The women with the highest PP12 levels had reported bleeding for a significantly longer time, suggesting that the major source of this protein, the decidua compacta, was active, certainly in as much as PP12 synthesis is concerned. Although these findings are of interest, they suggest that PP12 estimations are of no clinical value in the diagnosis or exclusion of anembryonic pregnancy.

High levels of CA 125 have previously been reported in aqueous extracts of first trimester decidua compared to non-pregnant endometrium or term decidua, suggesting that this tumour-associated antigen is a product of normal endometrium and decidua (Jacobs et al. 1988). A consistent pattern of a rise and fall in serum CA 125 levels during the first trimester of pregnancies with a retrospectively defined normal outcome has been demonstrated (Jacobs et al. 1990). CA 125 levels were higher in women with anembryonic pregnancy at 4–5 weeks and 6–7 weeks than in those with normal pregnancy outcome, both in spontaneous and assisted conception groups. two-thirds of samples obtained from women with anembryonic pregnancies from 4 to 8 weeks gestation has CA 125 levels that were greater than 2 standard deviations above the mean for pregnancies with normal outcome. These observations suggest that the presence of the fetus may suppress the release of CA 125 into the circulation in normal pregnancy. However, CA 125 estimations are unlikely to be of clinical value in the diagnosis of anembryonic pregnancy.

Alpha-fetoprotein (AFP), the major circulating protein in the early human fetus, is synthesized by the fetal liver and yolk sac. The association between elevated AFP levels and abortion is well established (Garoof and Seppälä 1974). However, Bennett et al. (1978) have demonstrated low maternal serum AFP levels in 10 women with anembryonic pregnancy presenting at 14–15 weeks gestation. We have recently determined maternal serum AFP levels in 21 women with anembryonic pregnancy (Stabile et al. 1989e). Fourteen women had normal AFP levels. In the remaining one-third of women, the levels of AFP were above the 95% limit of the normal range. In view of the meticulous ultrasound and histological studies which excluded the presence of fetal tissue, these unexpected findings have led us to postulate that these anembryonic pregnancies were in reality embryonic pregnancies in which the fetus was lost prior to the first consultation.

Conclusions

The so-called anembryonic pregnancy may well not exist at all. A better term for this condition might be embryonic arrest. The interval between arrest of embryonic development and clinical presentation will determine the sonographic features upon which the diagnosis may be based. This in turn will be reflected in the associated biochemical findings. There is no clear evidence of any early endocrinological differences between women with a fetus and those without. Indeed, trophoblastic protein synthesis appears to be independent of the presence of the embryo. The alternative hypothesis, that the embryo is present in patients with anembryonic pregnancy, albeit developing abnormally, and its trophic effect on the trophoblast diminishes as it undergoes resorption, is gaining wider acceptance.

References

Altman PL. Dittmer DS (1972) Biology data book 2nd edn. Federation of American Societies for Experimental Biology, Bethesda, Maryland

Aspillaga M. Whittaker P, Lind T (1986) Placental hormones and early pregnancy failure. Placenta 7: 458–459

Bennett MJ, Grudzinskas JG, Gordon YB, Turnbull AC (1978) Circulating levels of alpha-fetoprotein and pregnancy specific beta-1-glycoprotein in pregnancies without an embryo. Br J Obstet Gynaecol 85: 348–350

Chapman MG, Bolton AE, Mellows H, Grudzinskas JG (1984) Anembryonic pregnancy – a prospective study of placental biochemical parameters. Proceedings of the 5th international Congress of Placental Proteins, Annecy, p 102

Fujikira T, Froehlich LA, Driscoll G (1966) A simplified anatomic classification of abortions. Am J Obstet Gynecol 95: 902–905

Garoff L, Seppälä M (1974) Prediction of fetal outcome in threatened abortion by maternal serum placental lactogen and alphafetoprotein. Am J Obstet Gynecol 121: 257–261

Jacobs I, Fay TN, Stabile I, Bridges J, Oram DH, Grudzinskas JG (1988) The distribution of CA 125 in the reproductive tract of pregnant and non-pregnant women. Br J Obstet Gynaecol 95: 1190–1194

Jacobs I, Fay T, Yovich J et al. (1990) Serum levels of CA 125 during the first trimester of normal outcome, ectopic and anembryonic pregnancies. Human Reprod 5 (1): 116–122

Levi CS, Lyons EA, Lindsay DJ (1988) Early diagnosis of non-viable pregnancy with endovaginal ultrasound. Radiology 167: 383–385

Masson GM, Anthony F, Wilson MS, Lindsey K (1983) Comparison of serum and urine hCG levels with SP1 and PAPP-A levels in patients with first trimester vaginal bleeding. Obstet Gynecol 61: 223–226

McSweeney MB, Baber RJ, Gill RW et al. (1988) Prediction of IVF and GIFT outcome using transvaginal doppler assessment of ovarian blood flow. J Ultrasound Med 7: S73

Mikamo K (1970) Anatomic and chromosomal anomalies in spontaneous abortion. Am J Obstet Gynecol 106: 243–254

Nyberg DA, Laing FC, Filly RA (1986) Threatened abortion: sonographic distinction of normal and abnormal gestational sacs. Radiology 58: 397–400

Robinson HP (1975) The diagnosis of early pregnancy failure by sonar. Br J Obstet Gynaecol 82: 849–857

Rushton DI (1988) Placental pathology in spontaneous miscarriage. In: Early pregnancy loss: mechanisms and treatment. Proceedings of the 18th Study Group of the Royal College of Obstetricians and Gynaecologists, RCOG Publications, Peacock Press, Lancs, pp 149–157

Salem HT, Ghaneimah SA, Shaaban MM, Chard T (1984) Prognostic value of biochemical tests in

the assessment of fetal outcome in threatened abortion. Br J Obstet Gynaecol 91: 382–385
Schulman H. Fleisher A, Farmakides G, et al. (1986) Development of uterine artery compliance in pregnancy as detected by Doppler ultrasound. Am J Obstet Gynecol 155: 1031–1034
Stabile I, Campbell S, Grudzinskas JG (1987) Ultrasound assessment in complications of first trimester pregnancy. Lancet ii: 1237–1242
Stabile I, Bilardo C, Panella M, Campbell S, Grudzinskas JG (1988) Doppler measurement of uterine blood flow in the first trimester of normal and complicated pregnancies. Trophoblast Res 3: 301–307
Stabile I, Campbell S, Grudzinskas JG (1989a) Ultrasound and circulating placental protein measurements in complications of early pregnancy. Br J Obstet Gynaecol 96: 11–21
Stabile I, Campbell S, Grudzinskas JG (1989b) Doppler assessed uteroplacental blood flow impedance in the first trimester: physiological variation with site of measurement. J Obstet Gynaecol 9 : 177–179
Stabile I, Grudzinskas JG, Campbell S (1989c) Pulsed Doppler as applied to maternal circulation in normal and failed first trimester pregnancy. Echocardiography 6(3): 1–4
Stabile I, Howell R, Teisner B, Chard T, Grudzinskas JG (1989d) Circulating levels of placental protein 12 in complications of first trimester pregnancy. Arch Gynecol Obstet 246: 201–206
Stabile I, Olajide F, Chard T, Grudzinskas JG (1989e) Maternal serum alpha-fetoprotein levels in anembryonic pregnancy. Hum Reprod 4(2): 204–205
Whittaker PG, Stewart MO, Taylor A, Lind T (1989) Some endocrinological events associated with early pregnancy failure. Br J Obstet Gynaecol 96: 1207–1214
Yovich JL, Matson PL (1988) Early pregnancy wastage following gamete manipulation. Br J Obstet Gynaecol 95: 1120–1127
Yovich JL, Willcox DL, Grudzinskas JG, Bolton AE (1986) The prognostic value of beta hCG, PAPP-A, oestradiol and progesterone in early human pregnancy. Aust NZ J Obstet Gynaecol 26: 59–64

4. Embryonic Loss: Clinical Perspectives

J.L. Yovich

Introduction

For women conceiving after prolonged periods of subfertility, the early diagnosis of pregnancy is welcomed with an overwhelming sense of achievement. However, such enthusiasm should be tempered by the knowledge that early pregnancy wastage is high (25%–30%) and includes a 5%–6% risk of ectopic pregnancy (Yovich and Matson 1988; National Perinatal Statistics Unit [NPSU] 1988). Furthermore, late pregnancy complications such as preterm delivery and low birthweight are increased mainly, but not entirely, due to the markedly increased risk of multiple pregnancies if ovarian stimulation or in vitro fertilization (IVF)-related therapies have been applied (NPSU 1988; Yovich et al. 1990). For these reasons subfertile couples should be counselled at an early stage so that they can receive the diagnosis of pregnancy with cautious optimism.

The underlying causes of pregnancy wastage are likely to be an extension of those same factors underlying implantation disorders, namely embryo quality and uterine receptivity. However, the further advanced the pregnancy, the more likely that additional complex maternal factors will operate and embryo-based factors will be less relevant. In addition, from the clinician's standpoint, two questions are prominent:

1. Is it possible to make an early or predictive diagnosis of pregnancy outcome?
2. What therapeutic options may be considered given the earlier diagnosis of an abnormal pregnancy or the prediction of early fetal loss?

Diagnosis of Pregnancy

The placental hormone human chorionic gonadotrophin (hCG) remains the most useful substance to test for the early diagnosis of pregnancy, although a number of other proteins can be considered, namely Schwangerschaftsprotein 1 (SP1)

(Lenton et al. 1981), placental protein 14 (PP14) (Yovich et al. 1986a) and pregnancy-associated plasma protein A (PAPP-A) (Westergaard et al. 1983).

Beta-hCG is detectable between days 7 to 10 of the luteal phase in both spontaneous (Lenton and Woodward 1988) and IVF (Yovich et al. 1985a; Confino et al. 1986) conception cycles. However, many such cases may not show persisting rises nor reach the stage of either ultrasound (5th–8th week) or clinical (7th–10th week) diagnosis. Furthermore, hormone tests vary in both specificity and sensitivity hence laboratories must specify their reference standards (e.g. 25 mIU/ml beta-hCG detected by radioimmunoassay [RIA] set against the 2nd IS 61/6 equates with 52 mIU/ml on the first IRP 75/537). Increasingly, monoclonal enzyme-linked immunosorbent assays measuring colour or chemiluminescent endpoints are proving to have greater specificity and practical benefits than RIA, with coefficients of variation often under 5%.

However at this stage, for the aforementioned and other reasons there is a wide variation in the criteria applied for the diagnosis of pregnancy.

At PIVET, pregnancy diagnosis is based on the following criteria, arising from internal observations from more than 1600 clinically or histologically defined pregnancies and which is supported by independent observers (e.g. Lenton and Woodward 1988):

1. Quantitative serum beta-hCG $\geqslant$ 25 mIU/ml on or after day 16 of the luteal phase (dated from oocyte recovery or the day after LH surge)
2. Concomitant elevation of serum progesterone $\geqslant$ 31 nmol/litre and serum, oestradiol-17ß $\geqslant$ 620 pmol/litre
3. Beta-hCG continues to rise significantly on a further serum sample taken no less than 3 days later

If hCG injections have been used during the luteal phase, e.g. 1000 IU on days 4, 7, 10, and 13 (Yovich 1988), caution is required when interpreting the day 16 result. However the extensive experience at PIVET indicates that serum beta-hCG levels are almost never greater than 15 IU on samples collected 72 h or more after the injection and do not rise on the subsequent test if conception has not occurred.

Pregnancy Categories

Once pregnancy has been diagnosed, the following outcomes may occur:

Preclinical Pregnancy (Biochemical)

Any case which meets the above criteria for the diagnosis of pregnancy but does not reach completion of week 6, i.e. bleeding ensues when the beta-hCG level shows a fall, with subsequent levels <25 IU/ml. This may ensue after the completion of week 6 but if the event began at a prior stage and a clear sac is not demonstrable on ultrasound, it should still be categorized as a preclinical pregnancy loss.

Blighted Ovum (Anembryonic)

An intrauterine gestational sac is defined by ultrasound. However no clear fetal outline, fetal movements or fetal heart action is demonstrable within the sac which also needs to be differentiated from the pseudo-sac sometimes associated with ectopic pregnancies (Nyberg et al. 1983). The resolution of images from pelvic ultrasound is influenced by patient factors (e.g. the adverse effect of obesity), equipment characteristics (electronic phased array sector scanning preferred) and the scanning route (transvaginal technique may be preferable during early pregnancy, particularly for the retroverted uterus). The pregnancy may subsequently abort spontaneously or be evacuated electively following diagnosis.

Spontaneous Miscarriage

One or more viable fetuses are demonstrated within the gestational sac(s); i.e. fetal movements and/or heart action demonstrated but the pregnancy aborts before the 20th week.

Ectopic Pregnancy

Refers to any extrauterine pregnancy loss but the vast majority are intratubal. As previously noted this may be associated with an intrauterine pseudosac and increasingly, using transvaginal ultrasound, the intratubal pregnancy may be clearly defined, sometimes with a live fetus in situ. Occasionally combined intra- and extrauterine or heterotopic pregnancies will be diagnosed particularly in the high-risk situation of ovarian stimulation and/or IVF (Yovich et al. 1984, 1985b).

Other Early Pregnancy Losses

These include therapeutic pregnancy terminations, heterotopic pregnancies and hydatidiform molar pregnancies.

Advanced Pregnancies

Refers to those which advance beyond 20 weeks (dating is from LMP or adjusted LMP). Thereafter completed pregnancies are classified as births which are subcategorized as single or multiple, term or preterm, livebirths or stillbirths, perinatal losses (stillbirths and neonatal deaths) and normal or congenitally abnormal.

Histological confirmation of pregnancy will often but not always be obtained after pregnancy wastage. Preclinical pregnancies do not require curettage, improving ultrasound diagnostic skills means that suspected complete abortions or miscarriages may also not require curettage and many ectopics can now be treated by non-excision methods.

Pregnancy Outcomes

From the outset it appeared that pregnancies generated in women of subfertile marriages were at greater risk of early wastage than the normally fertile population. At PIVET all pregnancies diagnosed were therefore registered and outcomes tabulated in order to assess the wastage rates and determine any underlying factors with a view to potential therapeutic considerations.

Materials and Methods

Following the referral of couples to PIVET for infertility over a 7-year period, 1657 pregnancies have ensued and completed their clinical outcome by May 1989. Following a clinical and investigative assessment according to a defined protocol (Yovich and Grudzinskas 1990), treatments have included reconstructive tubal microsurgery, specific treatments such as surgical or hormonal management of endometriosis, ovarian stimulation for disorders of ovulation and a range of procedures involving gamete handling/manipulation i.e. donor insemination (DI); intrauterine insemination of husband's washed, precapacitated sperm (AIH); and certain IVF-related procedures – gamete intrafallopian transfer (GIFT), traditional IVF and embryo transfer (IVF-ET), pronuclear stage tubal transfer (PROST) and tubal embryo stage transfer (TEST). The methods have been fully described (Yovich et al. 1989a, 1990) Yovich and Grudzinskas 1990) and variants have included ovum donation and IVF surrogacy. The vast majority of women having ovarian stimulation and gamete manipulation procedures (but only a small number of those having unstimulated cycles) had close hormonal and ultrasound tracking throughout the conception cycle so that the LH surge and ovulation days were precisely documented for subsequent dating.

Once pregnancy was diagnosed, a serum sample was obtained from women each week (dated from luteal day 16) through to week 12 and analysed for quantitative beta-hCG, oestradiol-17ß (E2) and progesterone (P4). Current assays are performed using the Amerlite (Amersham, UK) system, and have been adjusted to the appropriate reference levels for the previous double antibody RIA (Diagnostic Products Corporation, LA, USA). The inter-assay variation for the Amerlite hCG-60 assay gave the following results – low range (7–12 IU/litre): 6.5%, medium range (25–38 IU/litre): 4.2%, higher range (186–278 IU/litre): 4.3%. Selected serum samples have also been analyzed for SP1, PAPP-A and PP14 using RIAs by courtesy of J.G. Grudzinskas (Joint Academic Unit of Obstetrics, Gynaecology and Reproductive Physiology, London Hospital Medical College, London) and M. Chapman (Department of Obstetrics and Gynaecology, United Medical Schools [Guy's] London).

Results and Discussion

Pregnancy outcomes from the respective treatment programmes are show in Fig. 4.1. Of the total 1657 pregnancies diagnosed, 1145 (69.1%) progressed to births with the delivery of 1613 infants. Early pregnancy wastage ranged from a low

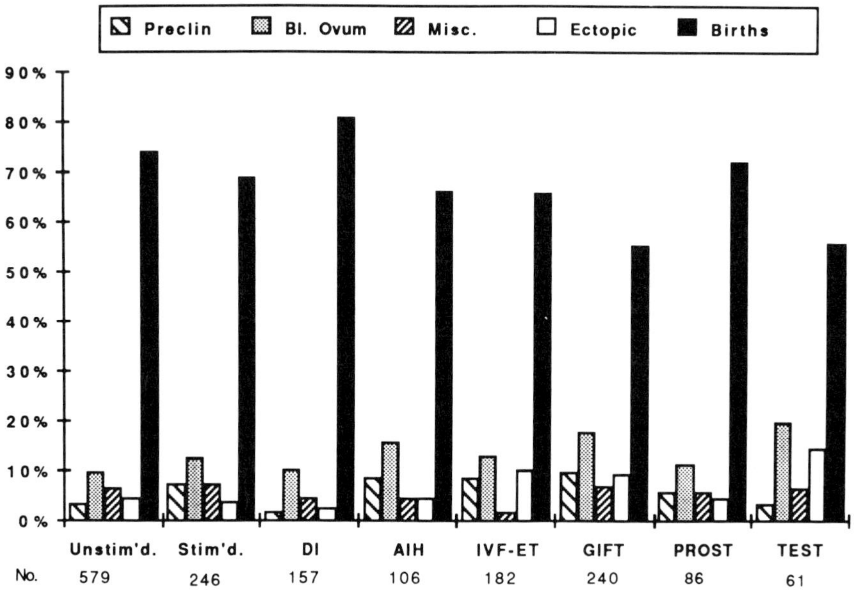

Fig. 4.1. Defined outcomes of 1657 pregnancies arising after various treatments for infertility over a 7-year period. Includes 5 heterotopic pregnancies categorized with ectopics, 12 therapeutic terminations categorized with spontaneous abortions and one hydatidiform mole categorized with blighted ovum pregnancies.

of 19% for DI to a high of 44.6% for GIFT. These findings are similar to a previous report from PIVET and are not related to age differences as the mean ages were similar in all programmes, ranging from 29.7 years in PROST to 32.7 years in GIFT (Yovich and Matson 1988). The better outcome for the DI programme may reflect the clear male-factor basis underlying the infertility (implying no female factor which might limit reproductive potential to conceive or carry a pregnancy) and the highly selected male gametes placed in the cervical canal (ensuring optimum embryo quality). With respect to the subcategories of pregnancy wastage the following interpretations can be made:

Preclinical Pregnancies

These comprised 6% (n=98) of all pregnancies and were highest in the GIFT programme. This latter finding was examined further and it was found that oligospermic patients treated by the modified GIFT protocol which involved transferring higher sperm numbers into the fallopian tubes (Matson et al. 1987) had early pregnancy wastage rates from combined preclinical and blighted ovum pregnancies of 56% (Yovich et al. 1989b). This finding is supported elsewhere (Rodriguez-Rigau 1989) and is likely to be due to polyspermic fertilization or other types of defective embryo which cannot be selected out in GIFT as with other IVF-related procedures. This is one of the reasons for developing the PROST and TEST procedures and regarding oligo/asthenospermia as contraindicated for GIFT.

The question of lingering exogenous hCG from luteal phase injections has been considered as a possible cause of false diagnosis of preclinical pregnancies in some patients. However, this is thought to be a rare phenomenon if it occurs and the finding of a 4% background rate of preclinical pregnancies in the unstimulated group (who also received no luteal phase injections of hCG) indicates that preclinical pregnancies are a real diagnostic category.

Blighted Ovum Pregnancies

This is the main category of early pregnancy wastage and ranged from 10% in women not receiving ovarian stimulation or having procedures involving gamete manipulation, to 20% for the TEST procedure. Previously we have commented on high blighted ovum pregnancy rates for AIH (Yovich and Matson 1988) and GIFT (see above) in relation to oligo/asthenospermia but this is unlikely to operate for TEST where embryos are preselected according to morphological criteria. Instead, the inclusion of post-cryopreservation embryos which may have suffered non-apparent damage, could explain the finding. With all IVF-related procedures it should be borne in mind that <25% of morphologically acceptable embryos have the capacity to implant even when maternal receptivity is optimal (Yovich et al. 1989a). It is likely that many IVF-generated embryos can begin the implantation process but not have the full capacity for normal post-implantation development.

Spontaneous Miscarriages

These comprised 6% (98 pregnancies) of outcomes and 32% of the combined group described in the past as "spontaneous abortions" (i.e. blighted ovum pregnancies and miscarriages; n=309). A high proportion of early miscarriages (6–12 weeks) were shown to have chromosomal aberrations on cytogenetic evaluation and later losses (12–20 weeks) were often multiple pregnancies.

Ectopics

Ectopic pregnancies were almost invariably tubal and comprised 6% (N=100) of outcomes. The rates were highest among patients with known or suspected tubal disease (Yovich 1990). In the TEST programme the highest rate of 14.8% was recorded and this was entirely among early cases included with past histories of fallopian tube reconstructions who failed to conceive spontaneously but had patency demonstrated in at least one tube (63 treatment cycles resulted in 23 pregnancies, 9 of which were ectopics [39%] with one arising after transcervical TEST). There was a similar background history of tubal disorders among the GIFT ectopics; as a result tubal transfer procedures are now totally contraindicated in any patient with any degree of tubal disease at PIVET. Ectopics are apparently an unavoidable problem in the IVF-ET group but may be minimized by careful uterine placement (Yovich et al. 1985c) which avoids deposition of embryos into the fallopian tubes where entrapment may occur if there are proximal endosalpingeal disorders or tubal dysfunction.

Heterotopic Pregnancies

Heterotopic pregnancies have occurred on five occasions. The hormonal data and abdominal ultrasound findings were misleading on each occasion by indicating parameters consistent with intrauterine pregnancy i.e. normal values for viable fetus and falling values for blighted ovum pregnancies. On an early occasion one woman presented in a state of clinical shock at 10 weeks with a ruptured tubal heterotopic pregnancy and subsequently miscarried her intrauterine twins almost 4 weeks later (Yovich et al. 1984). On each of the other occasions laparoscopy has been performed before the 9th week because of persisting vaginal bleeding (prune juice character) which did not cease following medroxyprogesterone acetate (MPA) therapy (see below). Persisting pelvic pain of a boring nature and localized to one iliac fossa has usually, but not always, been a supporting clinical symptom.

Hydatidiform Mole

This has occurred on only one occasion. The hormonal values were similar to the profile for blighted ovum (beta-hCG, E2 and P4 low and falling), the ultrasound features revealed the diagnostic snowstorm appearance and the histological findings after curettage indicated a degenerating hydatidiform mole.

Therapeutic Terminations

These have been performed on 12 occasions, almost invariably for genetic reasons following amniocentesis or chorionic villus sampling.

Late Pregnancy Outcomes

Data on large numbers of IVF-generated pregnancies indicates that the perinatal death rate is more than double that of the general community rates for singleton pregnancies and the risks are compounded by the high proportion of multiple pregnancies (NPSU 1988). The major problem is that of preterm delivery (12%–14% among IVF singleton pregnancies) and the problem is likely to be related to maternal factors rather than embryo characteristics or IVF techniques. The risk of singleton preterm delivery appears to be similar among subfertile patients regardless of the method of conception.

Multiple pregnancies are a consequence of ovarian stimulation and oocyte or embryo numbers transferred. IVF efficiency has improved in recent years due to improved ovarian stimulation methods; technical developments (e.g. in oocyte recovery and embryo transfer techniques); the introduction of tubal transfer procedures; increasing laboratory experience and expertise; and the use of luteal support regimens. Current data at PIVET indicates the risk of multiple pregnancy is 25%–30% when three embryos are transferred. This number is now set as the upper limit for oocytes and embryos. Pregnancy rates remain at 36% per treatment cycle with birthrates around 25% and it may well be time to consider further reductions in the maximum numbers transferred (Yovich et al. 1989a).

Fetal abnormality rates are not increased after fertility management (Yovich et al. 1988b) although one report suggests an increased incidence of spina bifida and transposition of the great vessels among IVF births and urinary tract malformations among GIFT births (NPSU 1988). Major recurrent abnormalities have not occurred among 1613 infants born following infertility treatments at PIVET.

Predicting Pregnancy Outcome

The evaluation of fetal wellbeing by a relatively simple serum test to reflect feto-placental function was inititally best achieved by human placental lactogen (hPL) estimations using RIA (Chard 1976). Low levels in the first trimester (>8 weeks)

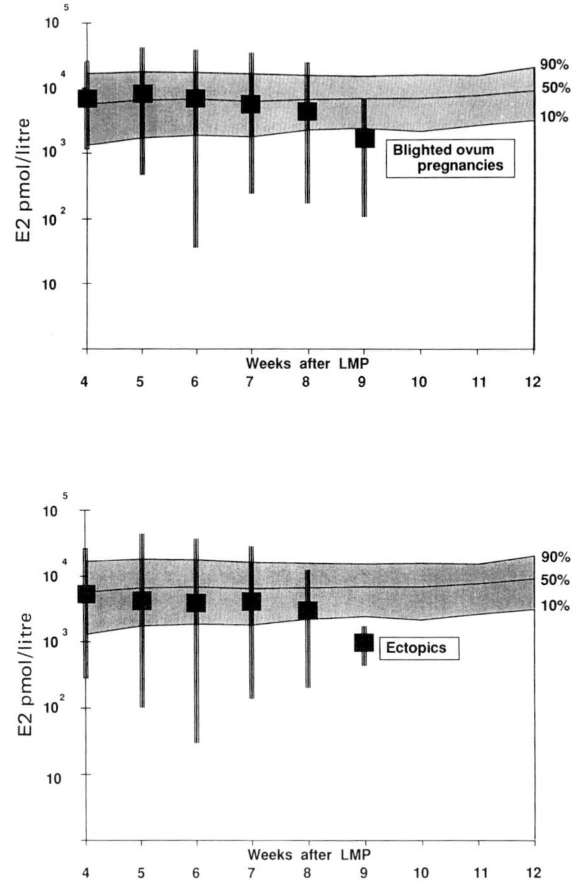

Fig. 4.2. Serial serum oestradiol-17ß (E2) estimations in women who had ovarian stimulation therapy, depicting profiles for normal singleton deliveries (shaded; n=100), tubal ectopic (n=52) and blighted ovum pregnancies (n=35). Filled boxes show observations around the mean and whiskers define the full range of observations at each week.

indicated a non-viable pregnancy and levels <4 μg/ml in late pregnancy indicated the fetus was at high risk from placental insufficiency leading to intrauterine growth retardation. However, clinicians were sceptical and preferred to place their confidence in the developing art of ultrasound at that time. Currently, there is a renewed interest in serum testing as a fine discriminator where ultrasound is at the limits of its diagnostic capacity (e.g. very early pregnancy) or as a screening test for time-consuming ultrasound examinations (e.g. genetic screening, the early detection of placental insufficiency) but mostly as a potential predictor of pregnancy outcome in both the early and late stages of pregnancy.

Early Pregnancy

Previous reports have addressed the question of the ability of placental hormone and protein measurements to provide a prognosis of pregnancy outcome (Yovich

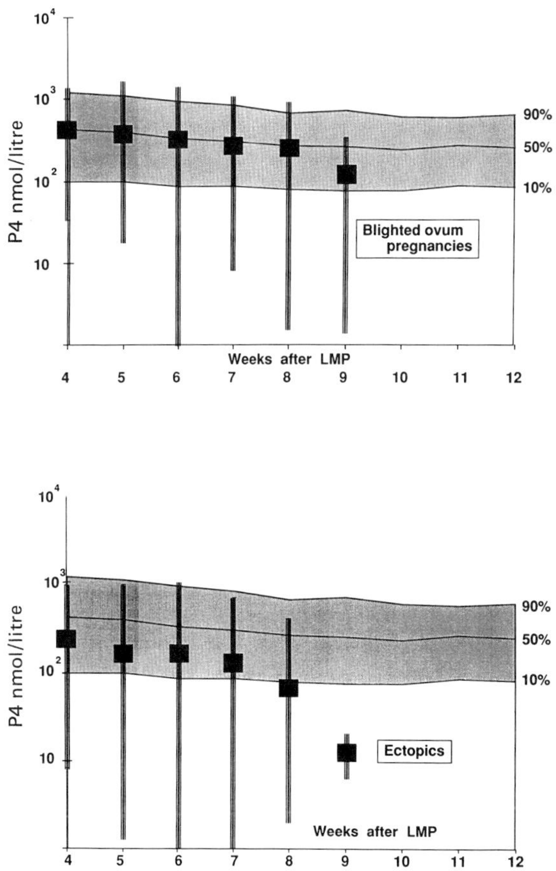

Fig. 4.3. Serial serum progesterone (P4) estimations in women who had ovarian stimulation therapy, depicting profiles for normal singleton deliveries (shaded; n=100), tubal ectopic (n=52) and blighted ovum pregnancies (n=35). Filled boxes show observations around the mean and whiskers define the full range of observations at each week.

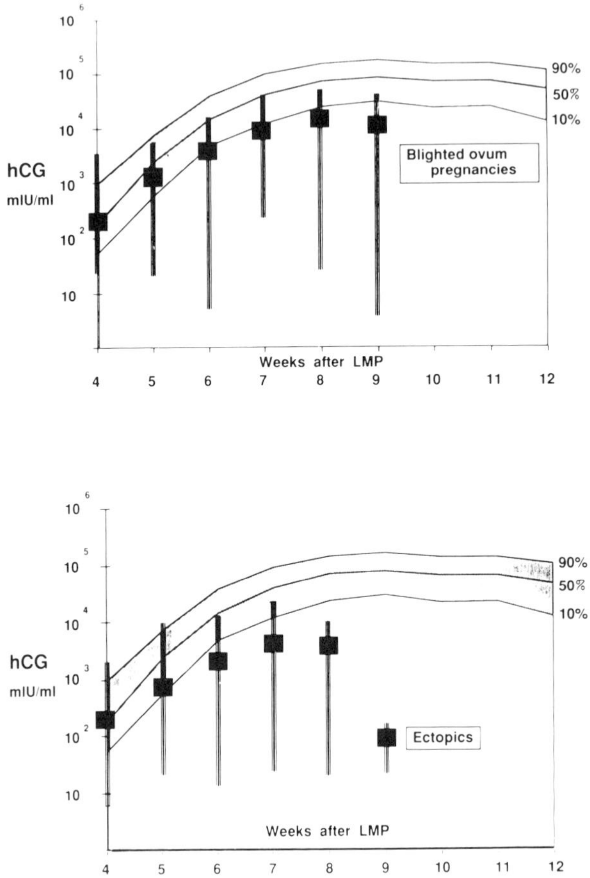

Fig. 4.4. Serial serum beta-hCG estimations in women who had ovarian stimulation therapy, depicting profiles for normal singleton deliveries (shaded; $n=100$), tubal ectopic ($n=52$) and blighted ovum pregnancies ($n=35$). Filled boxes show observations around the mean and whiskers define the full range of observations at each week.

et al. 1986a; 1986b). The most common clinical question concerns the differential diagnosis of spontaneous abortion and ectopic pregnancy. Serial estimations of E2 (Fig. 4.2), P4 (Fig. 4.3) and beta-hCG (Fig. 4.4) for 35 blighted ovum pregnancies and 50 ectopic pregnancies have been compared with the profiles from 100 normal singleton outcomes. All the cases had ovarian stimulation. In many patients the likelihood of pregnancy wastage was predictable at the time of pregnancy diagnosis by low levels of beta-hCG and sometimes low E2 and P4. For both ectopic and blighted ovum pregnancies, beta-hCG estimations provided the most sensitive indicator with significantly widening disparity from the norm with each advancing week. E2 and P4, whilst sometimes showing the same trend, did not become clearly diagnostic until a later stage when ultrasound information was also available. Furthermore, whilst ectopics tended to have lower beta-hCG levels, the profiles were not able to differentiate the two conditions until a late stage (8th and 9th week) when ectopic pregnancies almost invariable showed very low E2 and P4 levels, particularly the latter. This data supports other reports suggesting that low P4 levels are indicative of ectopics (Matthews et al. 1986) but only from the 8th week. This is probably related to the stage at which the ovarian contribution to circulating P4 wanes, revealing low trophoblastic activity. Absence of a clear gestational sac in utero at 8 weeks usually means ectopic pregnancy but the diagnosis is not always clear if a pseudosac or degenerating gestational sac is present when laparoscopy will be required to make the definitive diagnosis. Some studies suggest that PAPP-A may be a useful differentiating marker (Sinosich 1988; Jacobs et al. 1990a) as levels tend to remain elevated until late with blighted ovum pregnancies but are very low or absent with ectopics. SP-1 exhibits a profile similar to beta-hCG in anembryonic pregnancies (Yovich et al. 1986a) without any specific advantages (except perhaps when hCG therapy is being used during early pregnancy) and PP14 did not appear to provide a useful prognostic test in that category of wastage.

Late Pregnancy

To date we have concentrated on early pregnancy outcomes in the studies at PIVET and have not recognized any obvious connection between early pregnancy hormonal profiles of beta-hCG, E2 or P4 and late pregnancy complications. Profiles of beta-hCG, SP-1 and PAPP-A have been analysed with respect to plurality and these indicate higher levels during the first trimester of twin and triplet pregnancies (Jacobs et al. 1990b). It appears unlikely that late pregnancy outcomes such as preterm parturition and placental insufficiency will be predicted from early pregnancy profiles of hormones and proteins derived from the ovary, trophoblast or decidua. However, direct fetal and placental assessment by biophysical measurements such as ultrasound, Doppler and perhaps nuclear magnetic resonance imaging techniques will make increasingly greater contributions.

Therapeutic Implications

The value of making predictive diagnoses is to improve the therapeutic options. These may be categorized as preventive (pre-pregnancy), early pregnancy therapies and late pregnancy therapeutic strategies.

Preventive

Preventive treatments are considered at PIVET for cases of recurrent abortion (three or more) and such cases require comprehensive investigations to exclude underlying disorders.

Genetic Causes

Detailed banded chromosome analysis of leucocytes is checked from both partners.

Anatomical Causes

The detection of anatomical defects involves careful clinical evaluation of the woman along with hysterography, laparoscopy and hysteroscopy to check for evidence of fibroids, cervical incompetence, DES uterus/cervix, active pelvic endometriosis, genital tract infections and uterine abnormalities. With respect to the latter, uterine synechiae, a septate uterus and possibly bicornuate uterine abnormalities may be relevant.

Infective Causes

Serological tests are performed for antibodies in the detection of syphilis, brucellosis, toxoplasmosis and rubella. Endocervical swabs are cultured for aerobic and anaerobic bacteria and specific investigations are performed to exclude infection with *cytomegalovirus, Chlamydia trachomatis,* herpes virus, *Listeria monocytogenes* and *Mycoplasma hominis.* Mycobacterium tuberculosis also requires consideration depending upon clinical features and the patient's demographic background.

Maternal Disorders

Tests are performed for systemic lupus erythematosus – lupus anticoagulant and/ or cardiolipin antibody, ANF, C3 and C4; fasting blood sugar for diabetes; as well as screening for cardiovascular, renal and thyroid diseases. Other considerations such as exposure to anaesthetic gases, industrial chemicals and pesticides; the ingestion of antimetabolites and anticoagulants; and smoking/ alcohol history may also be relevant in individual cases. Fertility assessments should include evaluation of the luteal phase (see below).

Immunotherapy by Paternal Lymphocytes

It has been suggested that the absence of an essential maternal immunoregulatory response to the genetically foreign fetus is the cause of at least some cases of recurrent miscarriage (Taylor and Faulk 1981). It has been speculated that immunizing the woman with her husband's prepared lymphocytes will stimulate the appropriate maternal response; one controlled study (Mowbray et al. 1985) has suggested that this approach might be valid. Certainly women who recurrently miscarry often have negative mixed lymphocyte reactivity (MLR) which is positive in most women who have successfully completed a pregnancy. This test is used to screen patients into a double-blind control trial at PIVET, which is part of a multicentre study. It is not possible at this stage to make a prediction but so far the majority of failed pregnancies after immunotherapy (when the protocol detail is revealed) have occurred in women receiving their own (control) cells.

Early Pregnancy Treatments

Studies reported during the sixties indicated that hormone support therapy was probably not effective (Shearman and Garrett 1963; Goldzieher 1964; Klopper and MacNaughton 1965). Furthermore it was shown that 50%–60% of the fetuses obtained from women who experience spontaneous abortions have chromosomal abnormalities (Boué et al. 1975; Simpson 1980). However while the general rate of spontaneous abortions is considered to be 10%–15%, subfertile women who conceive are much more prone to abort their pregnancies (Lunenfeld and Insler 1978; Yovich and Matson 1988) and sometimes this was found to be caused by luteal phase defects (Jones 1976). In recent days two findings have influenced the current approach to hormone treatment during pregnancy. First, that pregnancies can be established and maintained in women without ovaries by simply providing exogenous oestradiol valerate and progesterone during the conception cycle and throughout the first trimester (Lutjen et al. 1984), and that high serum levels of progesterone should be maintained (Yovich et al. 1988a). Second, that after some ovarian stimulation treatments, the luteal phase may be severely shortened (Yovich et al. 1988a); this can be corrected by hCG injections to stimulate the corpus luteum or by using progesterone or the progestagen MPA.

Hormone Support Therapy

At PIVET, hormone support is provided for the following indications in the described regimens.

Ovarian Failure Pregnancies

Oral oestradiol valerate 2 mg t.d.s. is given in addition to Proluton 50 mg i.m.i. daily and progesterone pessaries (locally manufactured) 100 mg b.d. vaginally. (The ability of this current vaginal pessary to replace the injections altogether is being explored.) Placental production of E2 and P4 is usually, but not always adequate by the 8th week; the drug regimen is therefore continued to the 12th week and weaned over the ensuing fortnight.

Threatened Abortion

Women who present with fresh vaginal bleeding sufficient to cause staining (more than 3 cm on the underclothing) are offered MPA therapy within a trial testing its efficacy in reducing wastage from the spontaneous abortions of normal fetuses. Early data from this suggest a beneficial effect without causing the retention of abnormal fetuses or creating fetal abnormalities (Yovich et al. 1988b).

During the acute phase of bleeding, MPA tablets (Provera, Upjohn) are commenced 20 mg 4-hourly (120 mg/day) and women are advised to rest at home. As vaginal bleeding settles, the schedule is reduced to 20 mg q.i.d.; the patient can mobilize normally but should avoid coitus for 2 weeks. If beta-hCG levels remain elevated, MPA is continued and reviewed at the 8th week. With ultrasound confirmation of a viable pregnancy MPA is continued through to the 16th week and is weaned off over the ensuing fortnight. If ultrasound fails to confirm viability by the 8th week, the differential diagnosis of blighted ovum, missed abortion or ectopic pregnancy must be investigated.

Recurrent Abortion

In the belief that such cases may have a corpus luteum defect, hCG is used to maintain luteal activity and is usually supported by MPA. The regimen commences at the time of pregnancy diagnosis as follows:

5000 IU hCG i.m.i. twice weekly (e.g. Wed/Sun) to 10 weeks.
MPA 20 mg oral q.i.d. to 16 weeks, weaning over the ensuing fortnight.

In selecting MPA as the support progestagen for PIVET patients, we were influenced by previous observations that the drug did not cause significant congenital abnormalities and, in the case of virilization of one female infant amongst 170 newborn (Burstein and Wasserman 1964), only mild clitoral hypertrophy was noted. MPA is a substituted progesterone and therefore differs from the derivatives of the 19-nortestosterone group which have been used in the past and have been shown to have androgenic effects on the developing female fetus (Wilkins 1960). Female virilization has also been observed by the author associated with the use of both hydroxyprogesterone caproate and hydroxyprogesterone hexanoate. The orally active form of MPA was chosen rather than the depot form since the latter may occasionally maintain an elevated basal temperature and inhibit ovulation for several months after spontaneous abortion. Furthermore MPA is well absorbed orally and stable plasma concentrations around 27 nmol/litre are established on the regimens described (Yovich et al. 1985d). That study also examined the profile of steroid metabolites in maternal urine during the first trimester of pregnancy and showed no abnormal peaks on gas-liquid chromatography and mass spectrometry.

Genetic Abnormalities

These can be diagnosed by chorionic villus sampling for chromosome analysis and DNA probe analysis; amniocentesis for cytogenetic studies and alpha-fetoprotein (AFP) estimations; and midtrimester ultrasound scanning for anatomical abnormalities in high-risk patients. Several studies have shown the value of maternal serum estimations of AFP, unconjugated oestriol and beta-hCG to screen for Down's syndrome (see Chapter 11).

Ectopics

Only four of the 100 ectopic pregnancies presented in a ruptured state; two very early in the series and two others who were travelling and discontinued serial hormone monitoring. The benefits of the very early diagnosis of ectopic pregnancy are:

1. Avoidance of the life-threatening condition of rupture which is uncommon before the 7th week.
2. Early detection enables more conservative surgery to be considered (e.g. salpingotomy and microsurgical repair).
3. Unruptured ectopics may be treated without recourse to laparotomy.

Increasingly, unruptured ectopics are now treated by either laparoscopic aspiration (Pouly et al. 1986) or ultrasound-directed methods such as injection or the fetus of the gestational sac with methotrexate (Feichtinger and Kemeter 1987) or potassium chloride (Robertson et al. 1987); and needle aspiration (Davison and Leeton 1988).

Other Pregnancy Disorders

Serum hormones are generally in the normal range until the clinical event for those pregnancies which spontaneously miscarried. An ideal marker would discriminate between a normal and an abnormal fetus and thus allow rational hormone therapy. Similarly, the diagnosis of heterotopic pregnancy is difficult and may not be clear until tubal rupture. The diagnosis of non-heterotopic ectopics may be defined by the absence of PAPP-A in serum, but a positive marker is required for heterotopics because of the masking effect of the intrauterine pregnancy.

Late Pregnancy Treatments

During early pregnancy, the principles of management rest on the belief that most pregnancy losses are a consequence of embryo defects. Markers are sought to define the few cases of fetal loss which might be salvaged. However, in late pregnancy the principles of management assume that the fetus or fetuses are healthy and any treatment to restrict wastage is best directed towards assisting the maternal powers to carry the pregnancy to term. In this respect high-risk pregnancies such as high-order multiples are offered the following treatment at PIVET:

1. Maintain physical integrity of the cervix by the routine insertion of a cervical suture (Shirodkar type) as soon as a viable fetus is demonstrated (8th week).
2. Inhibit uterine contractility and irribility by MPA 20 mg q.i.d. orally throughout the pregnancy to 36 weeks if possible.
3. Reduce the risk of preterm labour by increasingly strict limitations of physical activity from 20 weeks gestation.

This regimen appears to be of benefit in reducing preterm delivery and perinatal mortality in triplet and higher order pregnancies (Yovich et al. 1989a). At PIVET it is now being applied routinely in the management of all multiples and other pregnancies categorized as high-risk for preterm labour.

Conclusions

Over the last two decades, major changes have occurred in the clinical management of early pregnancy complications. On the one hand the rapidly expanding use of assisted reproduction has been attended by an increased prevalence of blighted ova, ectopic pregnancies and spontaneous miscarriages. On the other hand, rapidly advancing diagnostic techniques (particularly serum assays and ultrasound) have enabled earlier diagnoses and thus allowed a more rational, elective approach to treatment. For example, blighted ovum pregnancies can be evacuated without waiting for clinical signs of abortion and ectopic pregnancies are increasingly being treated by non-laparotomy methods such as injection of the sac/fetus, or laparoscopic aspiration. The life-threatening clinical picture of ruptured ectopic pregnancy can be avoided in high-risk patients (e.g. those conceiving by assisted reproduction procedures) by serial monitoring of serum hormones and early pelvic ultrasound, preferably transvaginal. This, of course, is an expensive and relatively intensive protocol which can only be justified in selected circumstances. However it is possible to envisage a single blood test performed between the 6th and 8th week of all pregnancies which might indicate the potential viability of that pregnancy (e.g. by quantitative beta-hCG and steroid levels) as well as the likelihood of tubal pregnancy (e.g. from PAPP-A levels) and even genetic defects in apparently normal pregnancies. It also remains a useful research pursuit to attempt to define those potentially viable pregnancies which might benefit from hormonal support. Hopefully, even the prediction of late pregnancy complications such as preterm delivery might be possible using an early pregnancy serum marker and this would have important therapeutic implications during the first trimester.

Acknowledgements. Among the staff of PIVET Medical Centre, I wish to particularly acknowledge Paul Shenton, Sue Devine, Fiona O'Shea and Jim Cummins for their important contributions to this work.

References

Boué J, Boué A, Lazar P (1975) Retrospective and prospective epidemiological studies of 1500 karyotyped spontaneous abortions. Teratology 12: 11–26

Burstein R, Wasserman HC (1964) The effect of Provera on the fetus. Obstet Gynecol 23: 931–934

Chard T (1976) Human placental lactogen levels as a guide to fetal wellbeing. In: Klopper A (ed) Plasma hormone assays in evaluation of fetal wellbeing. Churchill Livingstone, Edinburgh pp 5–23

Confino E, Demir RH, Friberg J, Gleicher N (1986) The predictive value of hCG beta subunit levels in pregnancies achieved by in vitro fertilization and embryo transfer: an internatioal collaborative study. Fertil Steril 45: 526–531

Davison G, Leeton J (1988) Management of unruptured tubal pregnancy by aspiration of sac under ultrasound control. Lancet ii: 276

Feichtinger W, Kemter P (1987) Conservative treatment of ectopic pregnancy by transvaginal aspiration under sonographic control and methotrexate injection Lancet i: 381

Goldzieher JW (1964) Double-blind trial of a progestin in habitual abortion JAMA 188: 651–654

Jacobs IJ, Isaka K, Stabile I, Fay T, Yovich JL, Grudzinskas JG (1990a) Serum levels of placental proteins (hCG, SP1, PAPP-A) in anembryonic pregnancy, ectopic pregnancy and spontaneous abortion (submitted)

Jacobs IJ, Isaka K, Stabile I, Fay T, Yovich JL, Grudzinskas JG (1989a) Serum levels of placental proteins (hCG, SP1 PAPP-A) during the first trimester of twin and triplet pregnancies (submitted)

Jones GS (1976) The luteal phase defect. Fertil Steril 27: 351–356

Klopper A, MacNaughton M (1965) Hormones in recurrent abortion. J Obstet Gynaecol Br Cwlth 72: 1022–1028

Lenton EA, Grudzinskas JG, Gordon YB, Chard T, Cooke ID (1981) Pregnancy specific beta-1-glycoprotein and chorionic gonadotropin in early human pregnancy. Acta Obstet Gynecol Scand 60: 489–492

Lenton EA, Woodward AJ (1988) The endocrinology of conception cycles and implantation in women. J Reprod Fertil (Suppl) 36: 1–15

Lunenfeld B, Insler V (1978) Clinical use of human gonadotropins. In: Diagnosis and treatment of functional infertility. Grosse Verlag, Berlin pp 61–89

Lutjen P, Trounson A, Leeton J, Findlay J, Wood C, Renou P (1984) The establishment and maintenance of pregnancy using in vitro fertilization and embryo donation in a patient with primary ovarian failure. Nature 307: 174–175

Matson PL, Blackledge DG, Richardson PA, Turner SR, Yovich JM, Yovich JL (1987) The role of gamete intrafallopian transfer (GIFT) in the treatment of oligospermic infertility. Fertil Steril 48: 608–612

Matthews CP, Coulson PB, Wild RA (1986) Serum progesterone levels as an aid in the diagnosis of ectopic pregnancy. Obstet Gynecol 68: 390–394

Mowbray JF, Gibbings C, Liddell H, Reginald PW, Underwood JL, Beard RW (1985) Controlled trial of treatment of recurrent spontaneous abortion by immunization with paternal cells. Lancet i: 941–943

National Perinatal Statistics Unit (1988) IVF and GIFT pregnancies (Australia and New Zealand), Sydney, ISSN 1030–4711

Nyberg DA, Laing FC, Filly RA, Uri-Simmons M, Jeffrey RE (1983) Ultrasonic differentiation of the gestational sac of early intrauterine pregnancy from the pseudogestational sac of ectopic pregnancy. Radiology 146: 755–759

Pouly JL, Mahnes H, Mage G, Canis M, Bruhat MA (1986) Conservative laparoscopic treatment of 321 ectopic pregnancies. Fertil Steril 46: 1093–1097

Robertson DE, Smith W, Moye MA et al. (1987) Reduction of ectopic pregnancy by injection under ultrasound control. Lancet i: 974–975

Rodriguez-Rigau LJ, Steinberger E, Weidman ER, Smith KD, Ayala C, Gibbons WE (1989) Semen analysis and GIFT. In: Capitanio GL, Asch RH, De Cecco L, Croce S (eds) GIFT: from basics to clinics. Raven Press, New York, pp 235–244

Shearman RP, Garrett WJ (1963) Double-blind study of the effect of 17-hydroxyprogesterone caproate on abortion rate. Br Med J (Clin Red) i: 292–295

Simpson JL (1980) Genes, chromosomes and reproductive failure. Fertil Steril 33: 107–116

Sinosich MJ (1988) Pregnancy associated plasma protein-A: fact, fiction and future. In: Chapman M, Grudzinskas G, Chard T (eds) Implantation: biological and clinical aspects. Springer-Verlag, London, pp 45–81

Taylor C, Faulk WP (1981) Prevention of recurrent abortion with leucocyte transfusion. Lancet ii: 68–70

Westergaard JG, Sinosich MJ, Bugge M, Madsen LT, Teisner B, Grudzinskas JG (1983) Pregnancy-associated plasma protein A in the prediction of early pregnancy failure. AM J Obstet Gynecol 145: 67–69

Wilkins L (1960) Masculinization of female fetus due to use of orally given progestins. JAMA 118: 1028–1032

Yovich JL (1988) Treatments to enhance implantation. In: Chapman M, Grudzinskas G, Chard T (eds) Implantation: biological and clinical aspects. Springer-Verlag, London, pp 239–254

Yovich JL (1990) Tubal transfers: PROST and TEST. In: Proceedings of the international symposium on gamete physiology. California, 6–10 Nov. Plenum Press, New York (in press)

Yovich JL, Matson PL (1988) Early pregnancy wastage after gamete manipulation. Br J Obstet Gynaecol 95: 1120–1127

Yovich JL, Grudzinskas JG (1990) The management of infertility: a practical guide to gamete handling procedures. Heineman Medical Books, London (in press)

Yovich JL, Stanger JD, Tuvick A, Hahnel R (1984) Combined pregnancies following gonadotrophin therapy. Am J Obstet Gynecol 63: 855–858

Yovich JL, Stanger JD, Yovich JM, Tuvick AI, Turner SR (1985a) Hormonal profiles in the follicular phase, luteal phase and first trimester of pregnancies arising from in-vitro fertilization. Br J Obstet Gynaecol 92: 374–384

Yovich JL, McColm SC, Turner SR, Matson PL (1985b) Heterotopic pregnancy from in-vitro fertilization. J Vitro Fert Embryo Transfer 2: 146–150

Yovich JL, Turner SR, Murphy AJ (1985c) Embryo transfer technique as a cause of ectopic pregnancy in in-vitro fertilization. Fertil Steril 44: 185–189

Yovich JL, Willcox DL, Wilkinson SP, Polletti PM, Hahnel RA (1985d) Medroxyprogesterone acetate does not perturb the profile of steroid metabolites in urine during pregnancy. J Endocrinol 104: 453–459

Yovich JL, Willcox DL, Grudzinskas JG, Chapman MG, Bolton AE (1986a) Placental hormone and protein measurements during conception cycles and early pregnancy. In: Ludwig H, Thomsen K (eds) Gynecology and obstetrics, Springer-Verlag, Berlin Heidelberg, pp 854–857

Yovich JL, Willcox DL, Grudzinskas JG, Bolton AE (1986b) The prognostic value of hCG, PAPP-A, oestradiol-17ß and progesterone in early human pregnancy. Aust NZ J Obstet Gynaecol 26: 59–64

Yovich JL, Draper RR, Yovich JM, Edirisinghe WR, Cummins JM (1988a) Triplet pregnancy in a woman with primary ovarian failure following pronuclear stage tubal transfer (PROST). Infertility 11: 203–212

Yovich JL, Turner SR, Draper R (1988b) Medroxyprogesterone acetate therapy in early pregnancy has no apparent fetal effects. Teratology 38: 135–144

Yovich JL, Turner S, Yovich JM, Draper R, Jequier AM, Edirisinghe R, Cummins JM (1989a) In-vitro fertilization today. Lancet ii: 688–689

Yovich JL, Cummins JM, Bootsma B, Yovich JM (1989b) The usefulness of IVF and GIFT in predicting fertilization and pregnancy. In: Capitanio GL, Asch RH, De Cecco L, Croce S (eds) GIFT: from basics to clinics. Raven Press, New York, pp 321–332

Yovich JL, Draper RR, Turner SR, Cummins JM (1990a) The benefits of tubal transfer procedures. In: Ben-Rafael Z (ed) In vitro fertilization and alternate assisted reproduction. Plenum Press, New York (in press)

5. Embryo Biopsy

V.N. Bolton

Introduction

The development of a technique for embryo biopsy that will enable the diagnosis of genetic disorders in the preimplantation embryo would represent a major advance in prenatal diagnosis (McLaren 1985; Penketh and McLaren 1987; Whittingham and Penketh 1987). Currently, such couples are faced with a number of choices: they may opt to remain childless rather than risk giving birth to an affected child; they may embark on a pregnancy, and continue with it in the hope that the fetus is unaffected; they may conceive, and opt for prenatal diagnosis (by chorionic villus sampling at 8–12 weeks', by cordocentesis at 18–20 weeks', or by amniocentesis at 12–18 weeks' gestation), followed by termination of the pregnancy if the fetus is affected. This last choice may result in several cycles of conception and termination before an unaffected child is eventually conceived, or until the couple abandon all hopes of parenthood. However, if the diagnosis could be made during the preimplantation stage of embryonic development, followed by the transfer of unaffected embryos to the woman's uterus, these distressing choices would no longer be necessary. Preimplantation diagnostic techniques, if developed, would enable couples for whom terminations are unacceptable to embark on a pregnancy in the knowledge that their future child would not be affected by the disorder for which they are at risk.

The scale of the potential demand for preimplantation diagnosis is illustrated by the fact that genetic defects affect approximately 1% of live births, representing about 70 000 babies each year in the UK. Furthermore of the 250 000 spontaneous abortions per year in this country, more than half have recognizable chromosomal abnormalities. However, the present demand for prenatal diagnosis falls into two categories. The first, larger group is represented by women who are at relatively low risk of sporadic diseases e.g. older women and Down's syndrome. The second group consists of couples who have a known risk of transmitting a genetic disease to their children, the majority of whom have a 25% chance of an affected child in each pregnancy e.g. recessively inherited disorders such as thalassaemia, cystic fibrosis, and X-linked disorders such as Duchenne's muscular dystrophy and haemophilia. For example, at least 1000 pregnancies each year in the UK carry a 1 : 4 risk of cystic fibrosis. However, where the disorder is dominant, e.g. Huntington's chorea, the risk is as high as 50%.

It is for women in this latter group, who carry an X-linked disorder, and for whom the only guarantee of bearing an unaffected child is to undergo prenatal diagnosis and termination of all male fetuses, 50% of which will be unaffected, that prenatal diagnosis before implantation holds the most promise.

For preimplantation diagnosis to become a feasible, routine service, there are two basic requirements. First, it must be demonstrated that the process of embryo biopsy does not hinder the subsequent development of the conceptus. Second, it must be possible to remove sufficient material at biopsy to make a direct diagnosis which can be interpreted with confidence. Alternatively, at least some of the biopsied cells must be capable of proliferating in vitro, in order either to confirm the original, direct diagnosis or to provide sufficient material on which a diagnosis can be made.

Human Preimplantation Embryogenesis

In the ovary the oocytes are arrested in the metaphase of the first meiotic division. Shortly before ovulation, meiosis resumes, one set of chromosomes is expelled in the first polar body, and the second meiotic division begins. This is only completed at fertilization, with expulsion of the second polar body and formation of the diploid zygote.

The one-cell embryo undergoes a series of cleavage divisions, at each of which the cells (blastomeres) halve in size. Up to the 8- to 16-cell stage, the blastomeres appear spherical, with clearly defined outlines, but between the 16- and 32-cell stages, these cell outlines become less distinct, and the morula is formed. About 5 days after fertilization, when the embryo consists of 32 to 64 cells, a blastocyst forms, in which the outer trophectoderm cells are joined by tight junctions, enabling fluid to accumulate in the blastocoelic cavity. Those cells with no outside surface form the inner cell mass (ICM; Fig. 5.1). Implantation begins at about 6 days after fertilization, and the trophectoderm cells give rise to trophoblast

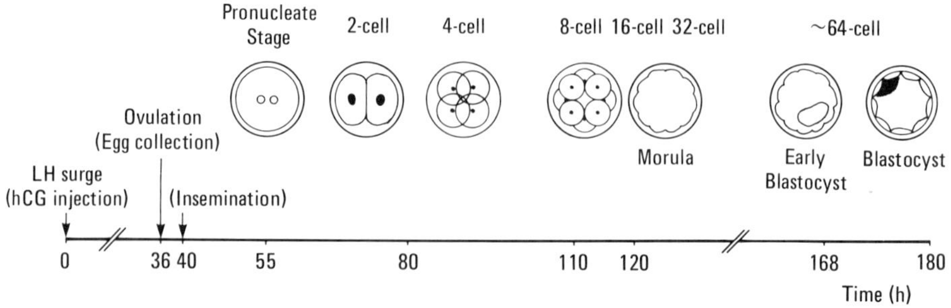

Fig. 5.1. Diagram illustrating human preimplantation embryogenesis to the fully expanded blastocyst stage.

and chorionic ectoderm, while the ICM yields all endoderm, mesoderm and embryonic ectoderm derivatives.

The fact that the mammalian embryo is "free-floating" in the reproductive tract up to the time of implantation has enabled the development of techniques for removing preimplantation embryos from the environment in vivo by uterine flushing, and maintaining them temporarily in vitro. Similarly, the technique of in vitro fertilization (IVF) exploits this "free-floating" phase of embryogenesis, with culture conditions in vitro attempting to mimic the environment in vivo. With increased experience and skill in the culture of human preimplantation embryos in vitro, the theoretical possibility of removing one or a few cells from the embryo, applying chromosomal (e.g. Down's), enzymatic (e.g. Lesch-Nyhan), or molecular (e.g. cystic fibrosis) diagnostic methods to biopsied cells, transferring embryos that are not affected by the disorder under investigation, and achieving a pregnancy is fast approaching a practical reality.

Sources of Embryos for Biopsy

Uterine Lavage

For normal, fertile women, preimplantation embryos could be collected from the uterine cavity after in vivo fertilization by transcervical uterine flushing (uterine lavage). This technique has been used following artificial insemination to collect preimplantation embryos from egg donors, which are then transferred to recipients with synchronized menstrual cycles (Buster et al. 1983; 1985; Buster 1985; Formigli et al. 1987). The method of transcervical flushing is similar to the technique developed for recovery of baboon embryos (Pope et al. 1980), and uses a double lumen catheter and continuous lavage (Sauer et al. 1988).

In 109 cycles of insemination and uterine lavage performed on 52 donors in natural cycles, 48 eggs and embryos were obtained, giving a recovery rate of only 44% (Buster et al. 1985; Formigli et al. 1987). Moreover, although lavage was performed consistently 5 days after the natural surge of luteinizing hormone (LH), the embryos were at various stages of development, ranging from 2-cell, through all cleavage stages, to morulae and fully expanded blastocysts (Table 5.1).

Table 5.1. Human preimplantation embryos recovered by uterine lavage

Stage of development	No. of embryos	Fate	Pregnancy	Outcome
Degenerate	4	Discarded	–	–
Unfertilized	6	Discarded	–	–
2- to 3-cell	2	Embryo transfer	0	–
4- to 7-cell	5	Embryo transfer	0	–
8- to 15-cell	12	Embryo transfer	3	1 ectopic 2 delivered
16- to 32-cell	2	Embryo transfer	0	–
Morula	6	Embryo transfer	2	1 abortion 1 delivered
Blastocyst	11	Embryo transfer	7	2 abortions 5 delivered

Data collated from Buster et al. 1985; Formigli et al. 1987.

Following transfer of individual embryos to the uteri of synchronized recipients, no pregnancies occurred with early cleavage stage embryos, whereas 9 of the 12 pregnancies resulted from transfer of morula and blastocyst stages.

These results provide the only data available on natural wastage during human preimplantation embryogenesis in vivo. Although the transfer of morula/ blastocyst stage embryos produced a relatively high pregnancy rate, the poor rate of recovery of embryos at this stage of development suggests that uterine lavage during natural cycles may not be a useful source of embryos for biopsy. Thus, for genetically at-risk couples wishing to undergo preimplantation diagnosis, it may be necessary to undertake multiple natural cycles of ovulation and lavage before first, a morula or blastocyst is retrieved, and second, it is shown to be free of the disorder under investigation. Ovarian hyperstimulation prior to lavage would increase the number of embryos retrieved from a single attempt, and thus the chance of identifying an unaffected morula or blastocyst. However, preliminary results with uterine lavage in hyperstimulated cycles have been disappointing (Sauer et al. 1989). From 6 donors who underwent 7 cycles of ovarian hyperstimulation and uterine lavage, a single morula was retrieved, which failed to produce a pregnancy following transfer to a recipient. Moreover, there were two retained pregnancies in this group; one was terminated, while the other was carried to term as a surrogate pregnancy.

These latter cases highlight further disadvantages of uterine lavage as a source of embryos for biopsy. In the natural cycle series, retained pregnancies occurred in 3 of the 109 cycles, infections in 2, unexplained abdominal pain in 1, and difficult catheterization in 4 (Buster et al. 1985; Formigli et al. 1987). In addition, since the procedure will necessarily be performed on women with patent fallopian tubes, fluid may be lost during lavage, with the theoretical risk of salpingitis due to the passage of bacteria from the cervix into the upper genital tract, and/or ectopic pregnancy.

Provided salpingitis or ectopic pregnancies do not result, the technique does have the advantage that it has no effect on the future reproductive potential of the patients. It causes minimal trauma, and therefore may be performed repeatedly with little consecutive risk. Embryos obtained by uterine lavage will be exposed to in vitro conditions for a minimal period, and therefore their viability will be minimally compromised. Finally, although a large number of embryos obtained in the series reported appeared to have undergone developmental arrest during cleavage, this may be the same proportion as observed in vitro, and furthermore, this may mean that those embryos which have developed to the blastocyst stage at lavage will have "selected" themselves, so that embryo biopsy and preimplantation diagnosis will be performed on embryos with the highest chance of implantation (Bolton et al. 1989, 1990).

In Vitro Fertilization

Techniques for IVF and embryo transfer for the treatment of infertility have improved over the last decade [Voluntary (Interim) Licensing Authority, 1986, 1987, 1988, 1989]. The introduction of ovarian hyperstimulation means that, in most cases, several embryos can be produced per treatment cycle, thus increasing the chance of pregnancy. Furthermore, ultrasound-guided techniques for follicle aspiration minimize the trauma of egg collection procedures, which can be

Table 5.2 King's College Hospital IVF pregnancies: 1 January 1988–31 July 1989; implantation rate per embryo

No of embryos transferred	No. of embryo transfers	Total no. embryos	No. (%) gestation sacs[a]	No (%) fetal hearts[a]
1	128	128	17 (13)	14 (11)
2	139	278	36 (13)	31 (11)
3	475	1425	219 (15)	201 (14)
Total	742	1831	272 (15)	246 (13)

[a]Excludes 10 ectopic pregnancies.

performed on an outpatient basis (Wren and Parsons 1989).

Despite these advances, the pregnancy rate per IVF treatment cycle remains low, even where up to three embryos are transferred. Indeed, data from the Assisted Conception Unit at King's College Hospital show that following transfer, only 15% of embryos implant and form a clinical pregnancy, with only 13% showing a fetal heart on ultrasound (Table 5.2). If later miscarriages are also taken into consideration, then up to 90% of embryo biopsy procedures performed for the purposes of preimplantation diagnosis on IVF-produced embryos might be spurious. Moreover, the biopsy procedure itself may damage the embryos and reduce their chances of implantation still further.

It has been suggested that the incidence of chromosomal abnormalities (monosomies, trisomies, heteroploidies, polyploidies) may be increased in embryos produced through IVF (reviewed by Bolton and Braude 1987), and may account for a significant proportion of this early embryonic loss. This represents an additional complication for preimplantation diagnosis, since embryos with gross chromosomal abnormalities may appear morphologically normal and, moreover, may well be free of the genetic disorder under investigation. Thus, despite genetic analysis of biopsied material, without routine karyotyping, embryos with such abnormalities may be considered suitable for transfer.

It should be noted that these data have been collated from infertile patients undergoing therapeutic IVF who, by definition, may be expected to produce a lower proportion of viable embryos than couples undergoing IVF solely for the purposes of preimplantation diagnosis. The majority of this latter group would be normal, fertile couples, whose chances of conception following such treatment may therefore be higher.

Biopsy Techniques

Disaggregation

The simplest method of embryo biopsy, requiring no specialized equipment, is by disaggregation of the cleavage stage embryo (Fig. 5.2a). The zona pellucida can be removed by digestion with an enzyme (e.g. pronase; 500 IU/ml), by dissolution using acidic solution (calcium- and magnesium-free acid Tyrode's solution, pH 2.5) (Nicolson et al. 1975), or by mechanical force using a fine pipette (Nijs and Van Steirteghem 1987; Nijs et al. 1988). Separation of the

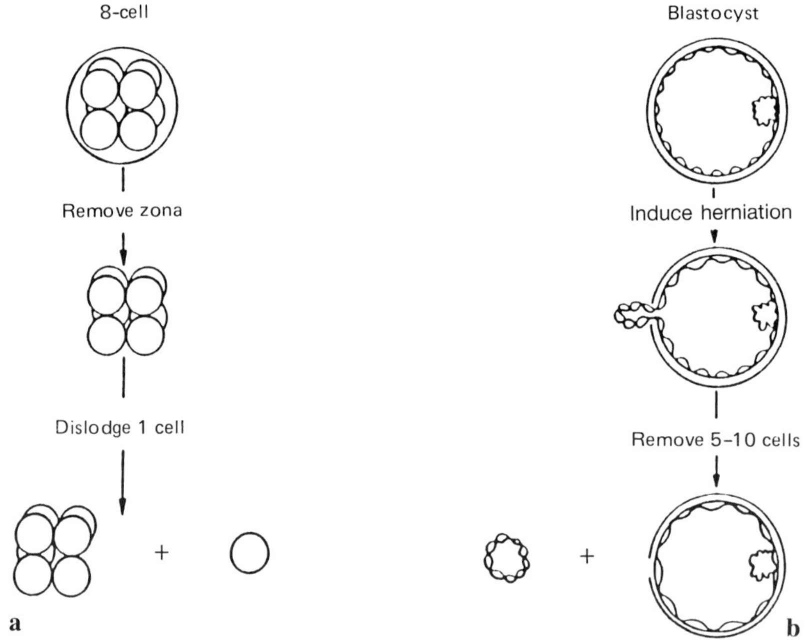

Fig. 5.2. Diagram illustrating embryo biopsy: **a** at the cleavage stage by disaggregation, **b** at the blastocyst stage by herniation.

blastomeres may be facilitated by preincubation in calcium-free medium (Monk et al. 1987b), pronase, or a chelating agent (EDTA-glycine; Nijs and Van Steirteghem 1987), and is achieved by gentle pipetting. A single blastomere may be retained for diagnosis, and the remaining blastomeres can be reaggregated by restoring the calcium concentration.

Micromanipulation

Micromanipulation can be used after embryo biopsy by disaggregation, in order to transfer the biopsied, reaggregated embryo into a host zona pellucida to facilitate further development (Willadsen 1979; Wassarman 1987). Alternatively, the biopsy procedure itself can be performed using micromanipulation, whereby the embryo is placed in calcium-free medium and held stationary using a glass holding pipette. A hole is made in the zona pellucida, either mechanically using a fine glass aspiration pipette (10–20 µm diameter) (Wilton and Trounson 1989), or by "drilling" using the same pipette filled with acid Tyrode's solution (Gordon and Talansky 1986; Handyside et al. 1989). Biopsy can then be performed by pushing an aspiration pipette through the hole, and aspirating a single blastomere from the cleavage stage (Wilton and Trounson 1989; Handyside et al. 1989; Fig. 5.3), or several cells from the blastocyst stage embryo (Gardner and Edwards 1968; Monk et al. 1987b). The aspiration pipette is then withdrawn from the

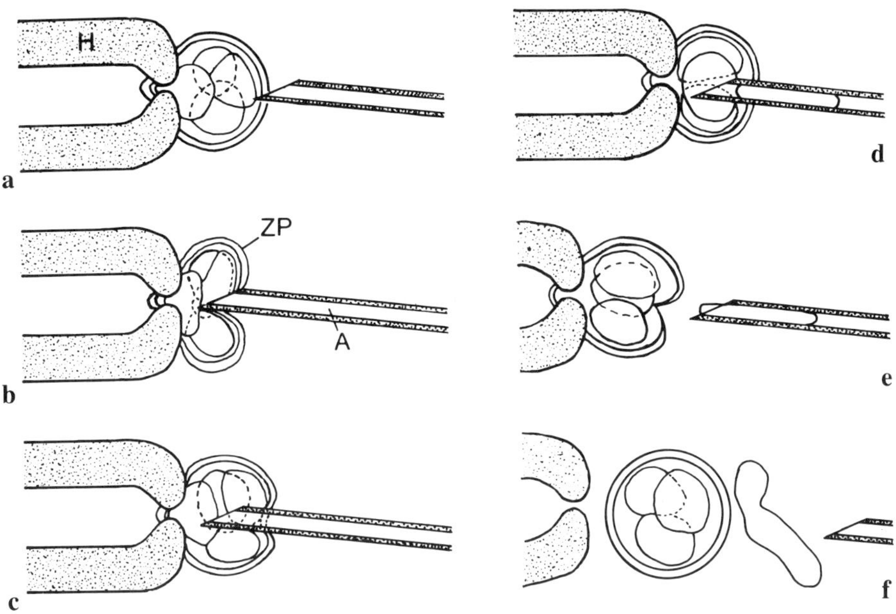

Fig. 5.3. Diagram illustrating biopsy of the cleavage stage embryo by micromanipulation. **a** The embryo is held stationary with the holding pipette (H). **b** The zona pellucida (ZP) is punctured by the aspiration pipette (A). **c** The aspiration pipette is inserted through the zona pellucida. **d** A single blastomere is drawn into the aspiration pipette. **e** The aspiration pipette is withdrawn. **f** The biopsied blastomere is expelled into the culture medium.

embryo, and the biopsied blastomere or cells are expelled into the culture medium. The entire biopsy procedure takes only 5–10 minutes (Handyside et al. 1989).

In the blastocyst, an alternative to performing biopsy by aspiration of cells is made possible from the observation that trophectoderm cells will herniate spontaneously through a hole in the zona pellucida (Monk et al. 1987b; Summers et al. 1988; Fig. 5.2b). Thus, following puncture or "drilling" of the zona, the blastocyst can be left to herniate in culture, and the herniated cells may be excised using glass needles or iridectomy scissors. This technique has the advantages of simplicity, together with the fact that it allows controlled herniation of trophectoderm at a point opposite the ICM, and therefore ensures biopsy of only extra-embryonic cells.

Animal Studies

Disaggregation

A number of studies have shown that disaggregation of cleavage stage embryos from different mammalian species results in loss of viability and subsequent abnormal development in vitro (Tarkowski 1959; Willadsen 1979; Willadsen & Fehilly 1983; Tsunoda and McLaren 1983; O'Brien et al. 1984; Rands 1986a; 1986b; Selwood 1986; Young and Foote 1987). For example, removal of the zona pellucida from 2-cell sheep embryos, followed by isolation of blastomeres and their insertion separately into host zonae, resulted in loss of 46% of the blastomeres during manipulation (Willadsen 1979). However, 88% of the surviving blastomeres formed late blastocysts when embedded in agar and transferred to ligated sheep oviducts.

In an evaluation of different techniques for the disaggregation of mouse 2-cell embryos and culture of isolated blastomeres, the zona was removed using pronase, acid Tyrode's, or mechanical force (Nijs and Van Steirteghem 1987; Nijs et al. 1988). The blastomeres were separated after treatment with pronase, a chelating agent, or calcium- and magnesium-free phosphate-buffered saline. Isolated blastomeres were cultured either naked, or after insertion into a host zona pellucida, and their fate is summarized in Table 5.3.

While more than 95% of control 2-cell embryos developed into blastocysts, and produced living fetuses following transfer to pseudopregnant recipients, between 17% and 23% of isolated blastomeres showed abnormal growth patterns, depending on the method of disaggregation. Abnormalities included double blastocoelic cavities, the development of trophoblastic vesicles (pseudoblastocysts with no ICM), and of disorganized groups of blastomeres. Moreover, although apparently normal blastocysts did develop from isolated blastomeres, the only fetuses that formed following the transfer of such blastocysts were following the insertion of blastomeres into a host zona, and then only in a small number of cases. Each of the isolation procedures investigated had a negative impact on the subsequent growth potential of the isolated blastomeres, although it was noted that where blastocyst formation did occur, the timing was identical to that of controls.

The abnormal development of isolated blastomeres from 2-cell embryos in the absence of a zona pellucida may be due at least in part to the inability of blastomeres at such early stages of development to adhere to each other (Johnson and Maro 1986). Without a zona to hold the blastomeres within the confines of a sphere, disorganized cleavage patterns result, and flattened groups or strands of cells form. Since none of these cells are "inside", trophoblastic vesicles, or even multiple blastocoelic cavities, will develop. Further problems associated with biopsy at the 2-cell stage follow from the fact that the embryo is literally halved in size. Since blastocyst formation appears to be a function of the number of cell cycles, rather than the number of cells present, the ratio of ICM to trophectoderm cells will be disrupted.

Table 5.3. Results of biopsy of the 2-cell mouse embryo by disaggregation

Procedure	No. cells	% developed normally	No. blastocysts transferred	No. living fetuses	%
Control	107	95	49	33	67
Bisected – host zona	1032	74	39	0	0
Bisected + host zona	88	70	20	5	25

Data from Nijs et al. 1988.

This concept is supported by results of a study in which one blastomere of an intact 2-cell mouse embryo was destroyed, and the blastocysts which developed were shown to contain a disturbed ratio of ICM to trophectoderm, with relatively few cells in the ICM (Rands 1985). Similarly, bisection of 8-cell mouse embryos after removal of the zona pellucida resulted in severely impaired development, with implantation and fetal development rates ranging from 0–40% and 0-12% respectively (Tsunoda and McLaren 1983; Ponzilius et al. 1987). In contrast, when a single blastomere was biopsied from mouse 8-cell embryos by disaggregation, fetal development was less severely compromised (Monk and Handyside 1987; Monk et al. 1987a). Thus, of 51 biopsied, zona-free embryos transferred to pseudopregnant recipients, 16 (31%) implanted and formed fetuses (Monk et al. 1987a).

Micromanipulation

Cleavage Stage

Aspiration of a single blastomere from 4-cell mouse embryos using the micromanipulation technique does not appear to affect adversely their subsequent development in vitro, with 94% (135/143) of biopsied embryos developing to the blastocyst stage compared with 98% (136/139) of controls (Wilton and Trounson 1989). After further culture for 24 hours, biopsied embryos were transferred to pseudopregnant recipients, and it was found that the implantation rate of biopsied embryos was reduced, compared with controls (mean ± SD: 53.1 ± 4.0 and 81.8 ± 8.4 respectively). However, those embryos which did implant showed normal fetal development.

It is possible that removal of 25% of the embryonic cell mass may be responsible for the relatively low implantation rate of biopsied 4-cell embryos observed in this study. However, the same group reported a further series, in which the survival rate of biopsied embryos was not significantly different from that of controls (Wilton et al. 1989; Table 5.4). Although biopsied embryos were left in culture for 40 hours before transfer in the latter study, the improved embryonic survival can almost certainly be attributed to improved operator technique during micromanipulation procedures in the second series.

Table 5.4. Results of biopsy of the 4-cell mouse embryo by micromanipulation

	No. of embryos per sample	No. (%) embryos surviving biopsy	No. of embryos transferred	No. (%) implantation site	No. % fetuses
Control	52	49 (94)	42	27 (64)	22 (52)
		NS		NS	NS
Biopsied	90	87 (97)	78	47 (60)	41 (53)

Data from Wilton et al. 1990.
NS: not significant.

Table 5.5. Results of biopsy of the marmoset blastocyst by herniation

Treatment	No. of			
	Embryos	Recipients	Pregnancies	Live young
Control	6	6	4	3
Day 9 biopsy	3	3	3	2
Day 10 biopsy				
(i) no CG	4	4	0	0
(ii) + CG	5	5	3	3

Data from Summers et al. 1988.
CG: chorionic gonadotrophin.

Blastocyst Stage

The birth of live young following trophectoderm biopsy by aspiration has been demonstrated in the rabbit (Gardner and Edwards 1968), mouse (Gardner 1971; Monk et al. 1987b), and cow (Mitchell 1977; Betteridge et al. 1981). Although the earliest studies reported a high rate of embryonic loss following biopsy, a high incidence of fetal death after implantation, and one anencephalic birth (Gardner and Edwards 1968), later studies have shown an improvement in techniques for excising trophectoderm (reviewed by Gardner 1985).

The first demonstration that trophectoderm biopsy can be applied to primate embryos without affecting adversely subsequent development came from a study using marmoset blastocysts (Summers et al. 1988). Herniation was induced by making a tear in the zona pellucida opposite the ICM on day 8 after fertilization, and the embryos were left for a further 24–48 hours in culture. Of those embryos left for 24 hours, 20% underwent herniation, while 50% herniated after 48 hours. The herniated cells were excised, the biopsied blastocysts were transferred to pseudopregnant recipients, and normal offspring were born (Table 5.5). However, for biopsied day 10 blastocysts, pregnancies followed only after administration of exogenous chorionic gonadotrophin (CG), presumably because the CG secreted by the reduced number of trophectoderm cells, after biopsy, was insufficient to support a pregnancy.

Human Studies

Disaggregation

Removal of the zona pellucida from human embryos at the 2-cell stage, and subsequent development of the separated blastomeres have been described (Edwards and Hollands 1988). Although the isolated blastomeres underwent cleavage, the resulting cells did not compact; instead, they formed a flattened array, and blastocyst formation did not take place. Similar results have been observed with early cleavage stage human embryos in this unit, where the zona pellucida was removed from 4-cell stage embryos, which were then left to develop in culture without disaggregation. The blastomeres cleaved in a disorganized manner, with multiple blastocoelic cavities developing (Fig. 5.4). However, removal of the zona from late 8-cell stage embryos resulted in the development of fully expanded blastocysts, which appeared normal at the level of the phase contrast light microscope (S. Hawes, unpublished observations).

These results suggest that biopsy by disaggregation may be possible in the human, but not before the 8-cell stage. However, this approach will not be successful in terms of biopsy for preimplantation diagnosis unless it is demonstrated that the absence of a zona does not impair embryo viability following transfer.

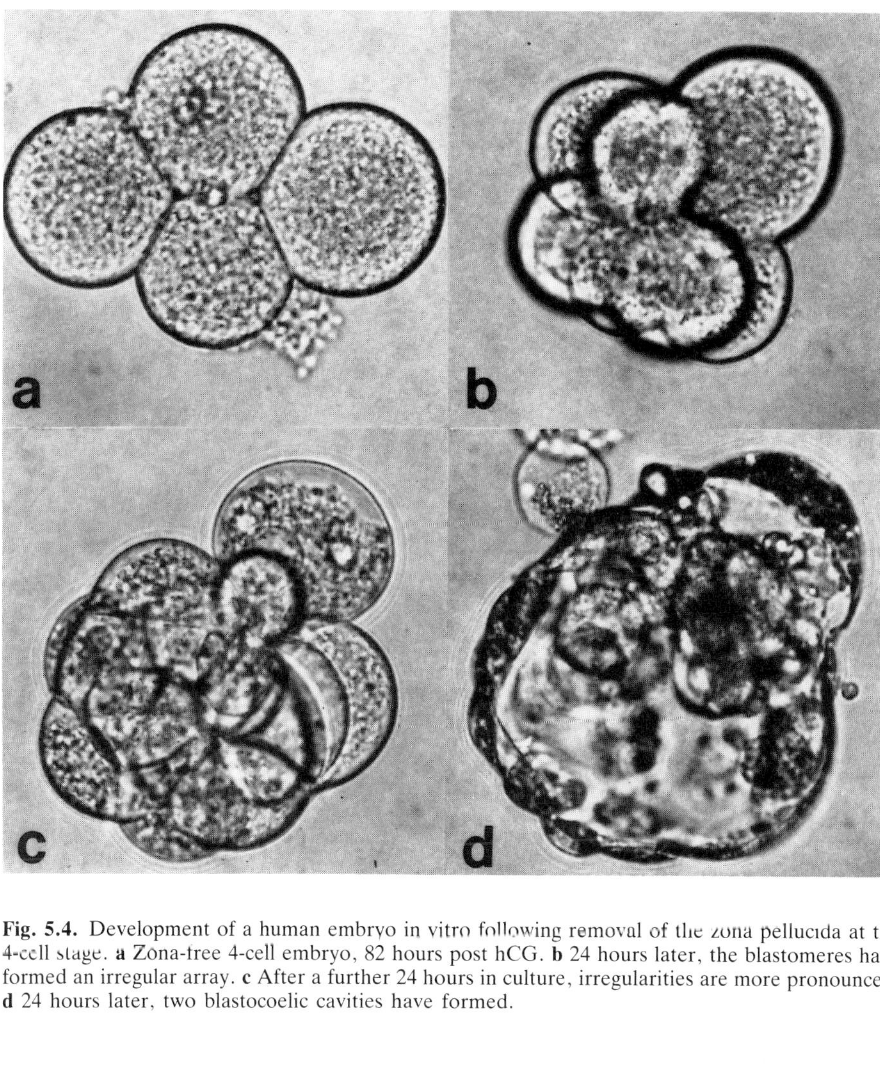

Fig. 5.4. Development of a human embryo in vitro following removal of the zona pellucida at the 4-cell stage. **a** Zona-free 4-cell embryo, 82 hours post hCG. **b** 24 hours later, the blastomeres have formed an irregular array. **c** After a further 24 hours in culture, irregularities are more pronounced. **d** 24 hours later, two blastocoelic cavities have formed.

Micromanipulation

Cleavage Stage

Using the "zona drilling" technique, biopsy of a single blastomere has been performed using human 6- to 10-cell stage embryos (day 3 after fertilization) (Handyside et al. 1989; Hardy et al. 1990). In the first study, 27 biopsied embryos were returned to culture, and 10 developed to the blastocyst stage by day 6 after fertilization. The viability of these blastocysts was assessed by counting cell numbers, the mean of which was found to be 35.6 (range 18–74) (Handyside et al. 1989). This compares with a mean cell number for intact, control blastocysts of 58.3 ± 8.1, and 84.4 ± 5.7 on days 5 and 6 respectively (Hardy et al. 1989). These results suggest that the biopsy procedure performed during cleavage results in reduced cell numbers in the blastocyst. The second study, by the same group, compared the development of biopsied and control embryos, and found that following the removal of 1 or 2 blastomeres, 33/45 (73%) embryos developed to the blastocyst stage, compared with 19/32 (59%) controls (Hardy et al. 1990). An examination of cell allocation to ICM and trophectoderm, and of glucose and pyruvate metabolism in control blastocysts compared with blastocysts developing after cleavage stage biopsy showed that cell numbers in both ICM and trophectoderm, and substrate uptakes are reduced after biopsy (Hardy et al. 1990). Whether or not these effects of biopsy are incompatible with subsequent implantation and pregnancy remains to be established.

Blastocyst Stage

In the only report describing embryo biopsy of a single human blastocyst, Edwards and Hollands (1988) used the herniation technique of Summers et al. (1988). Following the removal of a small number of mural trophectoderm cells, the biopsied blastocyst is reported to have partially collapsed, but subsequently hatched and produced hCG. Thus, the feasibility of blastocyst stage biopsy in the human remains to be confirmed.

Evaluation of Post-Biopsy Viability

The viability of animal embryos following biopsy during cleavage or blastocyst stages, as assessed by implantation, the formation of live fetuses, and the birth of normal offspring, has been described above. Ultimately, these provide the only real criteria by which to evaluate the feasibility of the biopsy technique. However, for the human embryo, viability studies involving embryo transfer are clearly not possible. It is therefore essential that post-biopsy viability is determined as far as possible through extensive studies in vitro.

The rate of blastocyst formation, evaluations of cell number and allocation, of metabolic activity (Handyside et al. 1989; Hardy et al. 1989), and of hCG production (Edwards and Hollands 1988) have been described for biopsied human embryos. The production of hCG by intact human blastocysts grown in vitro can be detected between day 7 and day 8 after fertilization, and the level appears to represent an indication of blastocyst viability (Fishel 1984; Lopata and Hay 1989). Thus, measurement of hCG secreted into the culture medium by biopsied blastocysts may be a useful tool in viability studies.

Additional information regarding the developmental potential of embryos biopsied during cleavage stages may be provided by observing the outgrowth of resulting blastocysts in vitro. Previous work using the mouse blastocyst (Robertson 1987; Monk et al. 1987b; Muggleton-Harris 1990) and preliminary data from the human blastocyst (Muggleton-Harris 1989) have shown that the proliferative potential of trophectoderm cells is limited compared with that of cells from the ICM. Thus, the ability of blastocysts to outgrow in vitro would demonstrate the presence or absence of an ICM; trophoblastic vesicles would not outgrow.

Validation of Diagnosis

The various diagnostic techniques that may be undertaken using biopsied material for the purposes of preimplantation diagnosis will be considered in detail elsewhere in this volume. It is important to note that the diagnosis may be made using a single cell, particularly if biopsy is performed during cleavage stages. Since the result will be used to decide whether or not to transfer a given embryo for the purposes of achieving a pregnancy, unless the diagnostic techniques are absolutely reliable, it is essential that the original diagnosis is confirmed using a larger amount of material. Attempts to induce proliferation in vitro of cells biopsied from human embryos have yielded promising results (Muggleton-Harris 1989) and the use of conditioned media, growth factors and substrates may improve this still further, so that the proliferated cells can then be used to repeat, and hopefully confirm, the original diagnosis.

Delayed Embryo Transfer

Following IVF, embryo transfer is normally performed on the second day after oocyte recovery, when embryos have developed to the 2- to 4-cell stage. Since it is likely that embryo biopsy will be performed either at the 6- to 10-cell (day 3) or blastocyst (day 5) stage, and since even with current techniques for rapid diagnosis, results are unlikely to be available before a further 6–8 hours have elapsed (Handyside et al. 1989), delayed embryo transfer represents another factor to consider in terms of the feasibility of preimplantation diagnosis.

Delayed embryo transfer can be achieved by cryopreservation of biopsied embryos, allowing a minimum of one menstrual cycle in which to obtain the diagnosis. Although techniques for cryopreservation of intact human embryos have improved considerably over the past 2 3 years (Van Steirteghem 1987; Mandelbaum et al. 1987; Cohen et al. 1988, 1989), no data are available regarding the post-thaw viability of biopsied, cryopreserved human embryos. There have

Table 5.6. Human IVF pregnancies following embryo transfer on day 2 or day 3 after fertilization

	DAY 2 (2- to 4-cell)		DAY 3 (6- to 10-cell)	
No. embryos transferred	No. of transfers	No. (%) of pregnancies	No. of transfers	No. (%) of pregnancies
1	52	5 (10)	41	5 (12)
2	79	9 (11)	56	9 (16)
3	156	38 (24)	114	33 (29)
Total	287	52 (18)	211	47 (22)

Data from van Os et al. 1989.

been few attempts to freeze animal embryos with an incomplete zona pellucida, and most have met with limited success (Kanagawa et al. 1979; Lehn-Jensen and Willadsen 1983; Heyman and Chesne 1984; Niemann et al. 1986). Indeed, although pregnancies have been achieved in the mouse following biopsy and ultra-rapid freezing of 4-cell embryos (Wilton et al. 1989), this technique has produced disappointing results with intact human embryos (Trounson and Sjoblom 1988; Trounson et al. 1988).

An alternative to cryopreservation is to delay the transfer of "fresh" embryos beyond day 2 after fertilization. Pregnancies have been reported following transfer of fresh, intact human embryos both on day 3 and day 5 after fertilization (van Os et al. 1989; Bolton et al. 1990). In the former study, a controlled trial showed no significant difference in the pregnancy rate for embryo transfers performed on either day (Table 5.6). This suggests that it will be possible to perform embryo biopsy early on day 3 and, provided results of the diagnosis can be obtained within 6–8 hours, to carry out embryo transfer later the same day (Handyside et al. 1989). The series in which embryo transfer was performed at the blastocyst stage, although smaller (5 pregnancies were established following the transfer of 49 blastocysts), suggests that it will be possible to carry out embryo transfers on day 5, following biopsy either the same day, or on day 3. For day 5 biopsies, this would have the advantages of blastocyst stage biopsy outlined above; for day 3 biopsies it would allow more time in which to undertake the diagnosis, and to induce proliferation of biopsied cells for confirmation. Moreover, by leaving cleavage stage biopsied embryos in culture, and only selecting those which underwent blastocyst formation in vitro for transfer, the chance of achieving a pregnancy may be increased (Bolton et al. 1990).

Concluding Considerations

Animal experiments suggest that there are two possible approaches to human embryo biopsy, one during cleavage, and the other at the blastocyst stage. Each approach has advantages and disadvantages. The advantages of cleavage stage biopsy include the fact that feasibility studies have already been undertaken; embryo transfer during cleavage is routine in therapeutic IVF; performing biopsy relatively early in preimplantation embryogenesis allows more time for diagnostic procedures. However, the cleavage stage embryo contains relatively few blastomeres, all of which are pluripotential, so that removal of a single blastomere may disturb the ratio of ICM to trophectoderm cells in the resulting blatocyst; cleavage stage blastomeres may undergo limited proliferation in vitro; the majority of cleavage stage embryos are "non-viable" and will undergo developmental arrest.

Blastocyst stage biopsy has the significant advantage that many more cells are present in the embryo, and therefore removal of several may have less effect on subsequent development; it is possible to remove extra-embryonic cells from the blastocyst; embryos which survive to the blastocyst stage in vitro may be those which are inherently viable; trophectoderm cells may be induced to undergo significant proliferation in vitro. However, unless cryopreservation is used, a maximum of 1–2 days is available for diagnostic procedures; the high rate of embryonic attrition in vitro may be due to suboptimal culture conditions; to date, the pregnancy rate following transfer of "fresh" blastocysts is disappointing.

Thus, while preimplantation diagnosis represents potentially one of the most important developments to follow from therapeutic IVF, there are many problems that require resolution before this technique can be introduced as a routine service in prenatal diagnosis. These relate first, to the high failure rate of IVF, since until the culture conditions in vitro for human preimplantation embryos are improved, and until accurate, objective criteria for assessment of human embryo viability are established, embryo biopsy will be performed in the majority of cases on embryos that are, either inherently or through exposure to trauma, incapable of surviving. Second, the technique, and timing, of biopsy itself require further investigation. Thus, although most efforts have concentrated on early cleavage stages, blastocyst stage biopsy probably holds the most promise for future success.

References

Betteridge KJ, Hare WCD, Sing EL (1981) Approaches to sex selection in farm animals. In: Brackett BG, Seidel SM (eds) New technology in animal breeding. Academic Press, New York, pp 109–125

Bolton VN, Braude PR (1987) Development of the human preimplantation embryo in vitro. In: McLaren A, Siracusa G (eds) Current topics in developmental biology 23: recent advances in mammalian development. Academic Press, London, pp 93–114

Bolton VN, Hawes, SM, Taylor CT, Parsons JH (1989) Development of spare human preimplantation embryos in vitro: an analysis of the correlations among gross morphology, cleavage rates, and development to the blastocyst. J IVF Embryo Transfer 6: 30–35

Bolton VN, Parsons JH, Wren ME (1990) In vitro fertilization and transfer of human preimplantation embryos at the blastocyst stage. Fertil Steril (in press)

Buster JE (1985) Embryo donation by uterine flushing and embryo transfer. Clin Obstet Gynecol 12: 815–824

Buster JE, Bustillo M, Thorneycroft IH, Simon JA, Boyers CP, Marshall JR, Louw JA, Seed RW, Seed RG (1983) Non-surgical transfer of in vivo fertilized donated ova to five infertile women: report of two pregnancies. Lancet ii: 223–224

Buster JE, Bustillo M, Rodi IA, Cohen SW, Hamilton M, Simon JA, Thorneycroft IH, Marshall JR (1985)Biologic and morphologic development of donated human ova recovered by non-surgical uterine lavage. Am J Obstet Gynecol 153: 211–217

Cohen J, Devane GW, Elsner CW, Fehilly CB, Kort HI, Massey JB, Turner TG (1988) Cryopreservation of zygotes and early cleaved human embryos. Fertil Steril 49. 283–298

Cohen J, Inge KL, Suzman M, Wiker SR, Wright G (1989) Videocinematography of fresh and cryopreserved embryos: a retrospective analysis of embryonic morphology and implantation. Fertil Steril 51: 820–827

Edwards RG, Hollands P (1988) New advances in human embryology: implications of the preimplantation diagnosis of genetic disease. Hum Reprod 3: 549–556

Fishel SB, Edwards RG, Evans CJ (1984) Human chorionic gonadotrophin secreted in preimplantation embryos cultured in vitro. Science 223: 816–818

Formigli L, Formigli G, Roccio C (1987) Donation of fertilized uterine ova to infertile women. Fertil Steril 47: 162–165

Gardner RL (1971) Manipulations on the blastocyst. Adv Biosci 6: 279–296

Gardner RL (1985) Origin and development of trophectoderm and inner cell mass. In: Edwards RG, Purdy JM, Steptoe PC (eds) Implantation of the human embryo. Academic Press, London, pp 151–178

Gardner RL, Edwards RG (1968) Control of the sex ratio at term in the rabbit by trasferring sexed blastocysts. Nature 218: 346–348

Gordon JW, Talansky BE (1986) Assisted fertilization by zona drilling: a mouse model for correction of oligospermia. J Exp Biol 239: 347–354

Handyside AH, Penketh RJA, Winston RML, Pattinson JK, Delhanty JDA, Tuddenham EGD (1989) Biopsy of human preimplantation embryos and sexing by DNA amplification. Lancet i: 347–349

Hardy K, Handyside AH, Winston RML (1989) The human blastocyst: cell number, death and allocation during late preimplantation development. Development 107: 597–604

Hardy K, Handyside AH, Markin K, Leese H, Winston RML (1990) Human preimplantation development in vitro is not adversely affected by biopsy at the 8-cell stage. Hum Reprod (in press)

Heyman Y, Chesne P (1984) Freezing bovine embryos: survival after cervical transfer of one half, one or two blastocysts frozen in straws. Theriogenology 21: 240

Johnson MH, Maro B (1986) Time and space in the early mouse embryo: a cell biological approach to cell diversification. In: Rossant J, Pedersen R (eds) Experimental approaches to mammalian embryonic development. Cambridge University Press, London, pp 35–65

Kanagawa H, Frim J, Kruuv J (1979) The effect of puncturing the zona pellucida on freeze-thaw survival of bovine embryos. Cam J Anim Sci 59: 623–626

Lehn-Jensen H, Willadsen SM (1983) Deep-freezing of cow "half" and "quarter" embryos. Theriogenology 19: 49–54

Lopata A, Hay DL (1989) The surplus human embryo: its potential for growth, blastulation, hatching, and human chorionic gonadotrophin production in culture. Fertil Steril 51: 984–991

Mandelbaum J, Junca AM, Plachot M, et al. (1987) Human embryo cryopreservation, extrinsic and intrinsic parameters of success. Hum Reprod 2: 709–715

McLaren A (1985) Prenatal diagnosis before implantation: opportunities and problems. Prenatal Diagn 5: 85–90

Mitchell D (1977) Sexing of embryos. In: Betteridge KJ (ed) Embryo transfer in farm animals. Monograph 16, Agriculture of Canada, Ottawa, p 26

Monk M, Handyside AH (1987) Sexing of preimplantation mouse embryos by measurement of X-linked gene dosage in a single blastomere. J Reprod Fertil 82: 365–368

Monk M, Handyside AH, Hardy K, Whittingham DG (1987a) Preimplantation diagnosis of deficiency in hypoxanthine phosphoribosyl transferase in a mouse model for Lesch-Nyhan Syndrome. Lancet ii: 423–425

Monk M, Muggleton-Harris AL, Rawlings E, Whttingham DG (1987b) Preimplantation diagnosis of HPRT-deficient male and carrier female mouse embryos by trophectoderm biopsy. Hum Reprod 3: 377–381

Muggleton-Harris AL (1989) Prolferation of cells derived from the biopsy of pre-embryos. Proc VIth World Congress on IVF and alternate Assisted Reproduction, Jerusalem, Israel

Muggleton-Harris AL (1990) Proliferation and growth potential of polar trophectoderm cells of the preimplantation mouse blastocyst. Development (in press)

Nicolson GL, Yanagimachi R, Yanagimachi H (1975) Ultrastructural localization of lectin-binding sites on the zonae pellucidae and plasma membranes of mammalian eggs. J Cell Biol 66: 263–274

Niemann H, Brem G, Sacher B, Smidt D, Krausslich H (1986) An approach to successful freezing of demi-embryos derived from 7-day bovine embryos. Theriogenology 25: 519–524

Nijs M, Van Steirteghem AC (1987) Assessment of different isolation procedures for blastomeres from two-cell mouse embryos. Hum Reprod 2: 421–424

Nijs M, Camus M, Van Steirteghem AC (1988) Evaluation of different biopsy methods of blastomeres from 2-cell mouse embryos. Hum Reprod 3: 999–1003

O'Brien JM, Critser ES, First NL (1984) Developmental potential of isolated blastomeres from very early murine embryos. Theriogenology 22: 601–607

Penketh R, McLaren A (1987) Prospects for prenatal diagnosis during preimplantation human development. Baillière's Clin Obstet Gynecol 1: 747–764
Ponzilius K-H, Nagai J, Marcus GH, Hackett AJ (1987) Survival of bisected mouse embryos after exposure to pronase and medium free of calcium and magnesium. Theriogenology 27: 859–867
Pope CE, Pope VZ, Beck LR (1980) Non-surgical recovery of uterine embryos in the baboon. Biol Reprod 23: 657–662
Rands GF (1985) Cell allocation in half- and quadruple-sized preimplantation embryos. J Exp Zool 236: 67–70
Rands GF (1986a) Size regulation in the mouse embryo: I. J Embryol Exp Morphol 92: 403–404
Rands GF (1986b) Size regulation in the mouse embryo: II. J Embryol Exp Morphol 98: 209–217
Robertson EJ (1987) Embryo-derived stem cell lines. In: Robertson EJ (ed) Teratocarcinomas and embryonic stem cells, a practical approach. IRL Press, Oxford, pp 71–112
Sauer MV, Anderson RE, Paulson RJ (1989) A trial of superovulation in ovum donors undergoing uterine lavage. Fertil Steril 51: 131–134
Sauer MV, Bustillo M, Gorrill MJ, Louw JA, Marshall JR, Buster JE (1988) An instrument for the recovery of preimplantation uterine ova. Obstet Gynecol 71: 804–806
Selwood L (1986) Cleavage in vitro following destruction of some blastomeres in the marsupial *Antechninus stuartii*. J Embryo Exp Morphol 92: 71–84
Summers PM, Campbell JM, Miller MW (1988) Normal in vivo development of marmoset monkey embryos after trophectoderm biopsy. Hum Reprod 3: 389–393
Tarkowski AK (1959) Experiments on the development of isolated blastomeres of mouse eggs. Nature 184: 1286–1287
Trounson A, Sjoblom P (1988) Cleavage and development of human embryos in vitro after ultrarapid freezing and thawing. Fertil Steril 50: 373–376
Trounson A, Peura A, Freeman L, Kirby C (1988) Ultrarapid freezing of early cleavage stage human embryos and eight-cell mouse embryos. Fertil Steril 49: 822–826
Tsunoda Y, McLaren A (1983) Effect of various procedures on the viability of mouse embryos containing half the normal number of blastomeres. J Reprod Fertil 69: 315–322
van Os HC, Alberda AT, Janssen-Caspers HAB, Leerentveld RA, Scholtes MCW, Zeilmaker GH (1989) The influence of the interval between in vitro fertilization and embryo transfer and some other variable on treatment outcome. Fertil Steril 51: 360–362
Van Steirteghem AC (1987) Survey of cryopreservation. In: Proc Vth World Congress on IVF and Embryo Transfer. American Fertility Society, Abstract 54, p 20
Voluntary (Interim) Licensing Authority (1986) The first report of the Voluntary Licensing Authority for human in vitro fertilization and embryology
Voluntary (Interim) Licensing Authority (1987) The second report of the Voluntary Licensing Authority for human in vitro fertilization and embryology
Voluntary (Interim) Licensing Authority (1988) The third report of the Voluntary Licensing Authority for human in vitro fertilization and embryology
Voluntary (Interim) Licensing Authority (1989) The fourth report of the Voluntary Licensing Authority for human in vitro fertilization and embryology
Wassarman PM (1987) The zona pellucida: a coat of many colors. Bioessays 6: 161–166
Whittingham DG, Penketh R (1987) Prenatal diagnosis in the human preimplantation period. Hum Reprod 2: 267–270
Willadsen SM (1979) A method for culture of micromanipulated sheep embryos and its use to produce monozygotic twins. Nature 277: 289–300
Willadsen SM, Fehilly CB (1983) The developmental potential and regulatory capacity of blastomeres from two-, four- and eight-cell sheep embryos. In: Beier HM, Lindner HL (eds) Fertilization of the human egg in vitro. Springer-Verlag, Berlin, Heidelberg, pp 353–357
Wilton LJ, Trounson AO (1989) Biopsy of preimplantation mouse embryos: development of micromanipulated embryos and proliferation of single blastomeres in vitro. Biol Reprod 40: 145–152
Wilton LJ, Shaw JM, Trounson AO (1989) Successful single-cell biopsy and cryopreservation of preimplantation mouse embryos. Fertil Steril 51: 513–517
Wren ME, Parsons JH (1989) Ultrasound directed follicle aspiration for oocyte collection. In: Chen C, Tan SL, Cheng WC (eds) Recent advances in the management of infertility. McGraw Hill, New York, pp 165–182
Young Y, Foote R (1987) Production of identical twin rabbits by micromanipulation of embryos. Biol Reprod 37: 1007–1014

6. Preimplantation Diagnosis by DNA Amplification

A.H. Handyside

Prenatal Diagnosis by DNA Analysis

As the molecular basis for an increasing number of inherited diseases is known, including recently the predominant deletion causing cystic fibrosis (Riordan et al. 1989), many genetic defects are now being diagnosed prenatally by DNA analysis (Cooper and Schmidtke 1987). With diseases in which the gene defects are relatively homogeneous, direct DNA analysis is often possible using cDNA probes; with other diseases involving heterogeneous defects or high rates of new mutations, closely linked markers, mainly restriction fragment length polymorphisms (RFLPs), are commonly used. Both of these approaches require a minimum of nanogram, and more usually microgram, quantities of fetal genomic DNA from a million or more cells (Old 1986). With the development of chorion villus sampling, a sufficient number of trophoblast cells can be recovered from the conceptus as early as 8 weeks of gestation (Rodeck 1984).

For preimplantation diagnosis, the small numbers of cells in human embryos at these early stages and limitations on the number that can be biopsied without seriously affecting the viability and development of the embryos prevent DNA analysis by these conventional approaches. The total number of cells in blastocysts 7 days after in vitro fertilization (IVF) – day 7, the maximum period embryos can be reliably cultured – is about 125, split between the outer trophectoderm with 80 and the inner cell mass (ICM), from which the fetus develops, with 45 cells (Hardy et al. 1989). Thus, irrespective of whether one or two cells are biopsied at the 8-cell stage on day 3, for example, and allowed to divide in culture, or a third of the trophectoderm cells are biopsied at the blastocyst stage, the maximum number of cells available is unlikely to exceed about 30 cells.

Strategy for Preimplantation Diagnosis

Among a variety of strategies for preimplantation diagnosis (Penketh and McLaren 1987), at present the most promising are:

1. Superovulation to increase the number of embryos screened in a single cycle
2. IVF and embryo culture
3. Biopsy of cell(s) from each 8-cell embryo early on day 3
4. Rapid diagnosis of the genetic defect
5. Transfer of selected biopsied embryos later the same day

As an alternative to IVF, preimplantation embryos could be recovered by uterine lavage after normal conception (Buster et al. 1985). However, the efficiency of embryo recovery after superovulation is low and the risks of ectopic pregnancies or of missing affected embryos have not been fully assessed.

Removal of even a single cell at the 2- or 4-cell stages on day 1 or 2 reduces the cellular mass of the embryo substantially (1/2 or 1/4 respectively) and may compromise their ability to form normal blastocysts with adequate numbers of ICM cells for fetal development. The cleavage rate, nutrient uptake and development of 8-cell embryos, however, is not adversely affected by removal of one or two cells (1/8 or 2/8) and numbers of cells in the trophectoderm and inner cell mass of blastocysts are only reduced proportionately (Hardy et al. 1990). On the other hand, culturing embryos (and/or cell biopsies) to more advanced stages with increased numbers of cells is limited by the mixed success of transfers later than day 3. We obtained no pregnancies following transfer of blastocysts on days 6 and 7 (Dawson et al. 1988). However, a few pregnancies have been reported after transfer of morulae and early blastocysts on day 5 (see Chapter 5).

Finally, another option, to cryopreserve embryos while the cell biopsies are allowed to divide in culture before diagnosis, is unattractive because current methods are less successful at cleavage stages than at the pronuclear stage and many are damaged or destroyed in the process (Testart et al. 1987). Also it is likely that biopsied embryos will be more susceptible to damage after freezing and thawing since the mechanical protection of the zona during this process may be reduced after drilling or making a slit for the biopsy.

Until these limitations are overcome, therefore, preimplantation diagnosis needs to be based on methods applicable to one or two cells biopsied from 8-cell embryos on day 3 and which can be completed within 12 hours. Rapid DNA analysis on small numbers or single cells has only recently been made possible with the introduction of a revolutionary new technique, the polymerase chain reaction (PCR), to amplify short segments of DNA up to 10^7-fold in a few hours (White et al. 1989).

DNA Amplification by the Polymerase Chain Reaction

PCR involves the enzymatic amplification of a DNA fragment using two oligonucleotide primers that flank the target sequence and hybridize to opposite strands oriented with their 3′ ends pointing towards each other. Repeated cycles of heat denaturation of the template, annealing of the primers and primer-directed extension by heat-stable DNA polymerase (derived from a thermophilic bacterium) result in the exponential accumulation of the specific target sequence.

Amplified fragments are generally short in the range of 100 to 500 basepairs (bp), although fragments up to 10 kilobasepairs (kb) have been successfully amplified. Amplification of unique sequences is possible from genomic DNA in crude extracts or cell lysates (after appropriate denaturation or inactivation of endogenous DNAses). Multiple pairs of primers have been used for simultaneous amplification of six different fragments of the dystrophin gene commonly deleted in Duchenne muscular dystrophy (Chamberlain et al. 1988). Many variants of the basic method are being developed, for example, for generating cDNA probes, sequencing and screening for mutations (Gyllenstein and Erlich 1988; Innis et al. 1988).

This combination of sensitivity, speed and versatility has led to increasingly wide application of PCR in prenatal diagnosis. In many cases, results can be available in a day compared with several weeks using conventional Southern blotting and hybridization procedures. In most cases, no more than 40 cycles taking 4 to 10 min to complete (about 3 to 7 h) give optimal yield of the amplified fragment.

One of the first applications in human genetics was to increase the sensitivity of detection of sickle cell anaemia enabling a diagnosis on as few as 75 cells from a small sample of fetal blood (Saiki et al. 1985, 1986). In this case, hybridization with radiolabelled allele-specific oligonucleotides (ASOs) were used to detect the defect, a single base change, in the amplified fragment of the ß-globin gene within 6 hours. The use of ASOs also eliminates any ambiguity arising from non-specific amplification of other target sequences.

Some examples of other methods which have been used for the detection of genetic defects in amplified DNA include:

1. The presence or absence of target DNA to detect a deletion of the ß-major haemoglobin gene in a mouse model of ß-thalassaemia (Holding and Monk 1989);
2. Differences in the size of the amplified DNA to detect the predominant deletion causing ß-thalassaemia in the Thai population (Winichagoon et al. 1989) (in this case a difference of only 4 bp)
3. The presence of allele-specific sites, by restriction endonuclease digestion or hybridization with ASOs, in a polymorphic locus linked to cystic fibrosis (Williams et al. 1988).

Problems with Single Human Embryo Cells

There are a number of potential problems associated with the application of DNA amplification for preimplantation diagnosis which need to be overcome. Some of these relate to how representative the DNA of cell biopsies is of the genotype of the fetus, and others are inherent in the use of PCR with small numbers or single cells.

Preimplantation embryos in vitro have a high incidence of cytoplasmic fragmentation, degenerate and dead cells (Hardy et al. 1989) and some are genetically mosaic (Papadopoulus et al. 1989). This could present a serious problem with single cell biopsies from cleavage stage embryos. For example, anucleate cytoplasmic fragments are occasionally large enough to be mistaken for normal cells. For diagnoses that depend on the presence or absence of the target sequence such as sexing by amplification of Y-specific repeat sequences, this could result in misdiagnosis (Fig. 6.1. lanes 8,9).

To safeguard against these problems, a number of precautions may be necessary. First, selection of normally fertilized embryos cleaving evenly and at the normal rate for biopsy should minimize the likelihood of selecting

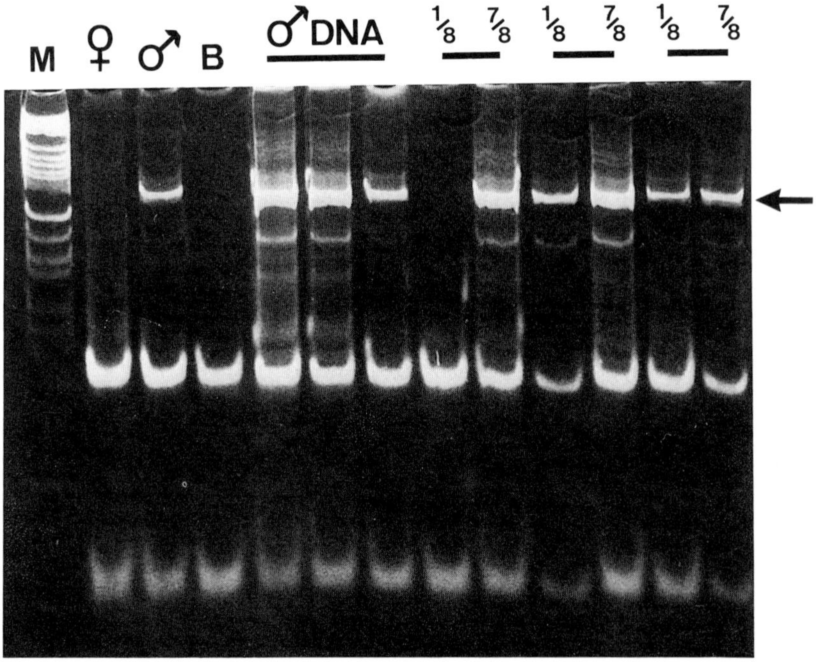

Fig. 6.1. Analysis of polymerase chain reaction products with oligonucleotide primers for a 149 bp fragment (arrowhead) of a 3.4 kb Y-specific repeat sequence by electrophoresis on a 12% polyacrylamide minigel and staining with ethidium bromide. Lane 1 (from left to right): DNA size markers; lanes 2,3: single cell biopsies; lane 4: control blank; lanes 5–7: dilutions of male genomic DNA–20 ng, 200 pg and 2 pg; lines 8–13: paired single cells and biopsied 8-cell male embryos.

Amplification is easily detected from as little as 2 pg of male genomic DNA (lane 7). Of the two single cell biopsies from a 6- and an 8-cell embryo from a couple at risk of transmitting X-linked adrenoleukodystrophy, the Y-specific fragment was absent in the first (lane 3) but present in the second and they were identified as male and female, respectively. Among three male embryos used to test the consistency of amplification from single cell biopsies, in two cases (lanes 10,11 and 12,13) amplification of the Y-specific fragment in the biopsied embryos themselves was also detected in the single cell. This would result in a false negative diagnosis. This embryo was partially fragmented and the biopsied cell may have been an anucleate cytoplasmic fragment. Amplification failure is unlikely in this case because of the presence of the shorter prominent "primer-dimer" fragment.

unrepresentative cells. Fragmentation, mosaicism and other abnormalities are most prevalent in abnormally fertilized or arrested embryos. Second, multinucleate or anucleate cells can be identified by examining the cells for nuclei using interference contrast or fluorescence microscopy with polynucleotide-specific fluorochromes. Preliminary work indicates that fluorochrome binding to nuclear DNA and brief exposure of cells to UV illumination do not interfere with PCR (Kontogianni and Handyside, unpublished observations). Fluorochrome labelling may also allow detection of any contaminating nuclei from cumulus cells or sperm which could occur when a hole is made in the zona pellucida by drilling with acid Tyrodes. Finally, biopsying two or more cells, if possible, would allow duplicate amplification which should increase the reliability of any diagnosis.

The remaining problems are those associated with PCR itself. Amplification of non-specific fragments or conversely sporadic amplification failure can occur with any set of primers under suboptimal conditions and the extent of the problem will vary for each set. Initially, it is essential to confirm amplification of the appropriate target with each set of primers, either using restriction sites to generate fragments of known size or hydridization with specific oligonucleotides. Co-amplification with a second set of primers has been suggested as a control for amplification failure (Ballabio et al. 1990). But this may be counterproductive as the conditions necessary for multiple PCR are a compromise and are unlikely to be optimal for the specific primers (Chamberlain et al. 1989). If hyperviable sites could be amplified (Jeffreys et al. 1988), a second set of control primers could be used to control for complete amplification failure and even contamination from unrelated individuals. With some primers, including those used for amplification of the Y-specific repeat (Fig. 6.1), the presence of a "primer-dimer" fragment resulting from self-priming and extension of the primers themselves provides a useful confirmation that amplification has been successful even in the absence of amplification of the specific target DNA.

Contamination of samples or reagents with spurious human DNA is relatively easy to eliminate by use of standard sterile techniques including autoclaving sample tubes, buffers and equipment. Carry-over contamination of the amplified fragment, however, is a more serious problem and can occur even when strict precautions are taken to separate preparative and product handling procedures (Kwok and Higuchi 1989). Digestion of oligonucleotides and carrier DNA with a restriction enzyme recognizing a site within the amplified fragment reduced contaminating target DNA and minimized background amplification (Handyside et al. 1989). Another approach which has been successful is to expose the PCR reagents including the DNA polymerase to UV light before adding them to the sample DNA (Sarkar and Sommer 1990). The longer double-stranded contaminating DNA is apparently more susceptible to UV damage and is degraded by the treatment leaving the short single-stranded oligonucleotide primers intact and without seriously affecting the DNA polymerase activity. However, if oligonucleotides are carefully prepared under sterile conditions, decontamination may not always be necessary (Fig. 6.1 lane 4).

To explore the possibilities of DNA amplification for preimplantation diagnosis, PCR has been used to amplify a variety of target sequences in unfertilized oocytes and cell biopsies from cleavage stage preimplantation embryos. Initially, a repeated sequence was amplified on the basis that this would increase the sensitivity of PCR for use with single cells. More recently, unique sequences have been successfully amplified from single cells by reamplifying the original product.

Chromosome-Specific Repeat-Sequences

Several families of tandemly repeated DNA sequences specific for individual human chromosomes have been identified raising the possibility that DNA amplification could be used for the detection of specific chromosomes. However, PCR is difficult to quantitate and amplification of chromosome-specific sequences is unlikely to be useful for the detection of abnormalities of chromosome number, including aneuploidy and translocations, unless the target sequence is also polymorphic. Recently, a variable number tandem repeat (VNTR) specific for chromosome 17 was amplified using oligonucleotides specific for the flanking sequences and shown to be highly polymorphic (Horn et al. 1989). If both parents were heterozygous for four different alleles, this would allow monosomy or trisomy 17 to be detected in their embryos by analysis of the size of the amplified fragments. The drawback, in this particular case, is that chromosomes 1 and 17 are the only trisomies not detected in spontaneous abortuses and are, therefore, probably eliminated at an early stage and less important for preimplantation diagnosis. With chromosomal abnormalities in general, it seems doubtful that DNA amplification will ever be able to match the range of genetic defects detectable by karyotype analysis of metaphase nuclei either using banding or in situ hybridization techniques.

With many X-linked diseases (now known to exceed 150) typically only affecting hemizygous males, the molecular basis of the disease is unknown and fetal sexing is the best available alternative to a specific diagnosis. Kogan et al. (1989) amplified a 149 bp fragment of a 3.4 kb sequence repeated about 800 to 5000 times on the Y chromosome which enables rapid sexing of fetal DNA from chorion villus samples. Using these primers, we consistently amplify enough target fragment for detection on ethidium bromide stained gels from as little as 1–2 pg of male genomic DNA (Fig. 6.1 lanes 5–7).

This sensitivity allows accurate sexing of human embryos from single cells biopsied at the 8-cell stage (Handyside et al. 1989). In 15 normally fertilized embryos (4 male and 11 female), the diagnosis was confirmed independently by in situ hybridization with a biotinylated Y-specific probe and fluorescent labelling of chromosomes with bis-acridine spermidine. In two out of four polypronuclear embryos, the Y repeat was detected by DNA amplification but in situ hybridization failed to detect the presence of a Y chromosome in the remaining nuclei. However, the majority of these abnormal embryos are dispermic and are often genetically mosaic with both triploid and diploid cells. With the exception of some rare X-linked diseases, such as Rett syndrome, only hemizygous males are affected and female embryos would be selected for transfer. Thus, the false positive amplification of the Y-specific fragment in these cases is less serious and would only have reduced the number of female embryos available for transfer. With three parthenogenetic embryos, in which cleavage had been initiated without fertilization, there was no amplification of the Y-specific fragment and the other methods confirmed the absence of a Y chromosome.

The Y-specific repeat is located in the heterochromatic region of the long arm of the Y chromosome (Cooke 1976). In some normally fertile males, this region is absent (Bobrow et al. 1971) and conversely, in rare cases can be translocated to autosomes and carried by normal females (Cooke and Noel 1979). As an alternative, the alphoid family of repetitive DNA present in the pericentromeric region of all human chromosomes exhibits significant chromosome specificity (Willard and Waye 1987). Amplification of Y- and X-specific alphoid repeats has recently been reported from small amounts of male and female dried blood (Witt and Erickson 1989). If the sensitivity of amplification of these repeats matches the Y repeat on the long arm and conditions can be found for co-amplification from both chromosomes, this would have the additional advantage of reducing misdiagnosis by controlling for amplification failures. The presence of the putative testis determining gene, the zinc finger Y (ZFY) gene, has been used for sexing by DNA amplification (Ebensperger et al. 1989). However, the ZFY gene can be translocated and a unique sequence is unlikely to be as sensitive as the chromosome-specific repeats.

Unique Sequences

DNA amplification of unique sequences in single cells was first achieved in single sperm and diploid fibroblasts (Li et al. 1988). However, amplification of a fragment of the ß-globin gene informative for sickle cell disease was only successful in 84% of single fibroblasts. Co-amplification of fragments from the low density lipoprotein receptor gene and HLA DQ alpha locus was only successful in a proportion of single spermatozoa providing unequivocal evidence that this was not caused by complete amplification failure or the accidental omission of cells from these samples. The incidence of these failures may be as high as 25% (Boehnke et al. 1989). If both alleles in single diploid embryonic cells are not consistently amplified, this would present a serious problem for reliable diagnosis. However, sperm nuclei have to be treated with alkali to achieve amplification at all. The DNA of nuclei from embryo cells may be more accessible after cell lysis and amplify more efficiently.

Amplification of two unique sequences, a small exon of the dystrophin gene which is frequently deleted in Duchenne muscular dystrophy and a sequence in strong linkage disequilibrium with cystic fibrosis (CS.7), has been demonstrated from single unfertilized human oocytes (Coutelle et al. 1989). Unfertilized oocytes are arrested in metaphase II of meiosis and retain a diploid set of chromosomes. Since care was taken to remove the first polar body, these unfertilized oocytes are equivalent in gene dosage to normal diploid cells. The amount of amplified fragment detected after the initial amplification was very low. However, with reamplification the DNA was easily detectable and allele-specific restriction sites could be analysed by digestion with appropriate enzymes. Of two oocytes from a woman heterozygous for two alleles at the CS.7 locus, one was also heterozygous but the other was homozygous for one allele. This may have resulted from crossing over during meiosis since the oocytes were in metaphase II. Equally, however, the same phenomenon of non-amplification of one allele, as observed with single sperm for different target fragments, may have occurred. Further studies will be necessary to assess the extent of fidelity of amplification in single embryo cells.

Recently, Holding and Monk (1989) have used a mouse model of ß-thalassaemia with a complete deletion of the ß-major haemoglobin gene for preimplantation diagnosis from single mouse embryo cells. After the first 10 cycles, they reamplified the initial fragment with non-overlapping nested primers to give a shorter fragment. With precautions for carry-over contamination, the incidence of false positives were eliminated. However, as with sperm and fibroblasts, 20% of single cell biopsies from embryos homozygous for the normal gene failed to amplify. This approach increases sensitivity (Mullis and Faloona 1987) and has the additional advantages that non-specific amplification is eliminated and cross-over contamination is reduced because the first set of primers cannot hybridize to the second DNA fragment. Reampliication with nested primers would also provide an opportunity to use allele-specific oligonucleotide primers or competitive binding of primers annealing to the wild-type or mutant sequences (Ballabio et al. 1990) which may simplify and speed up diagnosis after amplification.

Prospects for Preimplantation Diagnosis by DNA Amplification

DNA amplification is being used increasingly for prenatal diagnosis to a large extent because of the speed with which diagnoses can be performed, and as modifications of PCR are developed for the direct analysis of the presence of defects, such as competitive binding of fluorescently labelled primers, this trend is likely to continue. Many of these approaches may be adaptable for use with biopsies from early human embryos. The major constraints for preimplantation diagnosis, however, are those inherent in PCR itself when attempting to amplify from small numbers or single cells and the limits to which the preimplantation human embryo can be manipulated.

Amplification of repeated sequences is very sensitive and for this reason offers the best prospect for diagnosis while the number of biopsied cells is limited. We have recently started a clinical trial to biopsy and sex embryos by amplification of the Y-specific repeat for couples known to be at risk of X-linked disease and, in addition, with one or more previous terminations of affected pregnancies following conventional prenatal diagnosis. One woman, carrying a defect causing the severe neurological disease, adrenoleukodystrophy, had two normally fertilized embryos which reached the 6- and 8-cell stages and were biopsied early on day 3. DNA amplification from the single cells indicated one embryo of each sex (Fig. 6.1 lanes 2,3) and the female embryo was transferred later the same day. The biopsied male embryo, maintained in culture for a further four days, developed normally to the blastocyst stage and hatched out of the drilled zona in preparation for implantation. Most importantly, amplification from this biopsied embryo confirmed the male diagnosis.

Amplification of unique sequences is feasible from single oocytes and embryo cells with reamplification (Coutelle et al. 1989; Holding and Monk 1989). But a major problem remains the possibility of failure to amplify from both alleles at a single locus in diploid cells which is essential for accurate and reliable diagnosis and distinguishing carriers of genetic defects. Amplification from two cells biopsied from each embryo, either separately or together, may help to overcome this problem and this will have to be carefully evaluated before any attempt at diagnosis and transfer of cleavage stage embryos. Otherwise diagnosis by DNA amplification of unique sequences may have to wait for improvements in the success of other strategies which allow larger numbers of cells to be recovered from the preimplantation human embryo.

Acknowledgements. Approval for this work was granted by the local ethical committee of the Royal Postgraduate Medical School and the Interim Licensing Authority of the Medical Research Council and the Royal College of Obstetrics and Gynaecology. I would like to thank Professor Robert Winston for his enthusiastic support and Karin Dawson and the IVF team of the Wolfson Family Clinic, Hammersmith Hospital. This work is supported by the Muscular Dystrophy Group of Great Britain and Northern Ireland.

References

Ballabio A, Gibbs RA, Caskey CT (1990) PCR test for cystic fibrosis deletion. Nature 343: 220

Bobrow M, Pearson PL, Pike MC, El-Alfi, OS (1971) Length variation in the quinacrine-binding segment of human Y chromosomes of different sizes. Cytogenetics 10: 190–198

Boehnke M, Arnheim N, Li H, Collins FS (1989) Fine structure genetic mapping of human chromosomes using the polymerase chain reaction on single sperm: experimental design considerations. Am J Hum Genet 45: 21–32

Buster JE, Busillo M, Rodi IA, et al. (1985) Biologic and morphologic development of donated human ova recoved by non-surgical uterine lavage. Am J Obstet Gynaecol 153: 211–217

Chamberlain J, Gibbs RA, Ranier JE, Nyguyen PN, Caskey CT (1988) Deletion screening of the Duchenne muscular dystrophy locus via multiplex DNA amplification. Nucleic Acids Res 16: 141–156

Cooke HJ (1976) Repeated sequences specific to human males. Nature 262: 182–186

Cooke HJ, Noel B (1979) Confirmation of Y/autosome translocation using recombinant DNA. Hum Genet 67: 222–224

Cooper DN, Schmidtke J (1987) Diagnosis of genetic disease by recombinant DNA. Hum Genet 77: 66–75

Coutelle C, Williams C, Handyside AH, Hardy K, Winston RML, Williamson R (1989) Genetic analysis of DNA from single oocytes – a model for preimplantation diagnosis of cystic fibrosis. Br Med J 299: 22–24

Dawson KJ, Rutherford AJ, Winston NJ, Subak-Sharpe R, Winston RML (1988) Human blastocyst transfer, is it a feasible proposition? Hum Reprod suppl 145: 44–45

Ebensperger C, Studer R, Epplen JT (1989) Specific amplification of the ZFY gene to screen sex in man. Hum Genet 82: 289–290

Gyllensten UB, Erlich HA (1988) Generation of single stranded DNA by the polymerase chain reaction and its application to direct sequencing of the HLA-DQ alpha locus. Proc Natl Acad Sci USA 85: 7652-7656

Handyside AH, Pattinson JK, Penketh RJA, Delhanty JD, Winston RML, Tuddenham EDG (1989) Biopsy of human preimplantation embryos and sexing by DNA amplification. Lancet i: 347–349

Hardy K, Handyside AH, Winston RML (1989) The human blastocyst: cell number, death and allocation during late preimplantation development in vitro. Development 107: 597–604

Hardy K, Martin KL, Leese HJ, Winston RML, Handyside AH (1990) Human preimplantation development in vitro is not adversely affected by biopsy at the 8-cell stage. Hum Reprod (in press)

Holding C, Monk M (1989) Diagnosis of ß-thalasaemia by DNA amplification in single blastomeres from mouse preimplantation embryos. Lancet i: 532–535

Horn GI, Richards B, Klinger KW (1989) Amplification of a highly polymorphic VNTR segment by the polymerase chain reaction. Nucleic Acids Res 17: 2140

Innis MA, Myambo KB, Gelfand DH, Brow MAO (1988) DNA sequencing with Thermus aquaticus DNA polymerase and direct sequencing of polymerase chain reaction-amplified DNA. Proc Natl Acad Sci USA 85: 9436–9440

Jeffreys AJ, Wilson V, Neumann R, Keyte J (1988) Amplification of human minisatellites by the polymerase chain reaction: towards DNA fingerprinting of single cells. Nucleic Acids Res 16: 10953–10971

Kogan SC, Doherty M, Gitschier J (1987) An improved method for prenatal diagnosis of genetic disease by analysis of amplified DNA sequences. N Engl J Med 317: 985–990

Kwok S, Higuchi R (1989) Avoiding false positives with PCR. Nature 339: 237–238

Li A, Gyllensten UB, Cui X, Saiki RK, Erlich HA Arnheim N (1988) Amplification and analysis of DNA sequences in single human sperm and diploid cells. Nature 335: 414–419

Mullis KB, Faloona FA (1987) Specific synthesis of DNA in vitro via a polymerase-catalysed chain reaction. Methods Enzymol 155: 335–350

Old JM (1986) Fetal DNA analysis. In: Davies KE (ed) Human genetic diseases: a practical approach. IRL Press, Oxford, pp 1–17

Papadopoulos G, Templeton AA, Fisk N, Randall J (1989) The frequency of chromosome anomalies in human preimplantation embryos after in vitro fertilization. Hum Reprod 4: 91–98

Penketh R, McLaren A (1987) Prospects for prenatal diagnosis during preimplantation human development. In: Rodeck C (ed) Fetal diagnosis of genetic defects. Clinical obstetrics and gynaecology vol 1. Baillière Tindall, London, pp 747–764

Riordan J, Rommen JM, Kerem B-S, et al. (1989) Identification of the cystic fibrosis gene: cloning and characterisation of complementary DNA. Science 245: 1066–1073

Rodeck CH (1984) Obstetric techniques in prenatal diagnosis. In: Rodeck CH, Nicolaides KH (eds) Prenatal diagnosis. Proc 11th study group fo the Royal College of Obstetricians and Gynaecologists. RCOG, London, pp 15–28

Saiki RK, Scharf S, Faloona F, et al. (1985) Enzymatic amplification of ß-globin genomic sequences and restriction site analysis for diagnosis of sickle-cell anaemia. Science 230: 1350–1354

Saiki RK, Bugawan TL, Horn GT, Mullis KB, Erlich HA (1986) Analysis of enzymatically amplified ß-globin and HLA-DQ alpha DNA with allele-specific oligonucleotide probes. Nature 324: 163–166

Sarkar G, Sommer SS (1990) Shedding light on PCR contamination. Nature 343: 27 (scientific correspondence)

Testart J, Belaisch-Allart J, Lasalle B, et al. (1987) Factors influencing the success rate of human embryo freezing in an in vitro fertilization and embryo transfer program. Fertil Steril 48: 107–112

White TJ, Arnheim N, Erlich HA (1989) The polymerase chain reaction. Trends Genet 5: 185–189

Willard HF and Waye JS (1987) Hierarchical order in chromosome-specific human alpha satellite DNA. Trends Genet 3: 192–198

Williams C, Williamson R, Coutelle C, Loeffler F, Smith J, Ivinson A (1988) Same day, first trimester antenatal diagnosis for cystic fibrosis by gene amplification. Lancet ii: 102–103

Winichagoon P, Kownkon J, Yenchitsomanus P, Thonglairoam V, Siritanaratkul N, Fucharoen S (1989) Detection of ß-thalasaemia and haemoglobin E genes in Thai by a DNA amplification technique. Hum Genet 82: 389–390

Witt M, Erickson RP (1989) A rapid method for the detection of Y chromosomal DNA from dried blood specimens by the polymerase chain reaction. Hum Genet 82: 271–274

7. Transabdominal Chorion Villus Biopsy Versus Amniocentesis for Diagnosis of Aneuploidy: Safety Is Not Enough

R.J. Lilford, H. Irving, J.K. Gupta, P. O'Donovan and G. Linton

Introduction

Chorion villus sampling (CVS) is well established as the optimal diagnostic method for diagnosis of single gene defects. However, the majority of invasive diagnostic procedures are not performed for these conditions of high genetic risk but are carried out for diagnosis of aneuploidy. In this paper we attempt to answer the question: will chorion villus biopsy replace amniocentesis as the most widely used test for the prenatal diagnosis of Down's syndrome?

The answer to this question depends on two separate issues:

1. Whether the majority of women would select CVS.
2. Whether the majority of obstetricians will have the facilities to offer this test.

The first issue depends on both the relative safety (and accuracy) of CVS versus amniocentesis and also on how women view any trade-off between the convenience of CVS on the one hand and the safety (and accuracy) of amniocentesis on the other. To help answer these questions we present the result of 520 consecutive cases of transabdominal chorion villus biopsy, in terms of sampling success, diagnostic accuracy and pregnancy outcome, and discuss the reactions of women to these results.

The second issue, whether obstetricians will have the necessary facilities, will depend on the resources required for each procedure (relative cost-effectiveness) and to help answer this question we compare the time required to obtain and analyse chorion and amniotic fluid samples.

Patients and Methods

Method of Chorion Biopsy

The results of the first 520 consecutive transabdominal chorion villus biopsies with a minimum of 6 weeks follow-up at St James' University Hospital, Leeds, are reported. All but one of these patients have had either a termination of pregnancy or a follow-up scan 6 to 8 weeks after the procedure. The single remaining patient emigrated to Asia after a normal result and has been lost to follow-up. The technique of transabdominal chorion villus biopsy has been described in detail (Lilford and Maxwell 1984; Maxwell et al. 1986; Lilford et al. 1987). The safety of the procedure was assessed by measurement of the fetal loss rate among patients who did not go on to require termination of pregnancy. The accuracy of chorionic sampling is also assessed, with particular reference to chromosome analysis. The indications for this technique are given together with the gestational ages at which the procedures were performed.

Resource Implications

A detailed analysis was made of the clinic and laboratory time required to analyse 16 consecutive chorion biopsies and 17 amniocenteses. All the CVS were carried out at St. James' University Hospital, while the amniocenteses consisted of 11 at a district hospital (the Bradford Royal Infirmary) and 6 at the Leeds General Infirmary – also a teaching hospital. Pretest counselling was excluded since this should apply equally to both groups of patients, especially if chorion biopsy was to come into routine use. However the total time involved for the procedure was measured with a stopwatch for each patient and for each member of staff involved. Some patients underwent ultrasound scanning with a view to prenatal testing, but this was deferred for a week. In these cases, all time spent in the scan department, for the purpose of prenatal testing, was included. Two such patients were encountered in the amniocentesis group and one among patients having CVS. There were no failed procedures among these patients.

The costs of staff time were obtained from the hospital finance department in order to calculate the additional costs of CVS over amniocentesis. Staff involved in chorion biopsy were senior and therefore more expensive than those carrying out amniocentesis. For reasons that we shall discuss later, we believe that this is inherent in the nature of these techniques but we have also carried out a sensitivity analysis in which we assume that the same grade of staff were involved for each procedure. We therefore calculate the costs incurred by the staff who were actually involved and then repeat the exercise on the assumption that all clinical staff were of the same grade. Laboratory costs are also compared by quantifying the cost of laboratory staff time and reagents. Again we quantify this on the basis of seniority of staff who actually carried out the laboratory work, but then perform sensitivity analysis by recalculating this figure on the basis of staff of the same status.

Results

Safety and Accuracy of Chorion Villus Biopsy

The first 520 consecutive biopsies at St. James's Hospital have been analysed with respect to indications and short-term outcome, while the first 300 have been analysed in respect to gestational age at sampling and accuracy. Two hundred and seventy-seven of these were indicated on the basis of maternal age, 81 because of a previous aneuploidy and 11 for parental translocation. Twenty-three were done for fetal sexing, 3 for failed amniocentesis and 3 following biochemical screening for Down's. Enzyme analysis was the indication in 16 cases and in 87 cases the sample was submitted to gene probe diagnosis:

Cystic fibrosis	(26)
Muscular dystrophy	(26)
Thalassaemia/haemophilia	(21)
Other	(14)

Nineteen procedures were carried out because of anatomical findings on ultrasound examination known to be associated with aneuploidy.

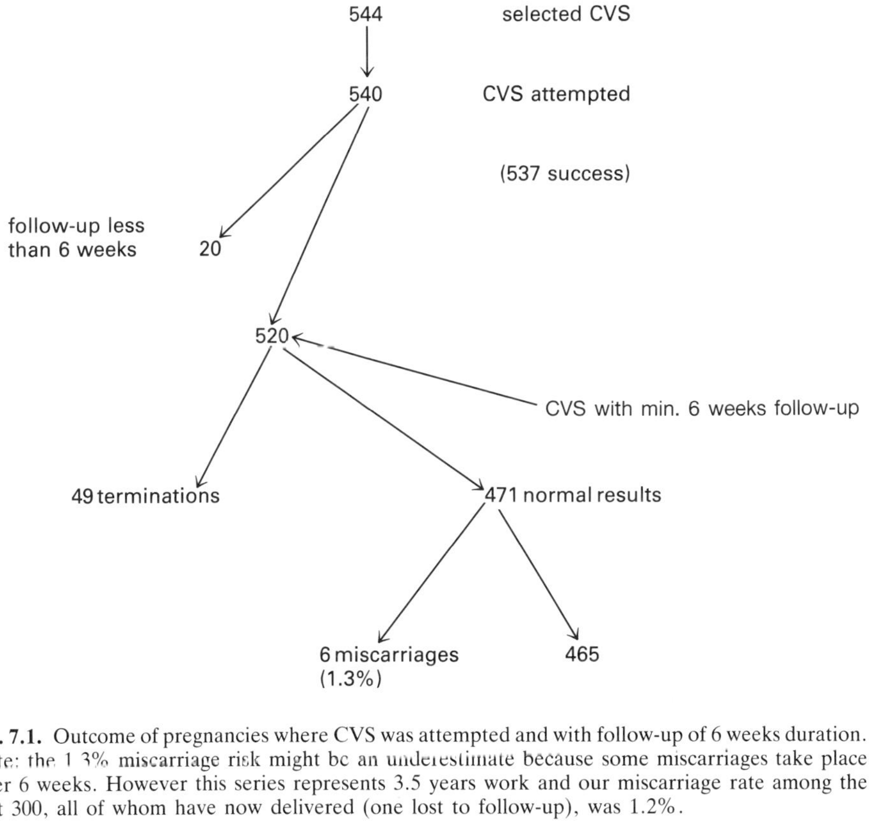

Fig. 7.1. Outcome of pregnancies where CVS was attempted and with follow-up of 6 weeks duration. Note: the 1.3% miscarriage risk might be an underestimate because some miscarriages take place after 6 weeks. However this series represents 3.5 years work and our miscarriage rate among the first 300, all of whom have now delivered (one lost to follow-up), was 1.2%.

The histogram of gestational ages of the first 300 patients in this series is shown in Fig. 7.1. The median gestational age for the series up to 300 was 11.9 weeks. Sixty-one procedures among the first 300 were carried out beyond 14 weeks gestational age. The mean gestational ages of the remaining 239 cases was 10.7 weeks.

Sampling was unsuccessful at the first attempt in 13 of the 520 cases. Repeat chorion biopsy was carried out in all but 3 of these and was successful in 2.

Termination of pregnancy was required in 49 cases (9.7%). One of these suffered intrauterine death prior to evacuation of the uterus. Seven of the remaining 471 cases with follow-up had undergone previous transcervical chorion villus biopsy at another hospital and one of these had already suffered ruptured membranes prior to the transabdominal procedure. This patient also miscarried. Four hundred and sixty-four patients with a normal result had not undergone previous transcervical sampling. Of these, 6 have miscarried prior to 28 weeks. Two of these miscarriages took place 7–9 weeks after the original procedure, and only 3 within 4 weeks. All but one of our cases have undergone follow-up ultrasound scan 6 to 8 weeks after the original procedure. There have been 2 fetal losses beyond 28 weeks, one from intrauterine growth retardation and one from a massive intrapartum abruption. The miscarriage rate (i.e. fetal loss prior to 28 weeks) was therefore 1.3% (95% confidence limits 0–2.1%) among 464 patients who did not have termination of pregnancy and who had not undergone previous transcervical sampling and with follow-up for at least 6 weeks. This rate of fetal loss between sampling and 28 weeks is not statistically different to the background rate of 1% to 2% (Wilson et al. 1984). One hundred and ninety-four patients have delivered. Six babies were premature (less than 34 weeks) and 3 of these have died. In each case the CVS was carried out late in the second trimester for fetal anomaly/growth retardation. For example, in one of these cases severe oligohydramnios preceded chorion villus biopsy, which was carried out because amniocentesis was impossible.

The samples which we obtained were suitable for diagnosis in all but one case where the patient was a carrier of a balanced translocation and where chorion culture failed and subsequent amniocentesis was necessary. Diagnostic answers were obtained in all other cases, although one sample was deemed insufficient for direct gene probe analysis and culture was necessary.

Placental mosaicism, either between culture and direct preparation, or between different cells obtained by direct analysis was found in 6 cases among the first 300 samples. Subsequent amniocentesis or fetal blood sampling was carried out in 4 of these. Details of these mosaics are given in Table 7.1.

One patient had a cytological false-positive diagnosis, in that a large euchromic marker chromosome on CVS was not confirmed in the fetus. This was not a clinical false-positive because the fetus had multiple abnormalities following termination of pregnancy. Two cases of Down's syndrome, one of 47XXY and one of 47XXX, were detected and confirmed after termination of pregnancy, which was requestd in each case. Two of these aneuploidies were found among patients requesting CVS for advanced age and the remainder following detection of structural abnormality. There were also two cases of unbalanced translocation in the fetuses of carrier patients.

One case which could be regarded a complete false-negative on direct and culture preparation has been encountered. This patient had CVS because of an ultrasound diagnosis of cystic hygroma and a normal 46XY karyotype was

Table 7.1. Mosaics among the first 300 consecutive CVS

No.	Indications for CVS	Direct karyotype	Culture karyotype	Fetal blood or Amnio	Outcome	Gest. age (weeks)
1	Failed amniocentesis/ maternal age	50XX+2C +2D/46XX	46XX	–	46XX term	18
2	Severe oligohydramnios/ growth retardation/ maternal age	46XY marker[a]	46XY marker[a]	–	Multiple abnor-malities of fetus, but 46XY	20
3	Maternal age	46XY 46XY/ 47XXY	46XY/ 47XXY	Klinefelter's mosaic term fetus	11	
4	Maternal age	46XY	46XX/ 46XX6q–[b]	46XY	46XY term	11
5	Maternal age	45XO	46XX	46XX 6XX term	11	
6	Haemophilia	92XXYY	46XY/ 92XXYY	46XY	46XY term	12

[a] Containing "euchromatin".
[b] Confirmed maternal cells by polymorphism banding. Culture instability due to fetal cells presumed to lead to loss of long arm of chromosome 6.

reported. The 4 kg baby had lax skin, Hirschprung's disease and hip dislocation and conventional chromosome analysis was normal, but culture in methotrexate (which extends the length of chromosomes), showed a small additional fragment on the long arm of chromosome 11. With hindsight this could then be seen on the other karyotype spreads. We believe that this small but important additional fragment would have been missed on amniocentesis, but technically this can be regarded as a false-negative result.

Staff time

Clinical Time

The time for all staff involved is shown in Table 7.2. The average operator time for CVS was 25 minutes compared with 6 minutes and 40 seconds for amniocentesis. For CVS the operator must be involved in preliminary scanning in order to choose the best angle of approach, whereas it is acceptable for the radiographer to select the biopsy site before the less exacting procedure of midtrimester amniocentesis. In addition, it is often necessary to ask the patient to empty or fill her bladder in order to optimize the uterine position prior to CVS. The total time involved in CVS was 97 staff minutes per procedure compared to 52.5 minutes for amniocentesis. The cytogeneticist attends for CVS and, as this is not really necessary, it could be excluded to give a total of 73 minutes staff time for CVS. Again the higher cost of CVS is related to the need for greater operator involvement rather than the total length of the procedure (25 minutes for CVS verus 25.5 minutes for amniocentesis).

If the cost of each unit of staff time is included, then the mean clinical cost

Table 7.2. Total staff-time and costs involved for the clinical procedures of CVS and amniocentesis

	Level of staff[a]	No of cases	Average time per case (min)	Cost of time (per h)	Total (£)	Grand total (£)
CVS	Consultant obstetrician	16	25.00	15.00	100.00	
(16)	Superintendent radiographer	12[b]	22.50	8.50	38.40	
	Consultant ultrasound	8[b]	28.50	15.00	57.20	
	Auxiliary nurse	15	23.16	2.50	14.50	
	Cytogeneticist	16	24.00	6.10	39.00	249
Amnio	Senior registrar	5	6.33	8.25	4.35	
(17)	Registrar	6	9.33	7.13	6.60	
	Clinical assistant	6	4.33	9.60	4.14	
	Superintendent radiographer	17	18.50	8.50	44.20	
	Staff nurse	17	26.16	4.30	32.30	92

[a] Based on 40-hour week, excluding overtime payments, on midpoint of scale without superannuation and NHS contributions.
[b] Staff doubled-up occasionally, once because the auxiliary nurse had left.

of each CVS is £15.60 compared to £5.39 for amniocentesis (Table 7.2). If the cytogeneticist's time at the sampling procedure is excluded, then the cost of CVS is reduced to £12.36. If, in addition, we assume that staff carrying out a particular function are the same grade, senior registrar for operator, superintendent radiographer grade for imaging and staff nurse to assist, then the comparative costs are £8.94 for CVS and £5.54 for amniocentesis.

Laboratory Time

When the processing of these chorion and amniotic fluid samples were timed in the cytogenetics laboratory, CVS was found to require almost twice as much time and to be more than twice as expensive in staff time and materials (£56 versus £26 per case; Table 7.3). More expensive culture medium (Chang) was used for culture of chorion villus biopsy and senior laboratory staff were involved. The most important difference was the analysis of chorion samples by both direct and long-term culture methods. Even if all cytogenetic staff are assumed to be the same (basic) grade, the cost of CVS per case is £44.20.

Analysis by the direct method alone would, in fact, be cheaper than amniocentesis and if detection of trisomies and major rearrangements and deletions were all that was required and if we were prepared to accept occasional false-negative diagnoses, then this method alone would suffice. However, the quality of direct metaphase-banding alone is not yet of a sufficiently high standard to give complete confidence in detecting small structural changes and one case of sex-chromosome aneuploidy would have been missed if we had relied on direct preparation alone. The use of long-term culture alone would make the test only slightly more expensive than amniocentesis, but the advantage of a rapid result would be lost and maternal cell contamination is a potential problem which occurred once in this series. It seems, therefore, that both direct preparation and culture are necessary.

Table 7.3. Laboratory times for processing of chorion and amniotic fluid samples in the cytogenetic laboratory (average staff-time in minutes)

CVS		
Booking in: initial preparation of tissue	5	
a) Direct preparation		
Harvesting and staining	45	
Analysis	120	170
b) Long-term culture		
Preparation and seeding of flasks	20	
4 changes of medium	20	
Harvesting, trypsinization and staining	65	
Analysis	120	225
		395[a]
Amniocentesis		
Booking in	5	
Setting up flasks	15	
Culture with changes of medium	20	
Harvesting, trypsinization and staining	65	
Analysis	120	
		225[b]

[a] This work was carried out by a senior cytogeneticist (paid £6.40 per hour or £42.20 per case). Hams F10 culture medium was used for two flasks (with four changes) and Chang medium for one flask (also with four changes). The cost of flasks and reagents was therefore £12.70 per case.

[b] A basic grade cytogeneticist carried out this work (£4.80 per hour or £18 per case). Hams F10 medium was used for four flasks with four changes costing £8.40 per case.

Additional Factors

We should stress that these results are useful for comparative purposes and show the staff time involved. Our calculations based on these underestimate the true total cost because they do not take into account factors common to both procedures, such as building, heating, electricity, hospital administration and short periods of rest for staff, nor laboratory administration, filing, sick-leave, answering the telephone and other factors which are more difficult to quantify. Only four terminations of pregnancy were carried out for aneuploidy among over 200 patients requesting prenatal diagnosis for maternal age and this is rather higher than one would expect from the age and risk profiles of all patients who undergo testing for advanced maternal age (some aneuploid fetuses abort at between 10 and 16 weeks gestational age). The approximate £150 additional cost of later termination of pregnancy when abnormalities are detected by amniocentesis would therefore have little impact on these comparative costs of CVS versus amniocentesis. Furthermore, some CVS patients (6 in our series) go on to amniocentesis anyway because of mosaicism (4 cases), failure to obtain a sample (1 case) or failed analysis of the sample. It is also impossible to quantify other wider economic factors, such as loss of earnings, because of the probably greater emotional impact of later termination of pregnancy. CVS is at an earlier stage of development than amniocentesis and costs will probably drop with time.

Discussion

The miscarriage rate of 1.3% for transabdominal chorion villus biopsy is similar to that for amniocentesis where total fetal loss rates vary from 0.5% to 3.5% (Simpson et al. 1975; The NICHD National Registry 1976; MRC Amniocentesis Working Party 1978; McMay and Whitfield 1984; Tabor et al. 1986). Furthermore the later mean gestational age at which amniocentesis is usually carried out may favour this technique in any direct comparison of miscarriage rates. However our 95% confidence limits extend to just over 2% and we must therefore accept that chorion villus biopsy *may* be up to twice as unsafe, in terms of miscarriage, as expertly performed amniocentesis. Although there were six cases of mosaicism, no complete false-negative or false-positive results have arisen in this study.

The world experience of chorion villus biopsy, reported to the Philadelphia register, is now 50 000. No untoward effects, apart from miscarriage, have yet been detected and rates of intrauterine growth retardation, prematurity and placental abruption do not appear to be increased. However, it is possible that, like the link between amniocentesis and pulmonary hypoplasia (Tabor et al. 1986), unexpected long-term consequences will be reported in the future. Complete false-negative or positive chromosome results i.e. false-positive or negative results on *both* direct preparation and culture have only been reported in two cases.

Two studies have examined the effect of probabilistic information on the choice between CVS and amniocentesis. Knott et al. (1986) found that half of all women would sacrifice up to a doubling in fetal loss rate in order to obtain the advantages of earlier diagnosis by CVS. We (Thornton et al. 1986) presented women with information similar to that contained in the MRC booklet for potential subjects in the CVS versus amniocentesis trial and then conducted a series of hypothetical "probability equivalent" multiple gambles (Pauker and Pauker 1977; Weinstein and Fineberg 1980). We confirmed that, among women who wish to have prenatal diagnosis, 50% would accept a doubling of the fetal loss rate (from 1% to 2%) in order to avail themselves of early diagnosis if their risk of Down's syndrome was one in 100. We performed 3 multiple gambles (amniocentesis versus nothing, CVS versus amniocentesis and CVS versus nothing) and we were, therefore, able to measure "coherence" – the ability of subjects to produce an answer on their third gamble, similar to that which would have been expected from their answers to the first two gambles (Keeney and Raiffa 1976; Llewellyn-Thomas 1982). The above findings were confirmed among a subset of "coherent" subjects i.e. those who understood the choices clearly.

The relative safety and accuracy of CVS therefore lie within the limits which most women would accept. These findings, taken by themselves, would suggest that chorion villus biopsy should largely replace amniocentesis. However, this presupposes that both tests are freely available, and that the only important consideration is consumer choice. This is not so; patients are denied many choices such as in vitro fertilization and cardiac transplantation because of resource limitations. The competing demands for medical resources are such that the increased resources required for chorion villus biopsy preclude widespread use of this technique as a screening test for Down's syndrome. The majority of Regional Health Authorities already have great difficulty servicing the existing number of requests for amniocentesis, let alone the more exacting requirements for chorion villus biopsy. The exact magnitude of the increased cost of chorion villus biopsy depends on whether more senior and therefore more expensive staff are required for the procedure and for the laboratory analysis. Although this factor may be slightly exaggerated in our study, both laboratory and clinical aspects of this test are more exacting than those required for amniocentesis. The most important factor, however, is the greater total amount of staff time involved. Our analysis of the costs of CVS versus amniocentesis does not constitute a complete health economics appraisal, as it does not take into account all the longer-term financial implications of each test. The relative costs of early versus late termination of pregnancy favours CVS while the cost of further investigations following ambiguous results favours amniocentesis. Nevertheless, these additional costs are rarely incurred in screening for Down's syndrome and the lower cost of amniocentesis is confirmed in both district and teaching hospitals.

Two other recent developments have a bearing on this discussion. The first of these is the possibility of first trimester amniocentesis. The miscarriage rate of this procedure has not yet been published and animal experiments show that pulmonary hypoplasia occurs to a greater degree when amniotic fluid is removed early in pregnancy (Heslop et al. 1984). This technique also requires a very precise ultrasound-directed biopsy method and therefore the clinical staff time is likely to be very similar to that required for transabdominal chorion biopsy. First trimester amniocentesis will also not overcome the problem of mosaicism because the amniotic fluid contains a very high proportion of trophoblast-derived cells in early pregnancy. The other important recent development is the refinement of risk prediction for Down's syndrome, by the use of biochemical markers (oestriol, chorionic gonadatrophin and alpha-fetoprotein) in maternal blood (see Chapter 17). Our existing knowledge of this subject is based on blood samples taken at 16 weeks gestational age. We anticipate that many women will wish to wait until 16 weeks gestational age and then determine their risk of Down's syndrome more accurately by biochemical screening. Unless the predictive accuracy of these biochemical markers may be confirmed in earlier pregnancy (see Chapter 12), the availability of these tests must be a further argument against widespread screening for Down's syndrome by means of chorionic sampling.

Our conclusions are that chorion biopsy is the test of choice for patients at high genetic risk. In most countries resource considerations, rather than the danger, inaccuracy or unacceptability of the test, will limit the use of this method for the majority of women wishing prenatal diagnosis for Down's syndrome.

Summary

Analysis of 520 consecutive transabdominal chorion biopsies followed up for a minimum of 6 weeks shows a miscarriage rate of 1.2%. Previous work by our group and others has shown that these results are well within the range that would be considered acceptable by most women wishing prenatal diagnosis of Down's syndrome. However, our measurements of clinical and laboratory staff time show that, even allowing for the reduced cost of early termination when required, CVS is likely to be a much more expensive test. This, together with the anticipated increased use of biochemical screening for Down's syndrome at 14–16 weeks gestational age, will limit the value of CVS for diagnosis of aneuploidy.

References

Heslop AF, Fairweather DVI, Blackwill RJ, Howard S (1984); The effect of amniocentesis and drainage of amniotic fluid on lung development in maca fascicularis during fetal and postnatal life. Br J Obstet Gynaec 91: 835–842

Keeney RL, Raiffa H (1976) Decisions with multiple objectives: preferences and value trade-offs, John Wiley and Sons, New York

Knott PD, Ward RHT, Lucas Mk (1986) Effect of chorionic villus sampling and early pregnancy counselling on uptake of prenatal diagnosis. Br Med J 293: 479·480

Lilford RJ, Maxwell D (1984) The development of a transcutaneous technique for chorion biopsy. Prenatal Diagnosis Group Newsletter: October, Queen Charlotte's Hospital, London

Lilford RJ, Irving HC, Linton G, Moran M (1987) Transabdominal chorion villus biopsy: 100 consecutive cases. Lancet i: 1415–1417

Llewellyn-Thomas H, Sutherland HJ, Tibshirani R, Ciampi A, Till JE, Boyd NF (1982) The measurement of patients' values in medicine. Med Decis Making 2(4): 449–462

Maxwell D, Lilford RJ, Czepulkowski BH, Heaton DE, Coleman DV (1986) Transabdominal chorionic villus sampling. Lancet i: 123–612

McMay MB, Whitfield CR (1984) Amniocentesis. Br J Hosp Med 31: 406–416

Medical Research Council Amniocentesis Working Party (1978) An assessment of the hazards of amniocentesis. Br J Obstet Gynaecol 85: Suppl 2

Pauker SP, Pauker SG (1977) Prenatal diagnosis: a directive approach to genetic counselling using decision analysis. Yale J Biol Med 50: 275–289

Simpson NE, Dallaire L, Miller JR, et al. (1976) Prenatal diagnosis of genetic disease in Canada – report of a collaborative study. Can Med Assoc J 115: 739–748

Tabor A, Madsen M, Obel EB, Philip J, Bang J, Nordgaard-Pedersen B (1986) Randomised controlled trial of genetic amniocentesis in 4606 low-risk women. Lancet i: 1287–1293

The NICHD National Registry for Amniocentesis Study Group (1976). Midtrimester amniocentesis for prenatal diagnosis. Safety and accuracy. JAMA 236: 1471–1476

Thornton J, Lilford R, Howel D (1986). The safety of amniocentesis. Lancet ii: 226

Weinstein MC, Fineberg HV, (eds) (1980) Clinical decision analysis. WB Saunders, Philadelphia

Wilson Rd, Kendrick W, Wittman BK, McGillvray BC (1984) Risk of spontaneous abortion in ultrasonically normal pregnancies. Lancet ii: 290

8. The Role of Echography in the Diagnosis of Fetal Chromosomal Defects

K.H. Nicolaides, R.J.M. Snijders and C.M. Gosden

Ultrasonography plays a central role in the diagnosis of fetal chromosomal abnormalities. It is used first, for accurate dating of pregnancy which is essential in the interpretation of maternal serum alpha-fetoprotein, human chorionic gonadotrophin and unconjugated oestriol; second, to enhance the safety and effectiveness of amniocentesis, placental biopsy or cordocentesis; and third, for examination of the external and internal anatomy of the fetus and the detection of major malformations, as well as more subtle ones which may be markers of chromosomal defects.

This chapter reviews the association between fetal malformations and chromosomal defects and reports the findings of cytogenetic analysis in 1262 fetuses with a wide range of malformations that were detected at ultrasound examination and were referred to our unit for further investigation during the past five years.

Brain Abnormalities

A transverse axial scan of the fetal head at the level of the cavum septum pellucidum will demonstrate the lateral borders of the anterior horns, the medial and lateral borders of the posterior horns of the lateral ventricles, the choroid plexuses, the third ventricle and the Sylvian fissures. The posterior fossa and cerebellum are visualized in the suboccipital bregmatic section.

Hydrocephalus

Congenital hydrocephalus has a birth incidence of 5–25 per 10 000 births. The majority of cases have no clear-cut aetiology and are probably due to a combination of genetic and environmental factors. Prenatal diagnosis is based

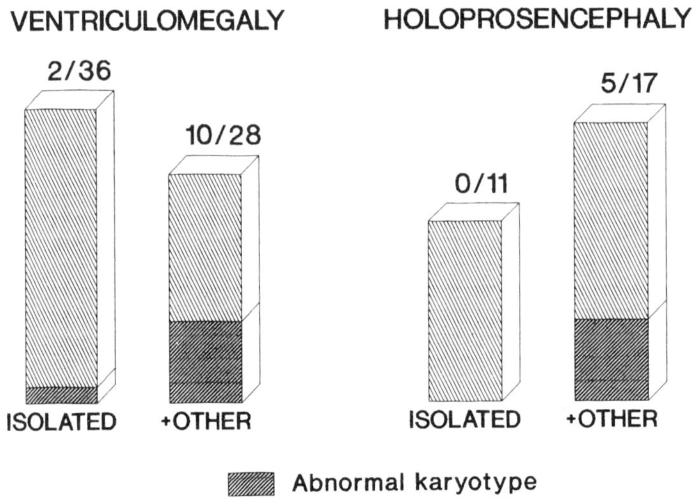

Fig. 8.1. Incidence of chromosomal defects in fetuses with hydrocephalus or holoprosencephaly in relation to the presence or absence of other additional malformations.

on the demonstration of an increase in the distance from the lateral wall of the anterior horn of the lateral cerebral ventricle to the midline compared to the width of the hemisphere (Campbell 1977). However, 5% of normal fetuses will have values above the 95th centile of the normal range, and serial measurements should demonstrate progressive ventricular dilatation before a definite diagnosis of hydrocephalus is made.

Chervenak et al. (1983) and Pilu et al. (1986) reported the presence of associated chromosomal defects in 11% and 30% of their respective series of fetuses with ventriculomegaly. In our series of 64 hydrocephalic fetuses (Fig. 8.1), there were 12 (19%) with chromosomal abnormalities including triploidy (n=4), trisomy 18 (n=2), trisomy 13 (n=1), trisomy 21 (n=1) and 48XYY+21 (n=1) 6p-(n=1), 47XY+gq(n=1). Chromosomal abnormalities were found in two of 36 (6%) with isolated hydrocephalus and in 10 of 28 (36%) fetuses with additional malformations.

Holoprosencephaly

This is a heterogenous group of cerebral malformations due to failure of cleavage of the forebrain. The majority of patients die in the neonatal period from complications associated with facial deformities including cyclops (blind ending proboscis, instead of a nose, above a single midline eye), ethmocephaly (proboscis above two closely situated orbits), cebocephaly (single nostril not communicating with the nosopharynx) and cleft lip. The small number of patients that survive suffer from mental retardation, epilepsy and spasticity. The risk of recurrence is approximately 6% although both autosomal dominant and autosomal recessive transmission has been described. Ultrasonographically, holoprosencephaly is recognized by a single, dilated midline ventricle, replacing the two lateral ventricles, as well as the associated facial defects.

In our series of 28 fetuses with holoprosencephaly (Fig. 8.1), 5 (18%) had associated chromosomal defects (trisomy 13, n=4; trisomy 18, n=1) and in all these cases there were additional malformations.

Choroid Plexus Cysts

Choroid plexus cysts are found in 2–20 per 1000 fetuses at 16–18 weeks' gestation but in more than 90% of cases they resolve by 25 weeks and are of no pathological significance (Chudleigh et al. 1984). However, if the cysts are associated with other malformations, they may indicate the presence of an underlying chromosomal abnormality (Nicolaides et al. 1986; Chitkara et al. 1988; Khouzam et al. 1989; Gabrielli et al. 1989; Thorpe-Beeston et al. 1990).

In our series of 33 fetuses with choroid plexus cysts and additional malformations Fig. 8.2), 19 (58%) had chromosomal defects including trisomy 18 (n=15), trisomy 13 (n=1), triploidy (n=1), and partial trisomy 21 (n=2). In 52 cases with isolated choroid plexus cysts including 39 where no antenatal karyotyping was performed, only one (2%) was chromosomally abnormal (trisomy 18). There are three additional reported cases in which choroid plexus cysts were the only antenatal finding where the fetuses had either trisomy 18 or trisomy 21 (Ricketts et al. 1987; Furness 1987, Ostlere et al. 1989).

Posterior Fossa Abnormalities

Cerebellar malformations are rare, but they may be associated with trisomy 15 and 18, hydrocephalus, spina bifida, encephalocoele or microcephaly. Cystic dilatation in the area of the cisterna magna, with partial or complete agenesis of the vermis, is found in the Dandy-Walker malformation (cystic dilatation of the fourth ventricle). The aetiology of the latter is unknown, although it may

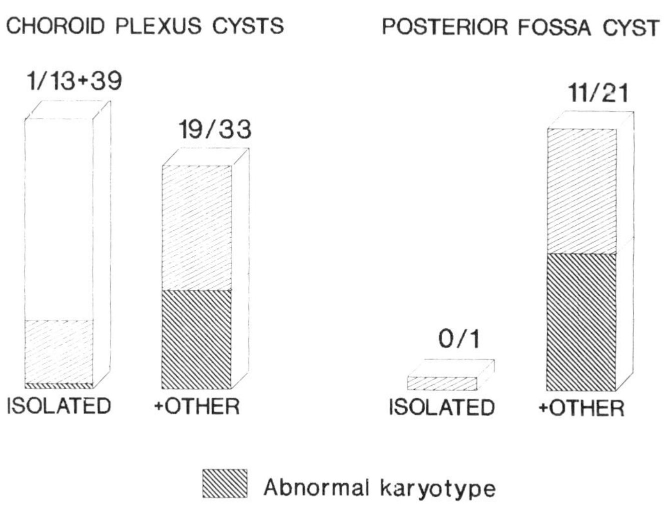

Fig. 8.2. Incidence of chromosomal defects in fetuses with choroid plexus cysts or posterior fossa cysts in relation to the presence or absence of other additional malformations.

occur as a part of Mendelian disorders such as Meckel's syndrome.

In our series of 22 fetuses with posterior fossa cysts and additional defects (Fig. 8.2), 11 (52%) had chromosomal abnormalities including trisomy 18 (n= 7), trisomy 13 (n=2), triploidy (n=1) and deletion 8q (n=1). In one fetus with an isolated cyst the karyotype was normal.

Skull, Face and Neck

Strawberry Skull

In 28 cases the fetal head was characteristically strawberry shaped. In all but one of the fetuses there were other malformations and in 24 (81%) there was an associated trisomy 18 (Fig. 8.3).

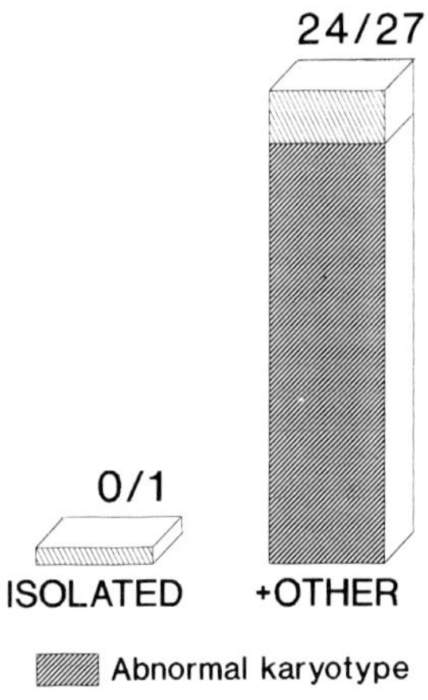

Fig. 8.3. Incidence of chromosomal defects in fetuses with strawberry-shaped head in relation to the presence or absence of other additional malformations.

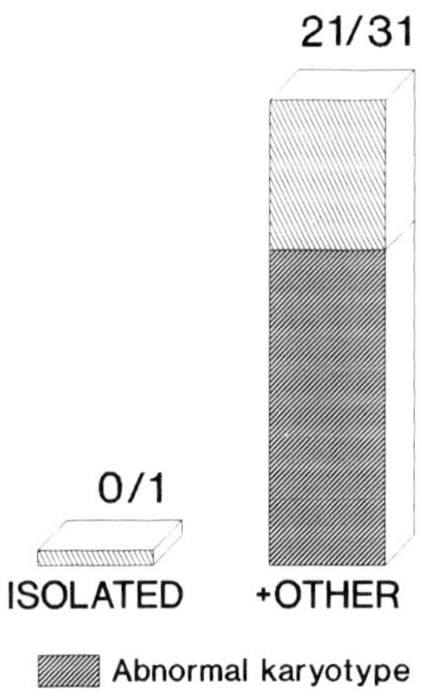

Fig. 8.4. Incidence of chromosomal defects in fetuses with facial cleft in relation to the presence or absence of other additional malformations.

Facial Cleft

Facial clefting, cleft lip and or palate, is one of the commonest congenital abnormalities found in approximately 1 : 700 livebirths. Both genetic and environmental factors are implicated in the causation of the defect. Chromosomal abnormalities are found in less than 1% of facial clefts (Pashayan 1983).

In our series of 32 fetuses with facial cleft (Fig. 8.3), 21 (66%) had chromosomal abnormalities (trisomy 18, n=10; trisomy 13, n=9; triploidy, n=1, partial trisomy 9, n=1).

Nuchal Oedema

Benacerraf et al. (1985a) noted the association between increased soft tissue thickening on the posterior aspect of the neck and trisomy 21. In a series of 1704 consecutive amniocenteses at 15–20 weeks' gestation in which there were 11 fetuses with trisomy 21, 45% of the trisomic and 0.06% of the normal fetuses had nuchal thickness >5mm (Benacerraf et al. 1985b).

In our series of 57 fetuses with nuchal oedema (Fig. 8.5), 28 (49%) had chromosomal abnormalities (trisomy 21, n=16; trisomy 13, n=3; trisomy 18, n=1, Turner's, n=3; 47XXY, n=1; deletions, n=2, triploidy, n=2).

Congenital Diaphragmatic Hernia

Congenital diaphragmatic hernia (CDH), with a birth incidence of 2–5 per 10 000, can be diagnosed by the ultrasonographic demonstration of stomach and intestines (90% of the cases) or liver (50%) in the thorax and the associated mediastinal shift to the opposite side. Polyhydramnios, ascites and other

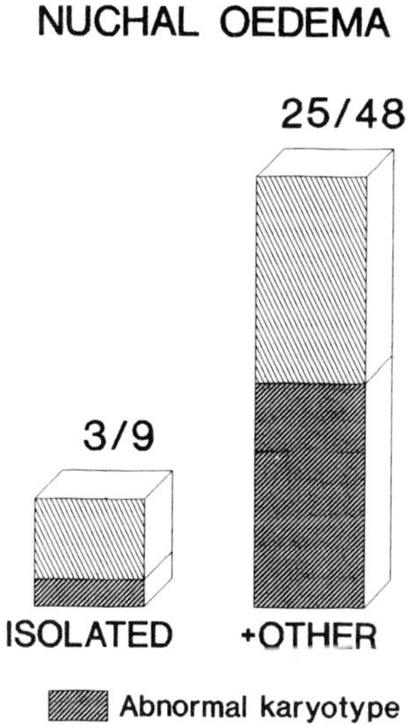

Fig. 8.5. Incidence of chromosomal defects in fetuses with nuchal oedema to the presence or absence of other additional malformations.

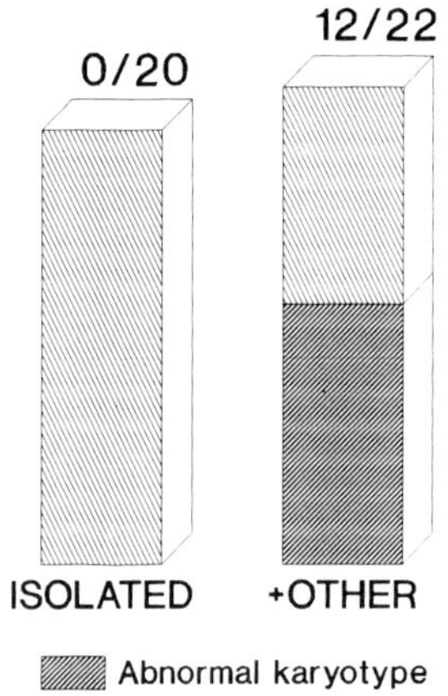

Fig. 8.6. Incidence of chromosomal defects in fetuses with congenital diaphragmatic hernia in relation to the presence or absence of other additional malformations.

malformations, predominantly craniospinal and cardiac, are often present.

Benacerraf and Adzik (1987) examined the incidence of associated malformations in cases of antenatally diagnosed CDH and found chromosomal abnormalities in 21% and major malformations in an additional 26% of 19 fetuses. Similarly, Thorpe-Beeston et al. (1989), reported chromosomal defects in 31% and major malformations in an additional 17% of 36 fetuses with CDH. In our extended series of 42 fetuses with CDH (Fig. 8.6), 12 (29%) had chromosomal defects, including trisomy 18 (n=7), trisomy 13 (n=3), triploidy (n=1) and deletion of the short arm of chromosome 9 (n=1). In all cases, in addition to the CDH there were other malformations such as choroid plexus cysts, posterior fossa cyst or holoprosencephaly, facial cleft, congenital heart defects, and digital abnormalities. None of the 20 fetuses with isolated CDH had chromosomal defects. The diaphragm develops from fusion of the septum transversum, the dorsal oesophageal mesentery, the pleuroperitoneal membranes and the body wall and is complete by 12 weeks' gestation. It is postulated that the aetiology of CDH in those fetuses with chromosomal abnormalities is developmental delay in the fusion of these components.

Congenital Heart Disease (CHD)

Gross structural abnormalities of the heart or major blood vessels which have actual or potential effects on the proper functioning of the heart are found in approximately 1% of livebirths and 2%–10% of stillbirths. While some of the defects resolve spontaneously (e.g. ventricular septal defect) and others are easily correctable (e.g. patent ductus), major structural abnormalities are either inoperable (e.g. hypoplastic left heart) or carry high operative risks (e.g. truncus arteriosus). The occurrence of CHD probably depends on the interplay of mutiple genetic and environmental factors (Nora and Nora 1978). Echocardiography has been applied successfully to the prenatal assessment of fetal cardiac function and structure and has led to the prenatal diagnosis of most moderate to major cardiac abnormalities (Allan 1984).

Detailed fetal echocardiographic studies are undertaken in specialized centres and are confined primarily to pregnancies at high risk of CHD. However, with improved expertise and increased availability of equipment in most obstetric ultrasound departments, it should be possible to incorporate basic echocardiography in the routine ultrasound screening programme performed for all pregnancies. Suspected anomalies can then be referred to specialized centres for further evaluation. Such a programme was undertaken in a recent study in France, where 460 fetuses of 20 000 pregnancies screened were thought to have CHD. This was confirmed in 70 patients. There were no false-positive diagnoses in the referral centre, and ony three defects were missed (Fermont et al. 1985).

Nora and Nora (1978) reported that heart defects are found in more than 99% of fetuses with trisomy 18, in 90% of those with trisomy 13, 50% of trisomy 21, 40%–50% of those with deletions or partial trisomies involving chromosomes 4, 5, 8, 9, 13, 14, 18 or 22 and in 35% of Turner's.

In our series of 90 fetuses with CHD (Fig. 8.7), 55 (61%) had chromosomal defects (trisomy 18, n=23; trisomy 21, n=9, trisomy 13, n=5, deletions/translocations, n=4; Turner's, n=9; 47XYY, n=1; triploidy, n=4). However, in 85 of the 90 cases with CHD there were other major fetal malformations such as posterior fossa cyst, exomphalos, diaphragmatic hernia, or renal defects.

Gastrointestinal Tract Defects

Sonographically, the stomach is identified as a sonolucent cystic structure in the upper left quadrant of the abdomen. This is a consistent finding and, in a recent review of more than 9000 fetal scans, the stomach was seen in 99% of the cases (Manning 1984). The bowel is normally uniformly echogenic until the third trimester of pregnancy when prominent meconium filled loops of large bowel are commonly seen. Oesophageal and gastrointestinal obstruction are often

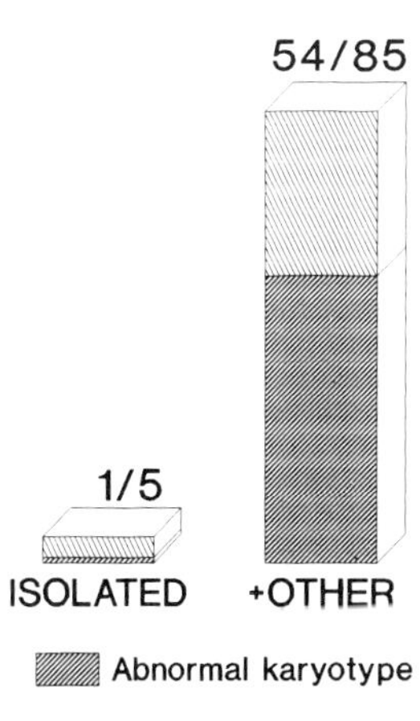

Fig. 8.7. Incidence of chromosomal defects in fetuses with congenital heart defects in relation to the presence or absence of other additional malformations.

diagnosed in the late second or third trimesters of pregnancy; the commonest indication for scanning is polyhydramnios, which is particularly common with higher obstructions.

Oesophageal Atresia

Oesophageal atresia is a sporadic condition found in 2–10 per 10 000 births and, in 90% of the cases, there is an associated tracheoesophageal (T-E) fistula (Holder and Ashcraft 1981). Both conditions result from failure of the primitive foregut to divide into the anterior trachea and posterior oesophagus. Normal development usually takes place between the third and fifth week of gestation and is complete by eight weeks. Prenatally the diagnosis of oesophageal atresia is suspected when, in the presence of polyhydramnios, repeated ultrasonographic examinations fail to demonstrate the fetal stomach. In the presence of a T-E fistula these signs are absent.

Other major abnormalities, mainly cardiac, are found in 50%–70% of the infants (Holder et al. 1964) and the fistula may be seen as part of the VATER association (Vertebral and Ventricular septal defects, Anal atresia, T-E fistula, Renal anomalies, Radial dysplasia and single umbilical artery) (Smith 1982). Associated chromosomal abnormalities were reported in 3%–4% of livebirths with oesophageal atresia. In our series of 17 fetuses (Fig. 8.8), 9 (53%) had chromosomal defects; including trisomy 18 (n=6), trisomy 13 (n=1), trisomy 21 (n=1) and partial trisomy 19 (n=1).

Duodenal Atresia

Duodenal atresia or stenosis has a birth incidence of 1 in 10 000 livebirths. In most cases the condition is sporadic, although a familial inheritance has been suggested by an autosomal recessive pattern in some families. At five weeks of embryonic life the lumen of the duodenum is obliterated by proliferating epithelium. The patency of the lumen is usually restored by the 11th week and failure of vaculization may lead to stenosis or atresia. The condition can readily be diagnosed sonographically by the characteristic "double-bubble" appearance

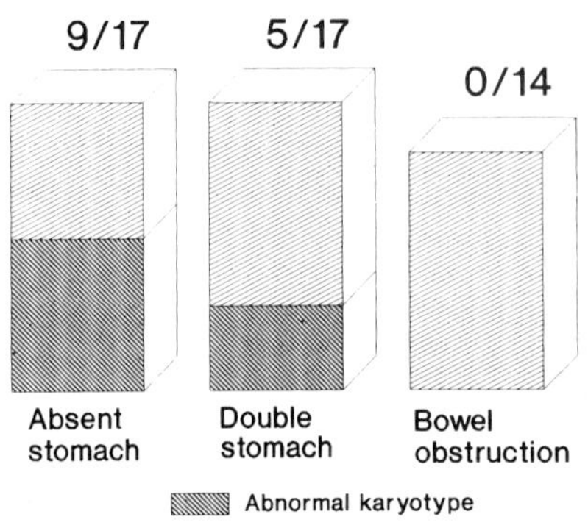

Fig. 8.8. Incidence of chromosomal defects in fetuses with gastrointestinal tract defects.

of the dilated stomach and proximal duodenum and the commonly associated polyhydramnios. However obstruction due to a central web may result in only a "single-bubble" representing the fluid-filled stomach. Continuity of the duodenum with the stomach should be demonstrated to differentiate a distended duodenum from other cystic masses including choledocal or hepatic cysts.

Approximately half of fetuses with duodenal atresia have associated malformations including: skeletal defects (vertebral and rib anomalies, sacral agenesis, radial abnormalities and talipes), gastrointestinal abnormalities (oesophageal atresia/T-E fistula, intestinal malrotation, Meckel's diverticulum and anorectal atresia), cardiovascular malformations (endocardial cushion defects and ventricular septal defects), and renal defects. In our series of 17 fetuses with duodenal atresia (Fig. 8.8), 5 (29%) had trisomy 21, 4 had congenital heart defects (24%) and 3 (18%) had renal malformations. Four of the trisomic fetuses and 2 of those with a normal karyotype had additional malformations. In contrast, only one of the 11 fetuses with isolated duodenal atresia had trisomy 21.

Bowel Obstruction

Jejunal and ileal obstructions are imaged as multiple fluid-filled loops of bowel in the abdomen and, in contrast to duodenal atresia, associated abnormalities are uncommon. Active peristalsis is often present and, if bowel perforation occurs, transient ascites, meconium peritonitis and meconium pseudocysts may ensue. Another presentation of small bowel obstruction is hyperechogenicity in the fetal abdomen. Anal atresia is associated with fluid-filled loops of bowel usually seen in the lower abdomen, but is not accompanied by polyhydramnios. Anal atresia may not present any antenatally detectable sonographic features.

In a combined series of 589 infants with a total jejunoileal atresia, additional abnormalities were found in 44% of cases (De Loreimier et al. 1969). Bowel abnormalities including malrotation of the bowel, imperforate anus, meconium peritonitis and ileaus, and omphalocoele or gastroschisis were present in 20% of the infants. Cardiovascuar or chromosomal anomalies were found in 7% of cases. In cases of anorectal atresia the incidence of associated defects is 70%–90%. The most commonly associated defects are genitourinary and include renal agenesis or dysplasia. Vertebral, cardiovascular and gastrointestinal anomalies have all been described. In our series of 14 fetuses with bowel obstruction (Fig. 8.8), there were no chromosomal defects.

Anterior Abdominal Wall Defects

Exomphalos

Exomphalos has an incidence of 2–4 per 10 000 births. The majority of cases are sporadic and the recurrence risk is less than 1%. However in some cases there may be a sex-linked or autosomal pattern of inheritance. Prenatal diagnosis is based on the demonstration of the midline anterior abdominal wall defect, the herniated sac with its visceral contents and the umbilical cord insertion at the apex of the sac. Embryologically, failure of fusion of the lateral ectomesodermal folds in the midine by the fourth week of gestation results in an isolated omphalocoele. Occasionally, there is an associated failure in the cephalic embryonic fold resulting in the pentalogy of Cantrell (upper midline omphalocoele, anterior diaphragmatic hernia, sternal cleft, ectopia cordis and intracardiac defects) or failure of the caudal fold in which case the omphalocoele may be associated with exstrophy of the bladder or cloaca, imperforate anus, colonic atresia and sacral vertebral defects (Cantrell et al. 1958).

Associated chromosomal defects are found in 35%–58% of infants with omphalocoele. In our series of 74 patients (Fig. 8.9), 28 (38%) had an abnormal karyotype including trisomy 18 (n=22), trisomy 13(n=4), triploidy (n=1) and Klinefelter's syndrome (n=1). Chromosomal defects were more common when the sac contained bowel only (16 of 25 cases) rather than liver (11 of 48 cases). All but one of the fetuses with chromosomal defects had either additional major malformations or more subtle markers of chromosomal defect including digital, facial or renal anomalies. Similarly, Nyberg et al. (1989) in a study of 26 fetuses with omphalocoele reported that the absence of liver from the omphalocoele sac or the presence of other malformations was associated with an abnormal karyotype.

Gastroschisis

In gastroschisis, with a birth incidence of 1 per 10 000, evisceration of the intestine occurs through a small abdominal wall defect located just lateral and usually to the right of an intact umbilical cord. The loops of intestine lie uncovered in the amniotic fluid and become thickened, oedematous and matted. Prenatal diagnosis

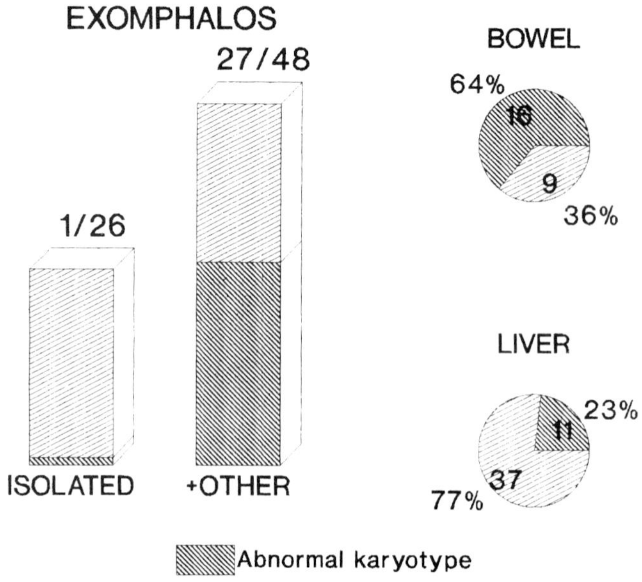

Fig. 8.9. Incidence of chromosomal defects in exomphalos (left) and in relation to the contents of the sac (right).

is based on the demonstration of the normally situated umbilicus and the herniated loops of intestine, which are free-floating. The vast majority of cases are thought to be sporadic, although there are examples of familial gastroschisis suggesting the possibility of an autosomal dominant mode of inheritance, with variable expression. Associated chromosomal abnormalities are rare, and although other malformations are found in 10%–30% of cases, these are mainly gut atresias, probably due to gut strangulation and infarction in utero.

Urinary Tract Defects

Using high-resolution ultrasound scanners, it is now possible to visualize the fetal kidneys as early as 10 weeks' gestation. The kidneys, located below the level of the stomach, on either side and anterior to the spine, are more sonolucent than the adjacent liver and contain a small echo-free central space, the renal pelvis. Both the renal length and circumference increase with gestation but the ratio of renal to abdominal circumference remains approximately 30% throughout pregnancy (Grannum et al. 1980). Urinary tract anomalies occur in approximately 2–3 per 1000 pregnancies.

Renal Agenesis

Bilateral renal agenesis has a birth incidence of 2 per 10 000. Although it may be secondary to a chromosomal abnormality or part of a genetic syndrome, such as Frazer's syndrome, more commonly it is an isolated finding. In non-syndromic cases, the risk of recurrence is approximately 3%. However, 13% of first degree relatives of affected infants have unilateral renal agenesis themselves and in these families the risk of recurrence is increased (Roodhooft et al. 1984). Antenatally, the condition is first suspected by the discovery of severe oligohydramnios and absent fetal bladder. Examination of the renal areas is often hampered by the "crumpled" position adopted by these fetuses and care should be taken to avoid the mistaken diagnosis of perirenal fat and large fetal adrenals for the absent kidneys. Doppler is proving to be an effective non-invasive technique for the distinction of renal agenesis from growth retardation as the cause of oligohydramnios.

Infantile Polycystic Kidney Disease

Potter type I renal dysplasia may occur sporadically but is more commonly inherited as an autosomal recessive condition. There is no reported association with chromosomal defects. Prenatal diagnosis is confined to the perinatal and probably the neonatal types and is based on the demonstration of bilaterally enlarged and homogeneously hyperechogenic kidneys. Although there is often associated oligohydramnios, this is not invariably so. These sonographic appearances, however, may not become apparent before 26 weeks' gestation and, therefore, serial scans should be performed for exclusion of the diagnosis.

Adult Polycystic Kidney Disease

Potter type II renal dysplasia is the common morphologic expression of autosomal dominant adult polycystic kidney disease (APKD) and other Mendelian disorders such as Meckel's syndrome. Prenatal diagnosis by ultrasonography is confined to a few case reports and the kidneys have been described as enlarged and hyperechogenic with or without multiple cysts. Unlike infantile polycystic kidneys, where there is a loss of the cortico-medullary junction, in APKD there is accentuation of this junction (McHugo et al. 1988). However, in counselling affected parents it should be emphasized that the prenatal demonstration of sonographically normal kidneys does not necessarily exclude the possibility of developing polycystic kidneys in adult life.

Potter Type II Renal Disease

This results from inhibition of the action of the ampulla of the ureteric bud with consequent hypodysplasia of collecting tubules and nephrons. The collecting tubules become cystic and the diameter of the cysts determines the size of the kidneys, which may be enlarged or small. Ultrasonographically, the former are recognized as large and multicystic and the latter as shrunken, irregular and hyperechogenic. The disorder can be bilateral, unilateral or segmental; if bilateral there is associated oligohydramnios and the bladder is either distended or "absent". The condition, which is generally sporadic, is thought to be a consequence of either developmental failure of the mesonephric blastema to form nephrons or early obstruction due to urethral or ureteric atresia. Associated multisystem malformations are often present both with bilateral and unilateral multicystic kidneys.

Obstructive Uropathies

The term "obstructive uropathy" encompasses a wide variety of different pathological conditions characterized by dilatation of part or all of the urinary tract. When the obstruction is complete and occurs early in fetal life, renal hypoplasia (deficiency in total nephron population) and dysplasia (formation of abnormal nephrons and mesenchymal stroma) ensue (Potter type II renal disease). On the other hand, where intermittent obstruction allows for normal renal develoment, or when it occurs in the second half of pregnancy, hydronephrosis will result and the severity of the renal damage will depend on the degree and duration of the obstruction.

Ureteropelvic Junction Obstruction (UPJ)

This is usually sporadic and although in some cases there is an anatomic cause, such as ureteral valves, aberrant lower pole vessels or fibrous adhesion, in most instances the ureteropelvic junction is patent and the underlying cause is thought to be functional. Prenatal diagnosis is based on the demonstration of hydronephrosis in the absence of dilated ureters and bladder; the amniotic fluid volume is usually normal.

Ureterovesical Junction Obstruction

This also causes hydronephrosis but in addition there is an associated hydroureter. The bladder is not distended but close inspection may reveal a ureterocoele within or adjacent to the bladder.

Urethral Obstruction

Incomplete or intermittent obstruction, due to posterior urethral valves, is associated with enlargement and hypertrophy of the bladder and varying degrees of hydroureters, hydronephrosis, oligohydramnios and pulmonary hypoplasia. Associated urinary ascites, observed in some cases, may be due to rupture of the bladder or transudation of urine into the peritoneal cavity.

Abnormal Karyotype

In our series of 480 fetuses with renal malformations (Fig. 8.10), where karyotyping was performed, abnormal chromosomes were found in 68 (14%)

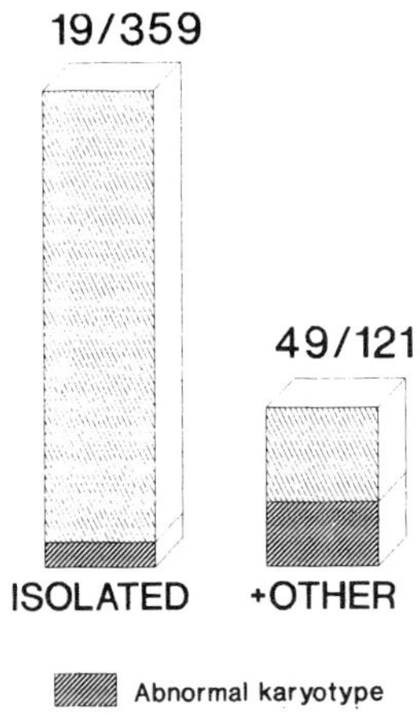

Fig. 8.10. Incidence of chromosomal defects in renal malformations, in relation to the presence or absence of other additional malformations.

cases. These include trisomies 8, 13, 18, 21 and 22 (n=49), deletions (n=9), triploidies or tetraploidies (n=4), and sex chromosome aneuploidies (n=6).

Chromosomal defects were found in:

1. 4 of the 22 fetuses (18%) with renal agenesis (trisomy 13, trisomy 18, partial trisomy 22 and Klinefelter's syndrome).
2. 12 of 129 (9%) with multicystic renal dysplasia (trisomy 13, n=4; trisomy 18, n=4; trisomy 21, n=1; triploidy, n=2; deletion 2q, n=1).
3. 52 of the 329 (16%) with hydronephrosis (trisomy 21, n=14; trisomy 18, n=12; trisomy 13, n=10; partial trisomy 8, n=1; deletions, n=8; Turner's, n=3; Klinefelter's, n=2; triploidy, n=1; tetraploidy, n=1).

In 359 cases the renal malformation was the only ultrasound finding; chromosomal defects were found in 19 (5%) of these fetuses. In contrast, 49 of the 121 (40%) with additional malformations were chromosomally abnormal (Fig. 8.10).

Skeletal Dysplasias

There is a wide range of rare skeletal dyplasias, each with a specific recurrence risk, morphology and implication for neonatal survival and qualty of life (Smith 1982; Romero et al. 1988). Prenatal diagnosis in families at risk of such anomalies necessitates expert genetic counselling if the ultrasonographer is to be alerted to the variation in dysmorphic expression that might be encountered. Our knowledge of the expression of these syndromes in utero is based on a small number of case reports, and therefore it is often necessary to extrapolate findings from the perinatal period when attempting prenatal diagnosis of individual conditions. In the event of identification of a skeletal dysplasia during routine ultrasound screening in a pregnancy not known to be at risk of a specific

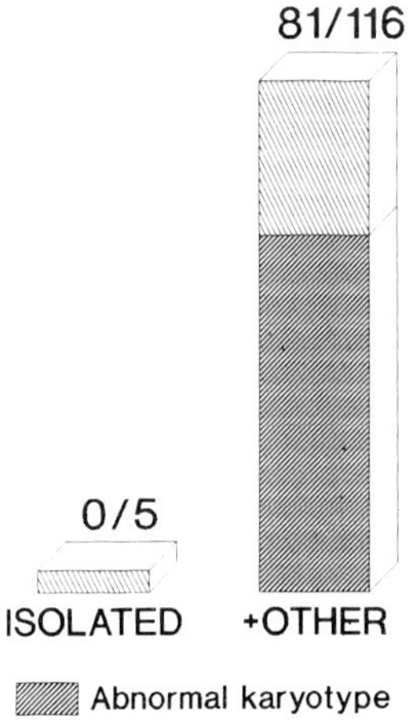

Fig. 8.11. Incidence of chromosomal defects in a variety of malformations of the extremities.

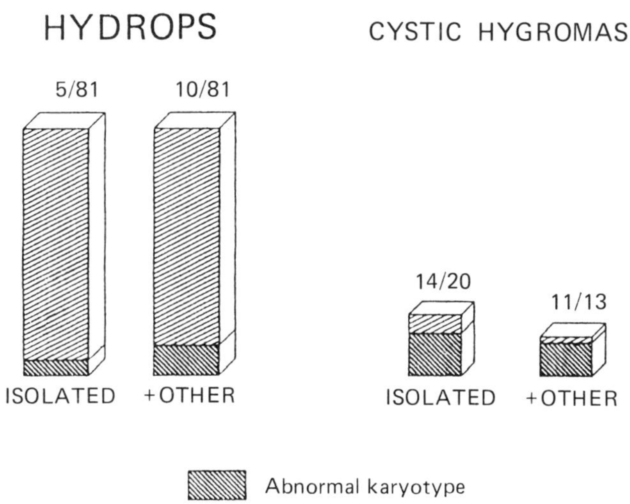

Fig. 8.12. Incidence of chromosomal defects in hydrops without (left), and with cystic hygromas (right), in relation to the presence or absence of other additional malformations.

syndrome, it is necessary to undertake a systematic examination in order to obtain the correct diagnosis. All four limbs must be evaluated, in terms of their length, shape, mineralization and movement, and the possible presence of associated abnormalities, particularly in the head, thorax and spine, should be determined. With the advent of high-resolution scanners, fetal fingers and toes can be seen and with meticulous examination abnormalities of numbers, shape, movement and attitudes can be recognized.

Characteristic abnormalities in the extremities are commonly found in a wide range of chromosomal defects and the detection of abnormal hands or feet at the routine ultrasound examination should stimulate the search for other markers of chromosomal defects. In our series of 121 fetuses with abnormal extremities (Fig. 8.11), 81 (67%) had chromosomal defects and in all cases additional malformations were detected (triploidy, n=22; trisomy 18, n=35; trisomy 21, n=10; trisomy 13, n=10; Turner's, n=1 ; deletions 4p or 8q, n=2; 47 XYY, n= 1). Clinodactyly was associated with trisomy 21, syndactyly with triploidy, overlapping fingers with trisomy 18, or deletions and polydactyly with trisomy 13. Rocker-bottom feet and talipes were found in trisomy 18 and 13 and sandal gap in trisomy 21.

Hydrops Fetalis

Hydrops fetalis, with an incidence of 3–10 per 10 000 births, is characterized by generalized skin oedema and pericardial, pleural, or ascitic effusions. This is a non-specific finding in a wide variety of fetal and maternal disorders, including haematological, chromosomal, cardiovascular, renal, pulmonary, gastrointestinal, hepatic and metabolic abnormalities, congenital infection, neoplasms and malformations of the placenta or umbilical cord (Potter 1943; Hutchison et al.

1982; Turkel 1982; Keeling et al. 1983; Nicolaides et al. 1985). With the widespread introduction of immunoprophylaxis and the decline in rhesus isoimmunization, non-rhesus causes have become responsible for at least 75% of the cases (Giacoia 1980; Machin 1981) and make a greater contribution to perinatal mortality (Anderson et al. 1983). While in many instances the underlying cause may be determined by detailed ultrasound scanning, frequently the abnormality remains unexplained even after expert post-mortem examination (Keeling et all 1983).

In our series of 195 fetuses with non-rhesus hydrops (Fig. 8.12), 33 had cystic hygromas. In 15 of the 162 (9%) without cystic hygromas, there were chromosomal abnormalities (trisomy 21, n=9; trisomy 13, n=1; partial trisomy 11, n=1; deletions, n=2; Turner's, n=1; tetraploidy, n=1). Chromosomal defects were found in 5 of the 81 (6%) fetuses with isolated hydrops and in 10 of the 81 (12%) with associated malformations.

Cystic Hygromas

Cystic hygromas are developmental abnormalities of the lymphatic system and are found most commonly around the neck. Although cystic hygromas may be isolated, in the majority of cases they are associated with hydrops fetalis. The ultrasound characteristics are those of a multiseptate, thin-walled cyst situated dorsolaterally in the cervical region. They are distinguished from an occipital encephalocoele or a cervical myelomeningocoele by the presence of a midline septum and the absence of a cranial or vertebral boney defect.

Chromosomal defects, particularly Turner's syndrome and multiple abnormalities, are common (Chervenak et al. 1983; Pearce et al. 1984; Nicolaides et al. 1985). In our series of 33 fetuses with cystic hygromas (Fig. 8.12), 25 (76%) had chromosomal defects (Turner's, n=23; trisomy 21, n=1; trisomy 18, n=1).

Small for Gestational Age

Analysis of blood samples obtained by cordocentesis from severely small for gestational age (SGA) fetuses has provided useful information on the cytogenetic, biochemical, metabolic and haematological status of such fetuses. Furthermore, it has provided end points for validation of the various non-invasive tests used in the assessment of fetal wellbeing. This section reviews the cytogenetic findings in 334 fetuses referred to our centre for further investigations because of suspected severe early-onset intrauterine growth retardation.

In all cases the fetal abdominal circumference, measured by ultrasonography, was at least 2 standard deviations (ranges=2–10) below the normal mean for gestational age. The amniotic fluid volume was subjectively assessed by ultrasonography to be normal in 122 of the 334 (37%) cases and reduced in 212 (63%) cases; in 103 of the latter there was oligohydramnios. Subsequently, the birth weight of these babies was always below the 10th centile and in 98% below the 5th centile for gestation and sex (Yudkin et al. 1987).

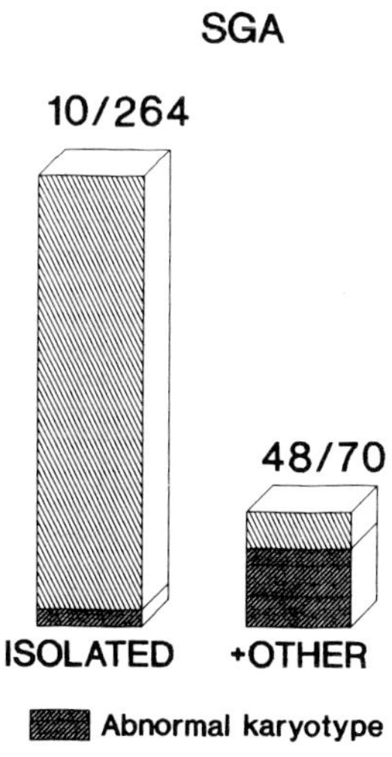

Fig. 8.13. Incidence of chromosomal defects in small for gestational age fetuses in relation to the presence or absence of other malformations.

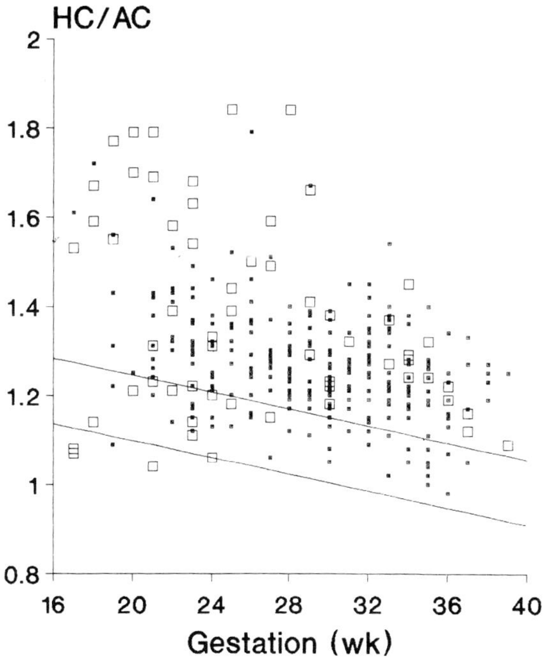

Fig. 8.14. Head circumference to abdomen circumference ratio in chromosomally (■) and abnormal (□) small for gestational age fetuses.

The fetal karyotype (Fig. 8.13) was normal in 276 cases and abnormal in 58 (triploidy, $n=21$; trisomy 13, $n=5$; trisomy 18, $n=16$; partial trisomy 19, $n=1$; trisomy 21, $n=5$; translocation trisomy 21, $n=1$; partial trisomy 22, $n=1$; deletion of the short arm of chromosome 4, $n=6$; unbalanced translocation involving chromosomes 4 and 15, $n=1$; balanced translocation involving chromosomes 5 and 11, $n=1$).

It is commonly stated that uteroplacental insufficiency is associated with asymmetrical fetal growth retardation while fetal genetic disease results in symmetrical growth retardation. However, our data indicate that certainly some chromosomal abnormalities are associated with severe asymmetry in growth and this is particularly marked in triploidy (Fig. 8.14).

Overall Results

A combined survey of 68 159 livebirths, revealed that 0.65% of newborns had a major chromosomal abnormality (Hsu 1986). There is a well-recognized association between fetal chromosomal defects and advanced maternal age. Thus, among livebirths the incidence increases exponentially from 0.5% for 35-year-old mothers to 1.6% at 40 years and 5.3% at 45 years; the corresponding incidences at the time of amniocentesis for maternal age are 0.8%, 2.5% and 8.3% respectively (Scheinemachers et al. 1982).

In our series of 1262 fetuses with malformations or growth retardation, 202 (16%) were found to be chromosomally abnormal. Chromosomal defects were found in 57 of the 916 (6%) fetuses with an isolated defect and in 145 of the 346 (42%) with more than one malformation (Fig. 8.15). The maternal age distribution of these fetuses is shown in Fig. 8.16. Though the risk of chromosomal defects was increased with maternal age, if karyotyping for fetal defects was undertaken only in women over 34 or over 29 years old then the respective pick-up rates of chromosomal defects would have been 26% and 51% (Fig. 8.17).

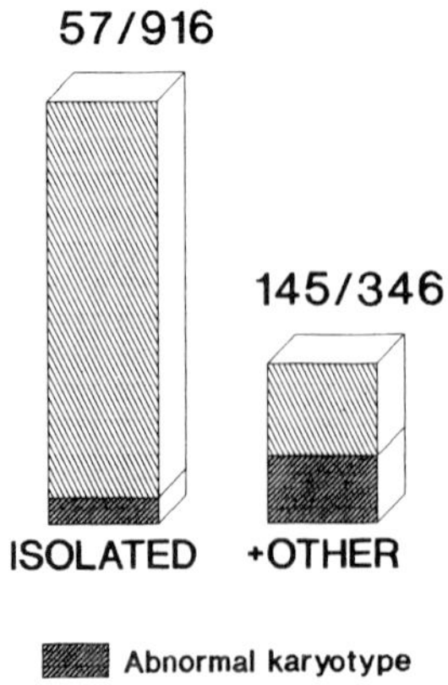

Fig. 8.15. Incidence of chromosomal defects in 1262 fetuses with a variety of malformations.

Conclusion

Severely growth retarded or morphologically deformed fetuses are often chromosomally abnormal. Certainly the incidence of chromosomal defects for ultrasonically detectable abnormalities (16% in this series) is much higher than the incidence reported in screening studies based on advanced maternal age.

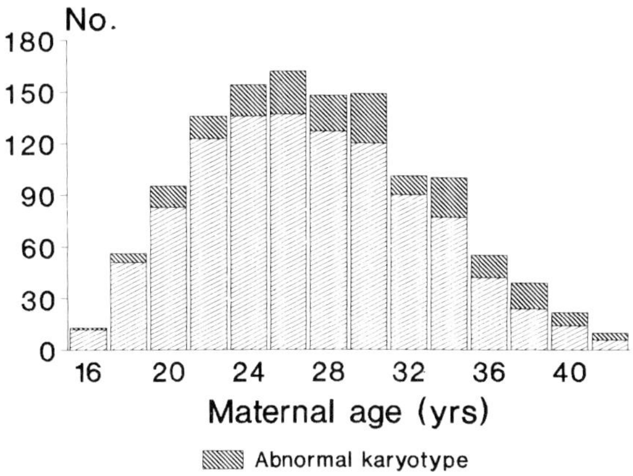

Fig. 8.16. Maternal age distribution of the chromosomally normal and abnormal fetuses.

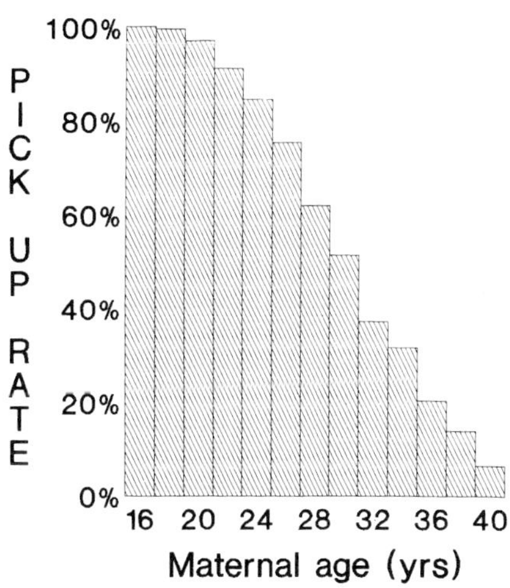

Fig. 8.17. Cumulative frequency of chromosomally abnormal fetuses in relation to maternal age.

The ultrasound diagnosis of a marker for a specific chromosomal defect should stimulate the search for other associated malformations and when these additional abnormalities are found the probability that the fetus is chromosomally abnormal is dramatically increased. The sensitivity of ultrasound screening for chromosomal defects remains to be determined.

References

Allan LD (1984). The prenatal detection of congenital heart disease. In: Rodeck CH, Nicolaides KH (eds) Prenatal diagnosis. Proceedings of the Eleventh Study Group of the Royal College of Obstetricians and Gynaecoogists. RCOG and John Wiley and Sons, Chichester, p 285

Anderson HN, Drew JH, Beischer NA, et al. (1983) Non-immune hydrops fetalis: changing contribution to perinatal mortality. Br J Obstet Gynaecol 90: 636.

Beischer NA, Fortune DW, Macafee J (1971). Non-immunologic hydrops fetalis and congenital abnormalities. Obstet Gynecol 38: 86

Benacerraf BR and Adzik NS 1987 Fetal diaphragmatic hernia: Ultrasound diagnosis and clinical outcome in 19 cases. Am J Obstet Gynecol 156:573

Benacerraf BR, Barss VA, Laboda LA (1985a). A sonographic sign for the detection in the second trimester of the fetus with Down's syndrome. Am J Obstet Gynecol 151: 1078

Benacerraf BR, Frigoletto FD, Laboda LA (1985b). Sonographic diagnosis of Down's syndrome in the second trimester. Am J Obstet Gynecol 153: 49

Campbell S (1977). Early prenatal diagnosis of neural tube defects by ultrasound. Clin Obstet Gynecol 20: 351

Cantrell JR, Haller JA, Ravitch MM (1958) A syndrome of congenital defects involving the abdominal wall, sternum, diaphragm, pericardium and heart. Surg Gynecol Obstet 107: 602

Chevenak FA, Isaacson G, Blakemore KJ et al. (1983) Fetal cystic hygroma: cause and natural history. N Engl J Med 14: 822

Chervenak FA, Duncan C, Ment LR et al. (1984) Outcome of fetal ventriculomegaly. Lancet ii: 179

Chitkara U, Cogswell C, Norton K, Wilkins IA, Mewfhalek K, Berkowitz RL (1989) Choroid plexus cysts in the fetus: A benign anatomic variant or pathologic entity? Report of 41 cases and review of the literature. Obstet Gynecol 72: 185

Chudleigh P, Pearce JM, Campbell S (1984) The prenatal diagnosis of transient cysts of the fetal choroid plexus. Prenatal Diagn 4: 135

DeLoreimier AA, Fonkalsrud EW, Hays DM (1969) Congenital atresia and stenosis of the duodenum and ileum. Surgery 65: 819

Fermont L, de Geeter B, Aubry MC et al. (1985) A close collaboration between obstetricians and paediatric cardiologists allows antenatal detection of severe cardiac malformations by 2D echocardiography. In: 2nd world congress of paediatric cardiology. Springer-Verlag, New York, p10

Furness ME (1987) Choroid plexus cysts and trisomy 18. Lancet 2: 693

Gabrielli et al 1989 S, Reece AR, Pilu G, Perolo A, Rizzo N, Bovicelli L & Hobbins JC (1989) The significance of prenatally diagnosed choroid plexus cysts. Am J Obstet Gynecol 160: 1207

Giacoia GP (1980) Hydrops fetalis (fetal oedema). A survey. Clin Pediatr 19: 334

Grannum P, Bracken M, Silverman R, Hobbins JC (1980) Assessment of fetal kidney size in normal gestation by comparison of ratio of kidney circumference to abdominal circumference. Am J Obstet Gynecol 136: 249

Holder TM, Ashcraft KW (1981) Developments in the care of patients with esophageal atresia and tracheoesophageal fistula. Surg Clin North Am 61: 1051

Hutchinson AA, Drew JH, Yu VYH et al. (1982) Non-immunologic hydrops fetalis: a review of 61 cases. Obstet Gynecol 59: 347

Keeling JW, Gough DJ, Iliff PJ (1983) The pathology of non-rhesus hydrops. Diagn Histopathol 6: 89

Khouzam MN, Hooker JG (1989) The significance of prenatal diagnosis of choroid plexus cysts. Prenat Diagn 9: 213

Machin GA (1981) Differential diagnosis of hydrops fetalis. Am J Med Genet 9: 341

Manning FA (1984) Ultrasound in prenatal diagnosis. In: Creasy RK, Resnik R (eds) Maternal fetal medicine: principles and practice. WB Saunders, Philadelphia, p 203

McHugo JM, Shafi MI, Rowlands D, Wever JB (1988) Prenatal diagnosis of adult polycystic kidney disease. Br J Radiol 61: 1072

Nicolaides KH, Rodeck CH, Lange I et al. (1985) Fetoscopy in the evaluation of unexplained fetal hydrops. Br J Obstet Gynaecol 92: 671

Nicolaides KH, Rodeck CH, Gosden CM (1986) Karyotyping in non-lethal fetal malformations. Lancet i: 284

Nora JJ, Nora AH (1978) The evolution of specific genetic and environmental counselling in congenital heart disease. Circulation 57: 205

Nyberg DA, Fitzsimmons J, Mack LA et al (1989) Chromosomal abnormalities in fetuses with omphalocele. Significance of omplhalocele contents. J Ultrasound Med 8: 299

Ostlere SJ, Irving HC, Lilford RJ (1989) A prospective study of the incidence and significance of fetal choroid plexus cysts. Pren Diagn 9: 205
Pashayan HM (1983) What else to look for in a child born with a cleft of the lip or palate. Cleft Palate J 20: 543
Piu G, Rizzo N, Orsini LF et al. (1986) Antenatal detection of fetal cerebral anomalies. Ultrasound Med Biol 12: 319
Pearce JM, Griffin D, Campbell S (1984) Cystic hygromata in trisomy 18 and 21. Prenatal Diagn 4: 371
Potter EL (1943) Universal oedema of the fetus unassociated with erythroblastosis. Am J Obstet Gynecol 46: 130
Ricketts NEM, Lowe EM, Patel NB (1987). Prenatal diagnosis of choroid plexus cysts. Lancet 1: 213
Romero R, Pilu G, Jeanty P, Ghidini A, Hobbins JC (1988) Prenatal diagnosis of congenital anomalies. Appleton, Lange, California, p 311
Roodhooft AM, Birnholz JC, Holmes LB (1984) Familial nature of congenital absence and severe dysgenesis of both kidneys. N Engl J Med 310: 1341
Scheinemachers DM, Cross PK, Hook EB (1982) Rates of trisomies 21, 18, 13 and other chromosome abnormalities in about 20 000 prenatal studies compared with estimated rates in livebirths. Hum Genet 61: 318
Smith DW (1982) Recognizable patterns of human malformation, 3rd edn. WB Saunders, Philadelphia
Thorpe-Beeston JG, Gosden CM, Nicolaides KN (1990) Prenatal diagnosis and chromosomal defects. (In press)
Turkel SB (1982) Conditions associated with non-immune hydrops fetalis. Clin Perinatol 9: 613
Yudkin PL, Aboualfa M, Eyre JA, Redman CWG, Wilkinson AR (1987) New birth weight and head circumference centiles for gestational ages 24–42 weeks. Early Hum Dev 15: 45

9. Embryoscopy: An Evolving Technology for Early Prenatal Diagnosis

E.A. Reece and J.C. Hobbins

Introduction

Endoscopic visualization of the embryo (embryoscopy) is a new and evolving technology. The concept of direct visualization of the embryo reflects not only an ongoing quest for improved diagnostic techniques, but also the potential for direct, targeted embryonic therapy. As we enter the last decade of this century, modern perinatology must address the concept that the embryo/fetus be regarded as a bona fide patient.

Embryoscopy is expected to play a significant role in this development. The technique, in brief, consists of using a rigid endoscope which is inserted through the uterine cervix and the chorion into the extracoelomic cavity under ultrasonographic guidance to permit embryonic visualization with the potential for prenatal diagnosis and treatment (Galliant et al. 1978; Cullen et al. 1989a).

The significance of these formidable advances is best realized when placed in a historical context. Fetal medicine is a new discipline, and its existence has to be credited to modern technology. Historically, the developing human fetus and its compartment were regarded as inaccessible, and pregnancy mysteriously resulted in a normal or anomalous infant. Evaluation of the fetus was neither considered nor possible except for assessment of fetal growth by increasing uterine size. Pregnancy management focused primarily on maternal care with the hope that the fetus would be an indirect beneficiary of such treatment.

Electronic fetal monitoring was the first of the major technological advances. The graphical display of fetal wellbeing, or the lack thereof, set the stage for prenatal evaluation. Ultrasonography greatly extended the possibilities for fetal evaluation. It became possible to assess fetal growth, behaviour and wellbeing, fetal anatomy, and even evidence of fetal physiology. With further improvement in ultrasound resolution, prenatal diagnosis of various developmental anomalies became possible (Hobbins et al. 1979; Manning et al. 1981; 1983; Bulic et al. 1987; Romero et al. 1987; Vergani et al. 1987; Curtis and Watson 1988; Green and Hobbins, 1988; Hill et al. 1988).

Table 9.1. First-trimester diagnostic techniques and their status

1. Chorionic villus sampling – successful and well established
2. Amniocentesis – safety not well established
3. MSAFP – efficacy not established
4. Ultrasound – limitations in resolution
5. Embryoscopy – evolving technology

Currently, ultrasonography is the mainstay of prenatal diagnosis of congenital structural anomalies. However, there is a changing trend in prenatal diagnosis. Women now request more information about their unborn child and require such information earlier in gestation. A variety of prenatal diagnostic techniques are available to address these concerns (Table 9.1). For those women who choose to have pregnancy terminations, such procedures are safer and associated with less maternal morbidity and mortality when performed earlier in the pregnancy. Hence, early prenatal diagnosis is feasible, socially desirable and medically sound. For chromosomal anomalies, DNA, and enzyme defects, early prenatal diagnosis is made possible by chorionic villus sampling. However, early detection of structural anomalies is hampered by the limits of ultrasound resolution. This new technology advances prenatal diagnosis into an era with the potential for even earlier diagnosis.

Procedure

Embryoscopy uses a rigid endoscope which is guided sonographically through the cervix and the chorion into the extracoelomic space. The tip of the endoscope

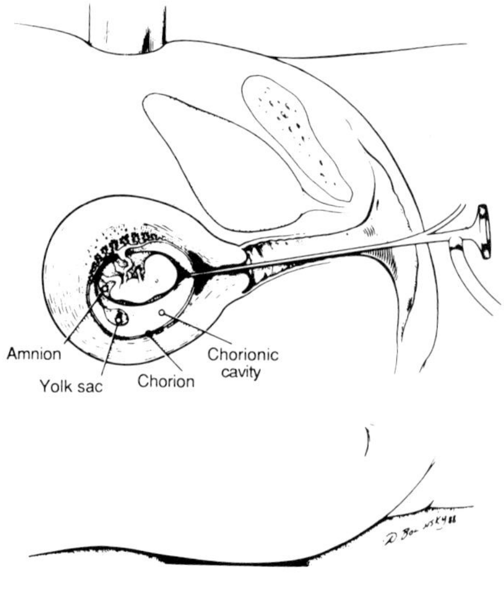

Fig. 9.1. Schematic drawing of the rigid endoscope passed through the cervix and chorion into the extracoelomic space where visualization of the conceptus is possible through the transparent amnion.

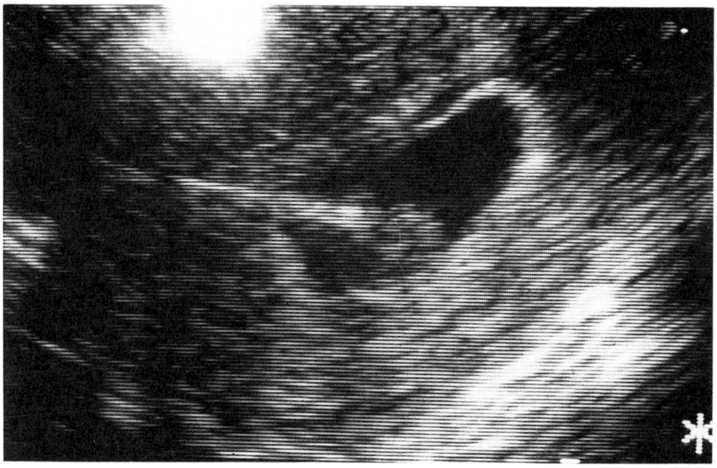

Fig. 9.2. Ultrasound picture which reveals the endoscope through the cervix and into the extracoelomic space. The endoscope is in close proximity to the embryo but separated by the amnion.

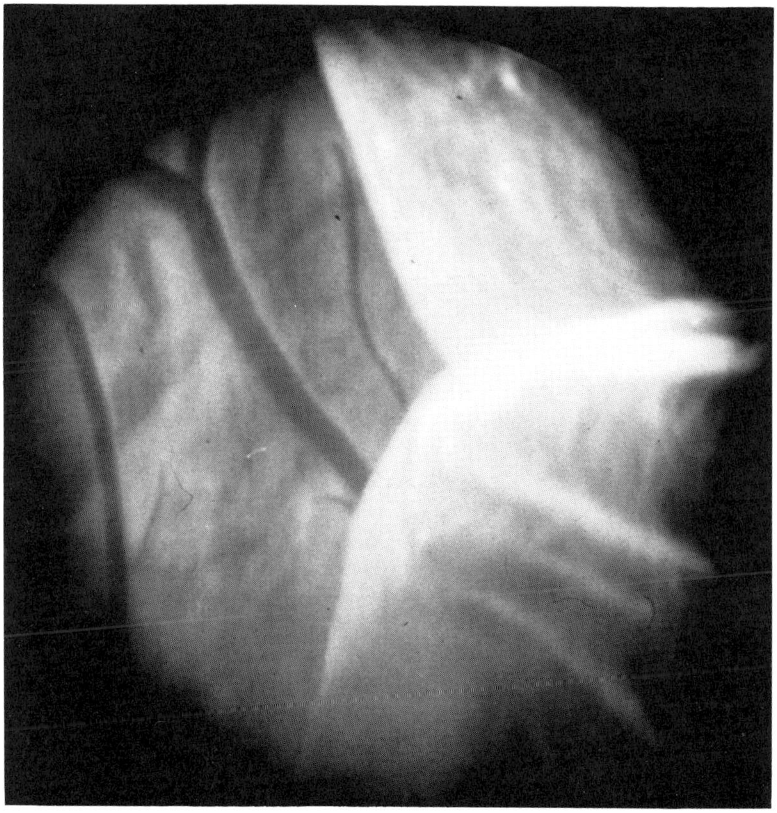

Fig. 9.3. Endoscopic view on video camera of the undersurface of the chorion and the intact amnion. Note the prominent vasculature.

is used to rupture the chorion leaving the amnion intact (Figs. 9.1 and 9.2). Rupture of the amnion is rare, but occurs after 11 weeks gestation when the chorion and amnion are fused. Visualization of the conceptus is enhanced by a bright halogen light source (Karl Storz, Culver City, CA). The conceptus can be seen directly through the endoscope or via a video camera and monitor (Fig. 9.3).

Potential disadvantages include the possibility of rupture of the amnion, fluid leakage, infection, and bleeding eventuating in pregnancy loss. Studies on continuing pregnancies will eventually reveal the frequency of occurrence or relative risks of these complications.

Our initial experience, reported elsewhere (Cullen et al. 1989a, b), reveals a 96% success rate in entering the extracoelomic space with conceptus visualization. Subsequently, our series has been expanded with a slightly higher success rate. Dumez has reported a similar success rate. He has also performed embryoscopy in over 50 continuing pregnancies, for the purpose of excluding head and limb anomalies, and reported two losses which occured at the start of his experience (Roume et al. 1985; Dumez 1988). Further experience will doubtless expand the indications for this procedure and will allow assessment of safety and determination of the risk of adverse effects. Table 9.2 lists the potential applications of embryoscopy.

Current Applications

Morphologic Evaluation

Embryoscopy can be performed as early as three weeks post-conception and continued through the first and into the second trimester. The procedure can be used to document developmental events. In this section, we will discuss the main features of both normal and abnormal development which are recognizable by embryoscopy.

Following conception, the embryonic period extends from weeks 4 through 8, when all major external and internal structures develop. This is the period of greatest susceptibility to the effects of teratogens which may result in developmental anomalies. By the end of this embryonic period, most definitive features are recognizable (Hamilton et al. 1964; Arey 1974; Moore 1988).

The embryo begins as a trilaminar disc which undergoes folding. This disc becomes cylindrical in shape due to rapid elongation and growth of the midline structures (including the neural tube and somites) at a rate greater than the margins of the disc. Folding of the neural tube longitudinally results in head and

Table 9.2. Potential applications of embryoscopy

1. Prenatal diagnosis of structural anomalies
2. Confirmation of early sonographic diagnosis prior to pregnancy termination
3. Early blood and/or tissue sampling
4. Embryo access for cell and/or gene therapy
5. The biology of embryonic development

tail regions, while transverse folding results in the body wall (Hamilton et al. 1964; Arey 1974). The fetal period begins after the 8th post-conceptual week and continues until delivery. This period involves growth and differentiation of the embryonic tissues and organs. Teratogenic insults at this time result in functional defects (Moore 1988).

The Head and Neck

The cephalic end of the fetus grows more rapidly than the rest of the body. This disproportion begins very early, with the highest number of somites clustering in the base of the head nurtured by a well-established blood supply. The brain and associated sense organs also develop early and remain disproportionately larger than other non-cephalic regions throughout embryonic life (Moore 1988). Prominent normal developmental milestones of the head and neck that can be observed externally are as follows (see Figs. 9.4 and 9.5):

Conceptional week 4: optic depression, optic evagination, and flexed branchial arches can be seen.

Conceptional week 5: the nasal pit, primitive mouth, and optic cups are recognizable.

CONCEPTIONAL AGE (WEEKS)	FACE		EXTREMITIES		ABDOMEN & GI TRACT
3.5		—		—	Foregut; yolk sac larger than amniotic sac
4.5	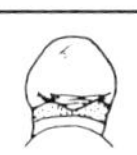	Fusion of mandible arches	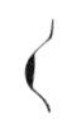	Arm bud	Formation of thyroid, liver and pancreas
5	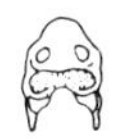	Olfactory placodes	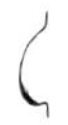	Leg bud	—
5.5	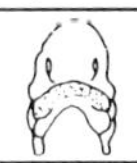	Nasal swellings	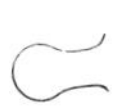	Hand plate; mesenchyme condensation; innervation	Intestinal loop into yolk stalk
6.5	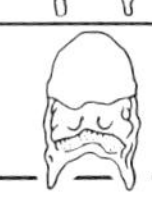	Primary palate	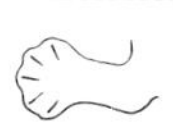	Finger rays; elbow	—
7.5		—	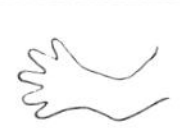	Fingers; tail regression complete by 12 wks	—
8		—	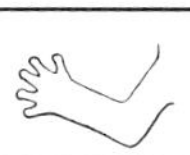	—	—
10		—		—	Gut withdrawal from cord

Fig. 9.4. External embryo/fetal development of the face, extremities, abdomen and gastrointestinal tract. (Modified and reprinted with permission from K. Moore: The developing human. Clinically oriented embryology. W.B. Saunders, 1985, pp 2–3.)

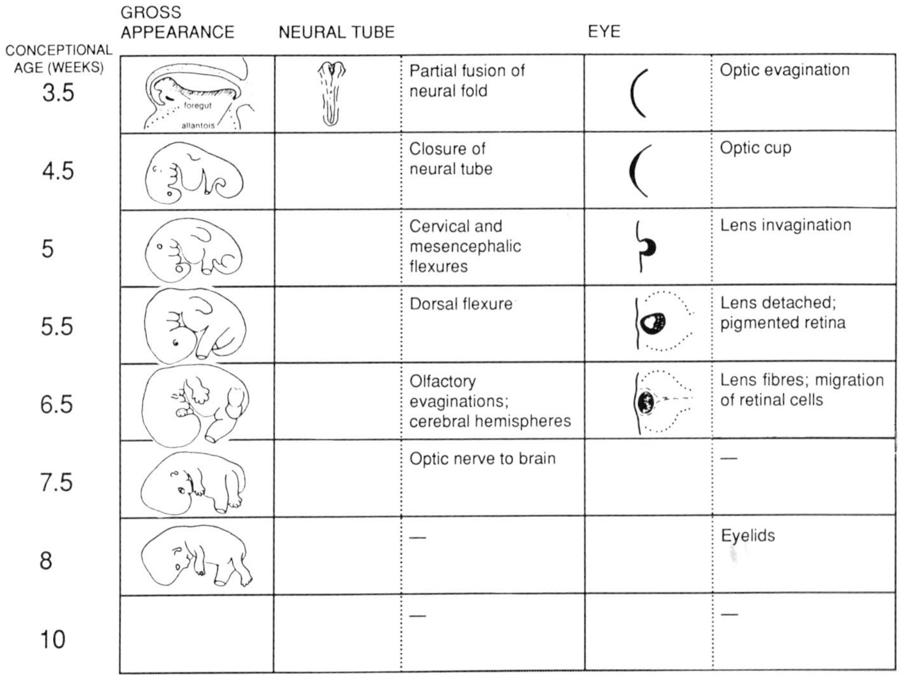

CONCEPTIONAL AGE (WEEKS)	GROSS APPEARANCE	NEURAL TUBE		EYE	
3.5	foregut, allantois		Partial fusion of neural fold		Optic evagination
4.5			Closure of neural tube		Optic cup
5			Cervical and mesencephalic flexures		Lens invagination
5.5			Dorsal flexure		Lens detached; pigmented retina
6.5			Olfactory evaginations; cerebral hemispheres		Lens fibres; migration of retinal cells
7.5			Optic nerve to brain		—
8			—		Eyelids
10			—		—

Fig. 9.5. External embryo/fetal development of the entire body, neural tube and eye. (Modified and reprinted with permission from K. Moore: The developing human. Clinically oriented embryology. W.B. Saunders, 1985, pp 2–3)

Conceptional week 6: the oral and nasal cavities are confluent, the upper lip is formed, and the head remains larger and flexed.

Conceptional week 7: all external and internal structures are present.

Conceptional week 8: the head is less flexed but retains its large size.

Conceptional week 9: the membranes fuse.

Conceptional week 10: the face has a normal human profile.

Embryoscopy has been used to witness many of these features during both the embryonic and fetal periods. The endoscopic view of the fetal face at 6 conceptional weeks reveals a prominent forehead, widely spaced eyes, and confluent oral and nasal cavities (Fig. 9.6). At 8 conceptional weeks, greater facial detail is seen (Fig. 9.7); and by 10 conceptional weeks, normal human facial features are recognized (Fig. 9.8).

Certain congenital malformations of the head and neck can be visualized in early pregnancy. Malformations of the head which may manifest externally include anencephaly, acrania, hydrocephaly, microcephaly and macrocephaly. However, those most likely to be diagnosable by first-trimester embryoscopy are anencephaly and acrania. Potentially diagnosable anomalies of the face include micrognathia and cleft lip. The latter is usually unilateral (left more often than right) but can be bilateral. The lip is often the only involved area, but the bony upper jaw may also be involved.

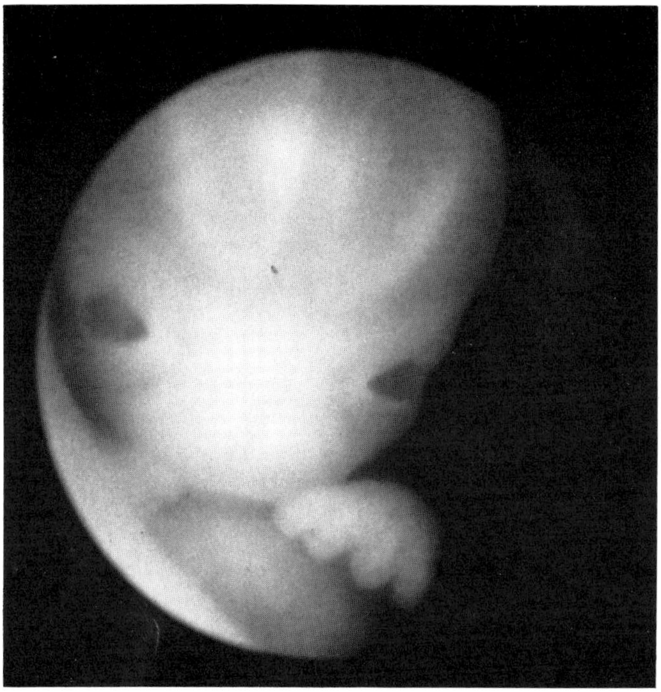

Fig. 9.6. Endoscopic view of the fetal face at 6 conceptional weeks of gestation. Note the prominent forehead, widely spaced eyes, and confluent oral and nasal cavities.

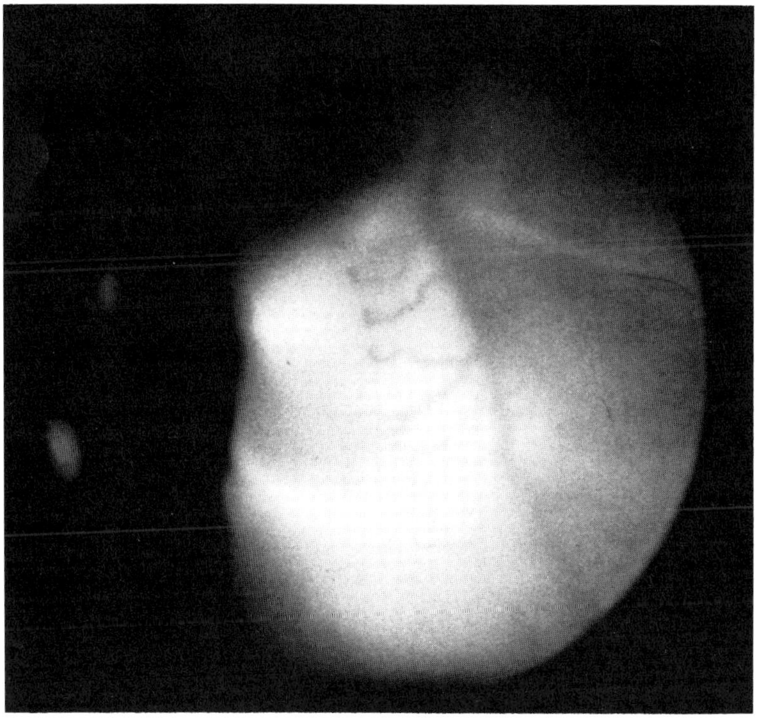

Fig. 9.7. Fetal face seen endoscopically at 8 conceptional weeks of gestation.

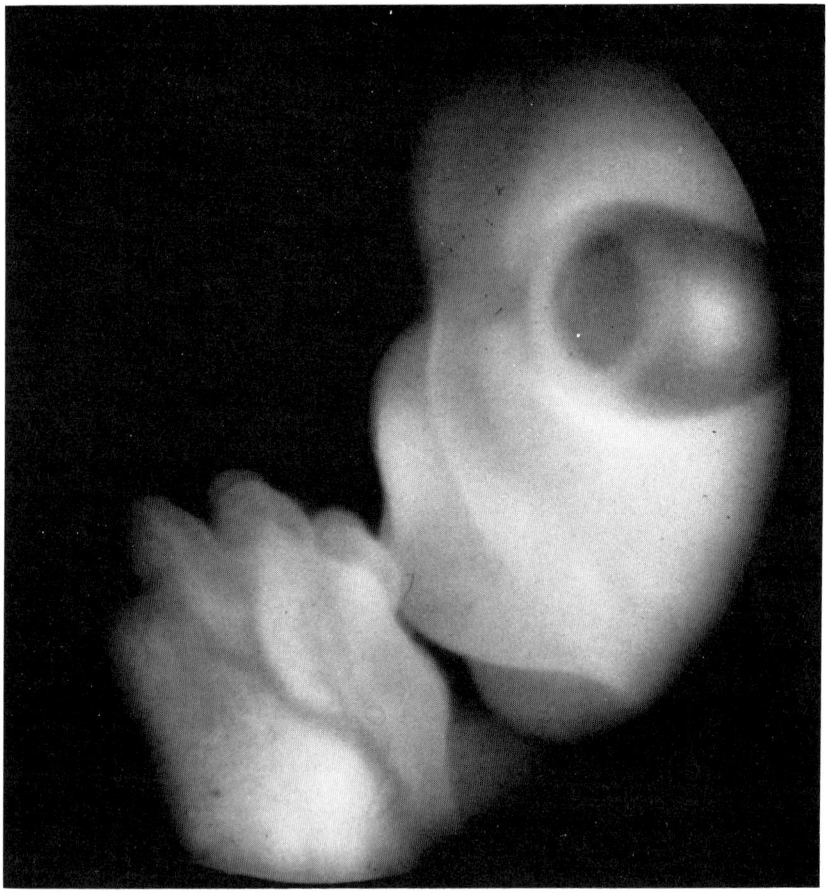

Fig. 9.8. Endoscopic view of fetal face at 10 conceptional weeks of gestation.

The eyes are initially located laterally and far from each other, but gradually this disproportion decreases as broadening of the head occurs (Hobbins and Mahoney 1974). Embryoscopy has the potential to diagnose hypertelorism and the absence of one or both eyes.

The ears develop around the first branchial groove and deepen to form the external meatus before shifting to a higher and more lateral position. Anomalies are often related to failure of upward shifting and also are potentially diagnosable using embryoscopy during early gestation.

The nose develops from a complex merging of the fronto-nasal bones with the maxillary processes; however, anomalies are not often seen.

The Trunk

The early embryo begins as a layered plate that undergoes infolding to produce a hollow cylinder, the trunk. In the dorsal region, the neural tube undergoes infolding to form a neural tube. The cephalic part of the neural tube rapidly

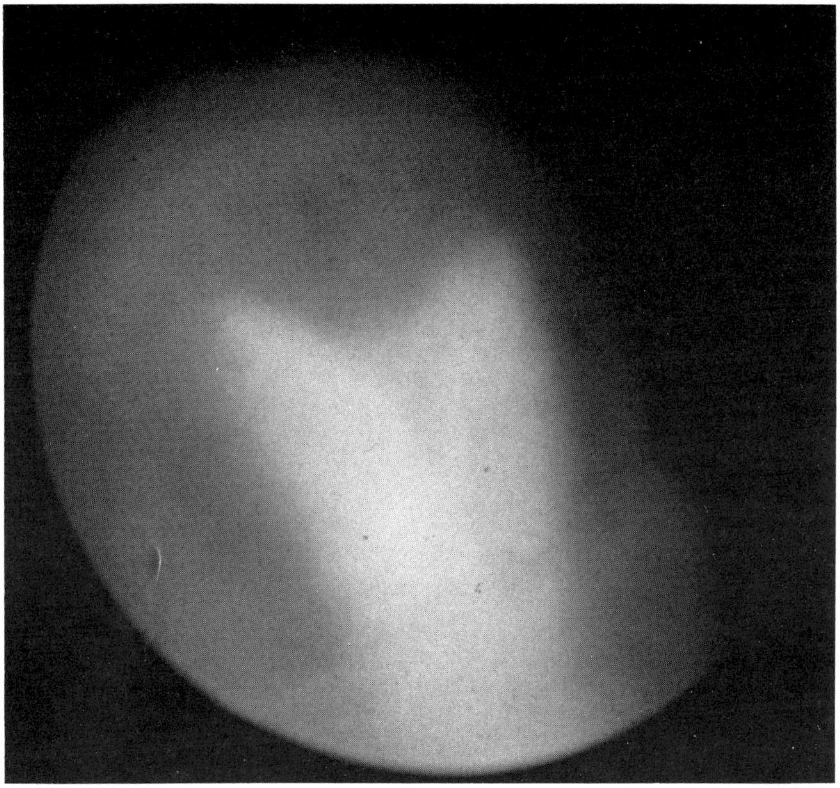

Fig. 9.9 The neural tube at 5 conceptional weeks of gestation with cephalic end open, seen via embryoscope.

grows to form the forebrain vesicle, the midbrain vesicle and the hindbrain vesicle. The ventricles are formed by the lumina of the neural tube. The future axial skeleton and muscles are represented by somites located in this dorsal region. Development of the internal organs adds to the form and shape of this cylinder (Hamilton et al. 1964; Moore 1988). Development of the gut occurs at a time when the abdominal cavity is still small; hence, herniation occurs in the body stalk at about 5 weeks. The gut remains extruded until about 10 weeks when reinsertion occurs followed by complete closure of the ventral wall.

These normal developmental events can be documented by embryoscopy. The neural tube is seen with the cephalic end open at about 5 conceptional weeks of gestation (Fig. 9.9); but by 7 conceptional weeks, there is complete closure of the neural tube (Fig. 9.10). The ventral hernia is seen as early as 4 conceptional weeks (Fig. 9.11); and by 8 conceptional weeks, the hernia is almost completely resolved (Fig. 9.12). Occasionally, the gut is seen to remain extruded after the 8th conceptional week.

Dorsal and ventral wall defects should also be diagnosable by embyoscopy. Anomalous development of the ventral wall can occur and may result from faulty wall closure resulting in gastroschisis or thoraco-gastroschisis with protrusion of the bowel and/or other organs. Omphalocele can be distinguished from

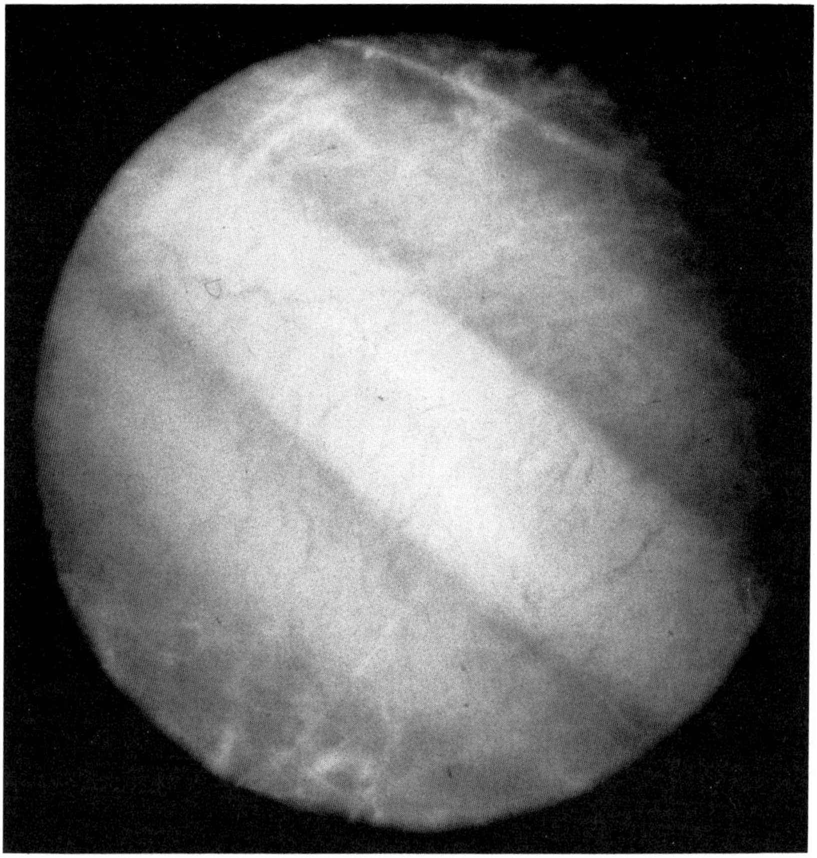

Fig. 9.10. Closed neural tube at 7 conceptional weeks gestation.

gastroschisis in that there is failed re-entry of the bowel contents from the body stalk. Faulty dorsal wall closure is associated with conditions such as spina bifida or rachischisis with or without herniation or neural elements (Moore 1988).

The Limbs

The normal development of limb buds is manifested first as lateral swellings or paddle-shaped structures in the late 4th conceptional week. Initially, arm buds are located far down on the body in the region of the lumbosacral somites. Flattening constrictions will demarcate foot and hand, leg and thigh, and forearm and arm regions. Hand-radial ridges, suggested by grooves, tell the location of digits. The lower limbs develop at a much slower rate. However, the thumbs and great toes separate early from the other digits in both upper and lower extremities. The upper limb buds appear first, develop first and attain normal appearance first. This disproportionate development is maintained until the second year of postnatal life when legs and arms become of equal length (Moore 1988).

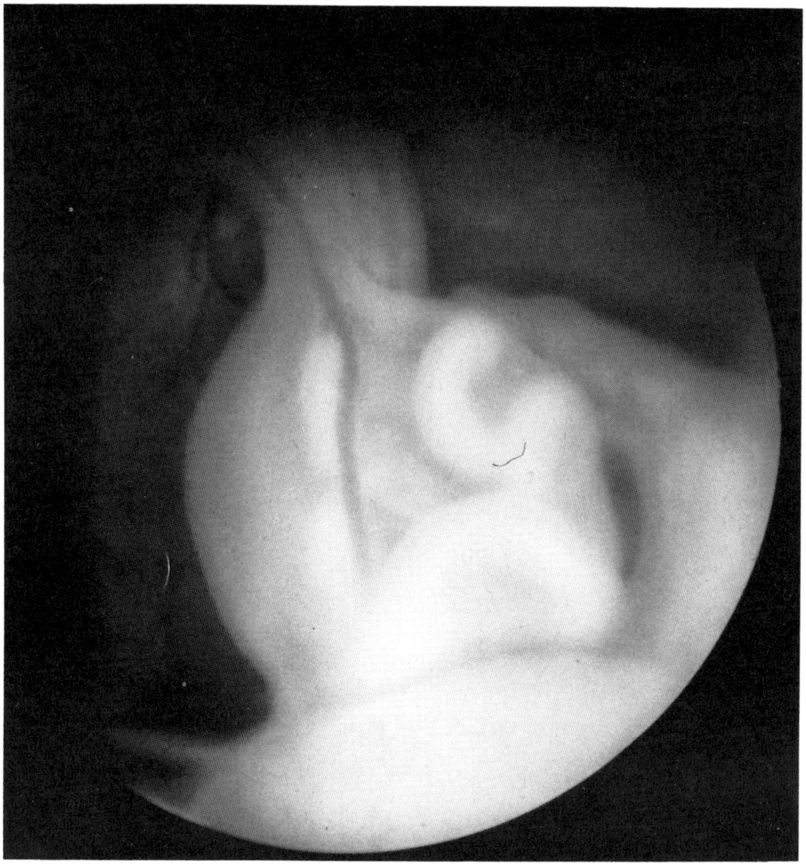

Fig. 9.11. Embryoscopic view of the ventral wall of embryo at 4 conceptional weeks depicting bowel in body stalk.

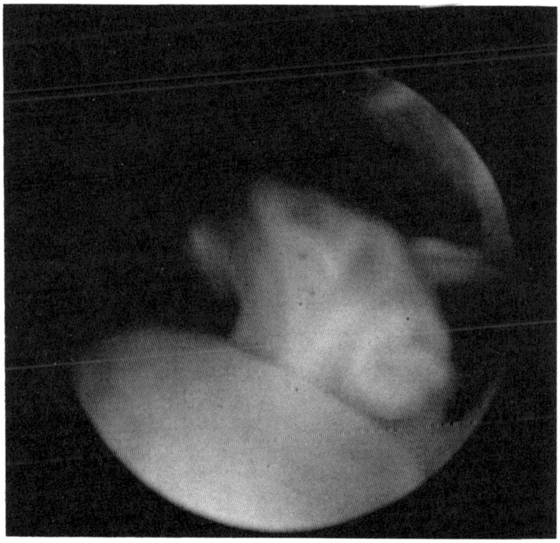

Fig. 9.12. Ventral wall of embryo at 8 conceptional weeks with hernia almost completely resolved, as seen via embryoscope.

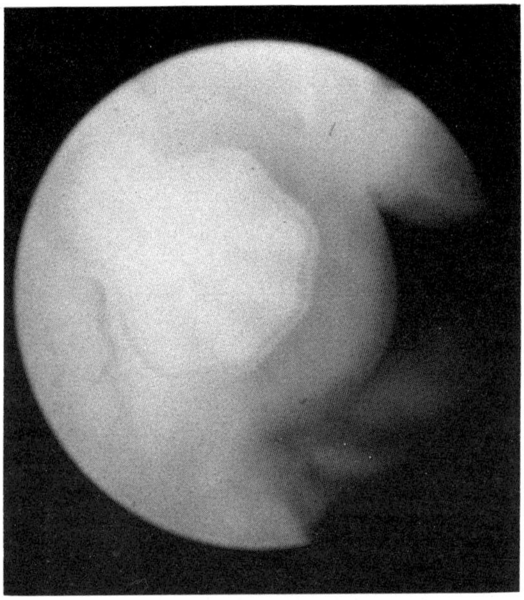

Fig. 9.13. Fetal hand seen endoscopically at 4 conceptional weeks gestation. Note the finger rays.

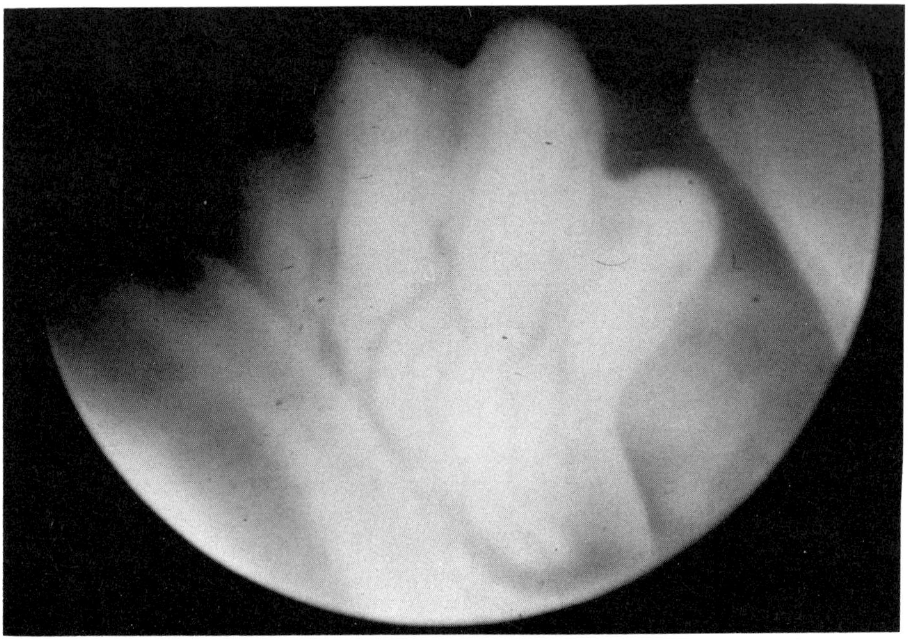

Fig. 9.14. Fetal hand with webbed fingers observed endoscopically at 6 conceptional weeks of gestation.

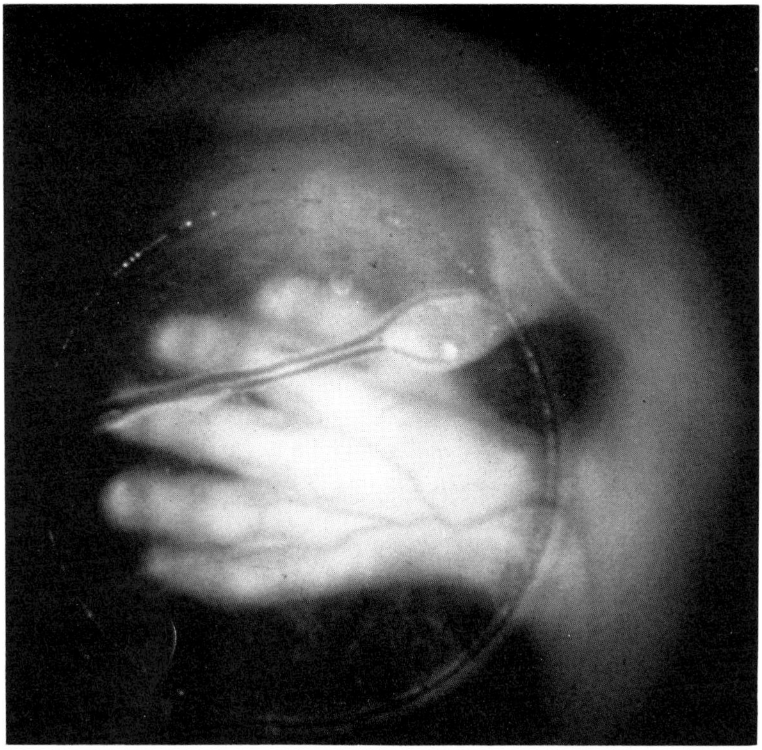

Fig. 9.15. Fully developed fetal hand observed endoscopically at 6 conceptional weeks of gestation.

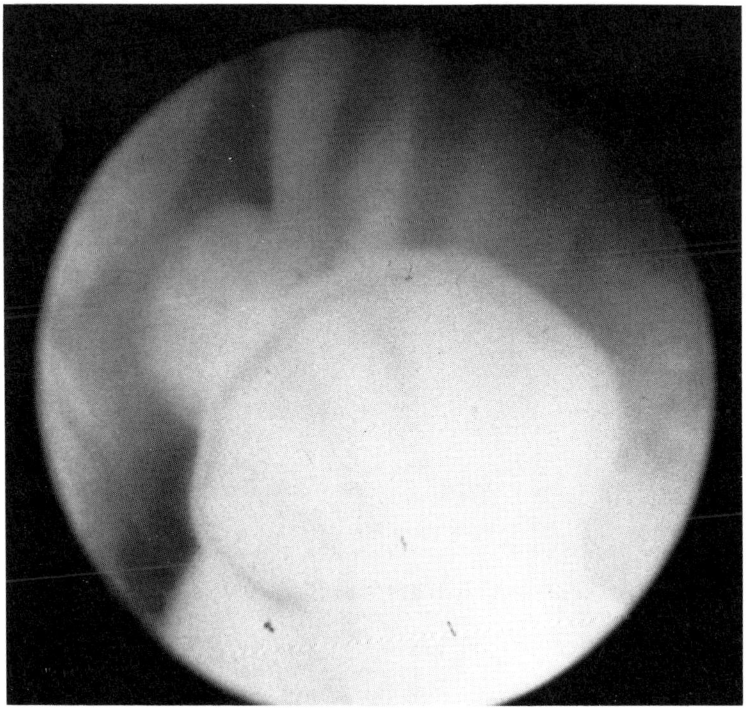

Fig. 9.16. Fetal foot seen via embryoscope at 7 conceptional weeks with toe rays.

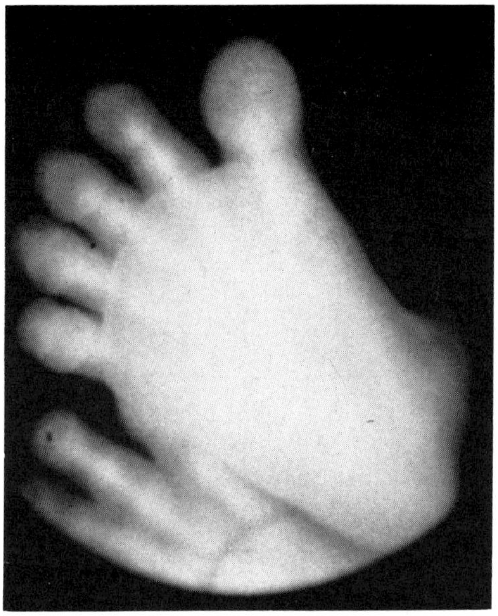

Fig. 9.17. Fully developed fetal foot at 9 conceptional weeks of gestation observed endoscopically.

Embryoscopy can once again document these normal events. The hand paddles are seen at 4 conceptional weeks with subtle demarcation of finger rays (Fig. 9.13); but by 6 conceptional weeks, webbed fingers are observed (Fig. 9.14). At 7 conceptional weeks, a fully developed hand is seen (Fig. 9.15). The developmental progression of the upper limbs can be as much as 2 weeks ahead of the lower extremities. For example, foot paddles and well-developed feet are seen 2 weeks later than the equivalent in the upper extremities – 6 and 8 conceptional weeks respectively (Figs. 9.16 and 9.17).

Embryoscopic visualization should show certain limb anomalies early in gestation such as hemimelia, phocomelia, sirenomelia, missing digits, lobster claw, polydactyly, syndactyly, brachydactyly, or club hand or foot (Moore 1988).

Other Structures

The yolk sac provides blood cells, gonadocytes, and epithelia for the digestive and respiratory tracts. After the yolk sac invaginates and contributes to the midgut, the extruded remnant of the yolk sac is non-functional.

Embryoscopically, the early yolk sac has a confluent and prominent vasculature (Fig. 9.18) in contrast to the yolk sac observed at 10 conceptional weeks where the blood vessels are smaller, more numerous and less prominent (Fig. 9.19). Anomalous development of the yolk sac has been described experimentally and has been associated with embryonic malformation (Pinter et al. 1986; Reece et al. 1985; 1989). These experiments were conducted during organogenesis. Clinical studies have examined the yolk sac after organogenesis (Reece et al. 1988). Embryoscopy will allow better information on the correlation between yolk sac and embryo development.

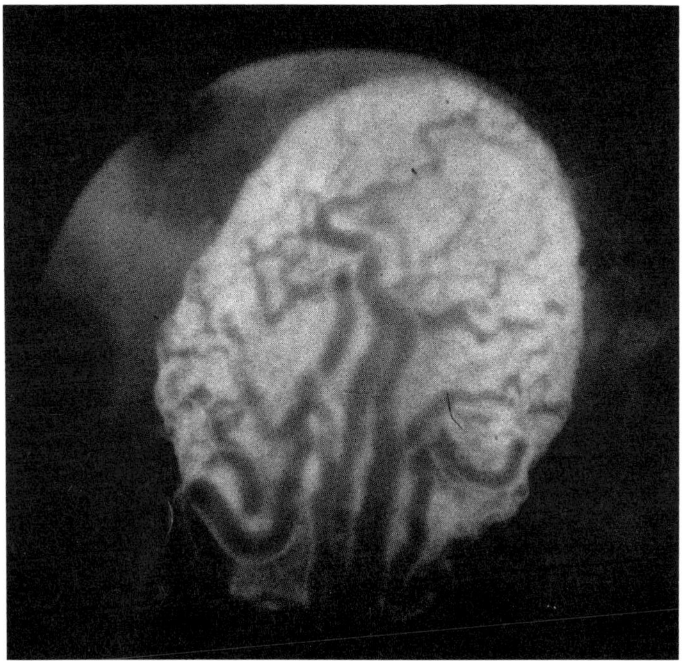

Fig. 9.18. The yolk sac at 6 conceptional weeks with prominent vasculature.

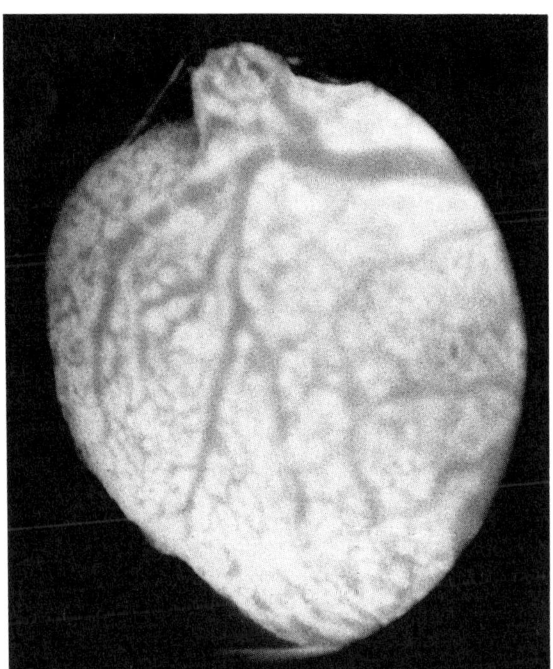

Fig. 9.19. The yolk sac at 10 conceptional weeks with minute and less prominent vessels.

Confirmation of Early Sonographic Prenatal Diagnosis

With the continued improvement in high-resolution ultrasound equipment, prenatal diagnosis has been extended to the early second trimester. When congenital anomalies are diagnosed and patients choose to undergo pregnancy termination, pathological confirmation and anatomic study are precluded following a destructive procedure. But verification of prenatally diagnosed anomalies is vital to ensure accurate patient counselling in subsequent pregnancies. Embryoscopy is now used to obtain a direct view of the embryo prior to evacuation and gives the opportunity for photographic documentation of the findings. This technology can document anomalies not recognized by ultrasound and confirms those abnormalities already identified sonographically.

The Future

Embryoscopic examination with the potential for embryonic therapy is an extension of existing diagnostic techniques as well as the beginning of a new era of first-trimester intervention. Fetal tissue sampling and gene therapy are future goals to which embryoscopy can be applied.

Tissue Sampling

First-trimester diagnosis of genetic diseases by organ tissue retrieval and/or embryonic blood sampling appear within reach. The evolution of techniques using gene probes for DNA analysis makes embryoscopy an attractive possibility for early prenatal diagnosis.

Diagnosis can be performed on the trophoblast via chorionic villus sampling between 9 and 12 menstrual weeks of gestation. However in almost 1% of cases, an additional fetal sample, such as fetal blood, is necessary to clarify initial aberrant chromosomal findings. In many cases such evaluation cannot be performed until the second trimester. Embryoscopic blood sampling in the first trimester may soon be feasible and would obviate this anxiety-laden period. Additional indications for fetal blood sampling include rapid prenatal diagnosis after the first trimester or early fetal blood typing in a mother with isoimmunization.

Gene Therapy

Rapid progress is being made toward human gene therapy (Anderson 1984; 1985). If this concept becomes a reality, embryoscopy will allow access to the human embryo at a time when it is immunologically "naive" and may therefore be receptive to grafts.

Embryoscopy opens a new era in fetal medicine. In the future more emphasis will be placed on the first trimester with direct biopsy of the embryo or the placenta, as in chorionic villus sampling, rather than on the amniotic fluid and fetus in the second and third trimesters. Embryoscopy should provide access to the entire conceptus, permitting both early diagnosis as well as the potential for early treatment. However, ethical questions will undoubtedly arise and will have to be addressed before the full potential of embryoscopy in fetal medicine is realized.

References

Anderson WF (1984) Prospects for human gene therapy. Science 226: 401

Anderson WF (1985) Human gene therapy: scientific and ethical considerations. J Med Phil 10: 275

Arey LB (1974) Developmental anatomy, 7th edn (revised). WB Saunders, Philadelphia

Beard RW, Filshie GM, Knight CA, Roberts GM (1979) The significance of the changes in the continuous fetal heart rates in the first stage of labor. J Obstet Gynaecol Br Cmwlth 78: 865

Bulic M, Podobnik M, et al. (1987) First trimester diagnosis of low obstructive uropathy. An indication of initial renal function of the fetus. J Clin Ultrasound 6: 715

Cullen MT, Reece EA, Viscarello RR, Hobbins JC (1989a) Transcervical endoscopic visualization of prenatally diagnosed anomalies prior to second trimester termination. Proc annual meeting of the society of gynecologic investigation, March 1989

Cullen MT, Reece EA, Whetham J, Hobbins JC (1989b) Embryoscopy: description and utility of a new technique. Am J Obstet Gynecol 162: 82–86

Curtish JA, Watson L, (1988) Sonographic diagnosis of omphalocele in the first trimester of fetal gestation. J Ultrasound Med 7: 97

Dumez Y (1988) Embryoscopy and congenital malformations. Proc international conference on chorionic villus sampling and early prenatal diagnosis, May 28–29, Athens, Greece

Galliant A, Lueken RP, Lindermann HJ (1978) New instruments and new methods. A preliminary report about transcervical embryoscopy. Endoscopy 10: 47

Green JJ, Hobbins JC (1988) Abdominal ultrasound of the first trimester fetus. Am J Obstet Gynecol 159: 165

Hamilton WJ, Boyd JD, Mossman HW (1964) Human embryology, 3rd edn. W. Heffer & Sons Ltd, Cambridge

Hill LM, Thomas ML, et al. (1988) Sonographic assessment of the first trimester fetus. A cautionary note. Am J Perinatol. 5: 13

Hobbins JC, Mahoney MJ (1974) Progress toward in utero diagnosis of hemoglobinopathies: technique for obtaining fetal blood. N Engl J Med 290: 1065–1067

Hobbins JC, Grannum PAT, Berkowitz RL, et al. (1979) Ultrasound in the diagnosis of congenital anomalies. Am J Obstet Gynecol 134: 331

Hobbins JC, Grannum PAT, Romero R, Reece EA (1985) Percutaneous umbilical blood sampling. Am J Obstet Gynecol 152: 1–6

Hogge WA, Schomberg SA, Golbus MS (1986) Chorionic villus sampling: experience of the first 1000 cases. Am J Obstet Gynecol 154: 2349

Hon EH (1968) An atlas of fetal heart rate patterns. Harty Press, New Haven, CT

Hon EH, Quilligan EJ (1967) The classification of fetal heart rate. Conn Med 31: 779

Mahoney MJ, Hobbins JC (1977) Prenatal diagnosis of chondroectodermal dysplasia (Ellis-Van Creveld Syndrome) with fetoscopy and ultrasound. N Engl J Med 297: 258

Manning FA, Hill LM, Platt LD (1981) Qualitative amniotic fluid volume determination by ultrasound: antepartum detection of intrauterine growth retardation. Am J Obstet Gynecol 139: 254

Manning FA, Lange FR, Morrison J, Harman CR (1983) Determination of fetal health: methods for antepartum and intrapartum fetal assessment. Curr Prob Obstet Gynecol 7: 1

Martin AO, Simpson JL, Rosinsky B, et al. (1986) Chorionic villus sampling in continuing pregnancies. II. Cytogenetic reliability. Am J Obstet Gynecol 154: 1353

Moore KL (1988) The developing human. Clinically oriented embryology, 4th edn. WB Saunders, Philadelphia

Pinter E, Reece EA, Leranth CZ, et al. (1986) Yolk sac failure in embryopathy due to hyperglycemia. An ultrastructural analysis of the yolk sac differentiation associated with embryopathy in rat conceptuses under hyperglycemic conditions. Teratology 33: 363–374

Reece EA, Pinter E, Leranth CZ, et al. (1985) Ultrastructural analysis of malformations of the embryonic neural axis induced by hyperglycemic conceptus culture. Teratology 32: 363–374

Reece EA, Scioscia AL, Pinter E, et al. (1988) Prognostic significance of the human yolk sac assessed by ultrasonography. Am J Obstet Gynecol 1598: 1191–1194

Reece EA, Pinter E, Leranth CZ, et al. (1989) Yolk sac failure in embryopathy due to hyperglycemia: horseradish peroxidase uptake in the assessment of yolk sac dysfunction. Obstet Gynecol 74: 755–762

Romero R, Pilu G, Jeanty P, Ghidini A, Hobbins JC (1987) Prenatal diagnosis of congenital anomalies. Appleton & Lange, Norwalk, CT

Roume J, Aubry MC, Labbe F, Dumez Y, Aubry JP, Henrion R (1985) Prenatal diagnosis of limb and digital abnormalities. Evaluation of the activity of the Port Royal University Clinic from 1979 to 1983. J Genet Hum 33: 457–461

Sievers S, Hagenbusch M, Eckert M (1983) Management of pregnant women with thalassemia minor. Fortschr Med 101: 687–688

Vergani P, Ghidini A, et al. (1987) Antenatal diagnosis of fetal acrania. J Ultrasound Med 6: 715

10. Sexing the Pre-embryo

J.D. West

Preimplantation Diagnosis

The advent of therapeutic procedures for infertility, such as in vitro fertilization (IVF) and gamete intrafallopian transfer (GIFT), has allowed access to the preimplantation stages of human development. These early embryos or pre-embryos (McLaren 1986) have only a small number of cells (between one and several hundred) but each cell is genetically identical to any cell of the later conceptus. As such the pre-embryo is potentially a source of cells for prenatal diagnostic tests of human genetic diseases. The possibility of very early prenatal diagnosis (preimplantation diagnosis) has been considered for several years (McLaren 1985; Penketh and McLaren 1987; West et al. 1987; Monk 1988; West 1989; Handyside et al. 1989) and we now stand on the brink of the first clinical applications.

Human pre-embryos are now routinely cultured to the 4–6 cell stage during the course of IVF and later stages (e.g. blastocysts) can be flushed from the reproductive tract and returned for implantion into the uterus (e.g. Buster et al. 1985). If one or more cells could be safely removed from such a pre-embryo without compromising the pre-embryo's potential for further development it would be possible to carry out prenatal diagnosis at the preimplantation stage. It would then be possibe to transfer to the uterus only those pre-embryos that were not genetically affected, thus avoiding the need for therapeutic abortion of affected conceptuses identified at later stages of development. Realization of this technique requires

1. The development of a safe method of removing a cell (or cells) from human pre-embryos.
2. The use of cryopreservation of pre-embryos if the genetic test takes several days (such methods are now available and would enable unaffected pre embryos to be transferred to the patient at an appropriate time in a subsequent menstrual cycle).
3. The development of genetic tests that are accurate and sufficiently sensitive for a reliable diagnosis.

Recent experiments suggest that pre-embryos could be biopsied either by removing a portion of trophectoderm that is induced to herniate through the overlying zona pellucida (Papaioannou 1986; Summers et al. 1988) or by dislodging a cell from a pre-embryo at about the 8-cell stage (Handyside et al. 1989) and this is discussed fully in another chapter. Several types of genetic test are now being evaluated for use in preimplantation diagnosis. These include chromsome analysis (e.g. Angell et al. 1988), biochemical assays (e.g. Monk 1988) and molecular tests involving either in situ hybridization (West et al. 1987, 1988; Jones et al. 1987; Penketh et al. 1989) or amplification of target DNA by the polymerase chain reaction (Handyside et al. 1989; Coutelle et al. 1989). This chapter will consider possible tests for distinguishing between male and female pre-embryos. Other molecular tests will be discussed in another chapter.

Reasons for Sexing the Pre-embryo

Identification of male and female pre-embryos by preimplantation diagnosis would allow the selection of female pre-embryos to be returned to the mother for further development in cases where only males were at risk for an X-linked genetic disease. This would then avoid the conception of affected sons. In time, highly sensitive specific tests, suitable for preimplantation diagnosis, will undoubtedly become available for many X-linked genetic disorders. For these disorders, use of the specific test would allow both female and unaffected male pre-embryos to be identified and returned to the reproductive tract.

Possible Methods of Sexing the Pre-embryo

The usual method of distinguishing between a male and female conceptus is by cytogenetic analysis of metaphase chromosomes to determine whether a Y chromosome is present. This karyotypic analysis is a routine prenatal diagnostic procedure and yields a wealth of information in addition to chromosomal sex. Although several weeks are required (for cell culture) this is a very reliable means of sexing the fetus. However, karyotyping is dependant on having good quality metaphase preparations and this would be very difficult to achieve routinely when the test sample comprised only a small number of cells. For this reason other techniques would probably have to be used for preimplantation diagnosis of sex.

A number of alternative methods, that do not require metaphase preparations, are available for sexing the conceptus. These either detect the two X chromosomes in female cells or identify the presence of the Y chromosome in males.

The sex chromatin method depends on the presence of visible sex chromatin (Barr body) after the inactivation of one of the two X chromosomes in XX female cells. Unfortunately this method is unreliable because only about 30% of XX cells have identifiable sex chromatin and it is possible to confuse other chromatin with sex chromatin in interphase nuclei. In any case, this method is unsuitable for pre-embryos before the time of X-chromosome inactivation.

The long arm of the human Y chromosome (Yq) has a region that can be seen to fluoresce by ultraviolet microscopy, after treatment with quinacrine dihydrochloride or spermidine *bis*-acridine. Fluorescent spots (F-bodies) can be seen in interphase nuclei and these have been used to identify the presence of the Y chromosome in interphase nuclei. Unfortunately, this again is not sufficiently reliable for routine purposes both because some men have Y chromosomes that lack the fluorescent region (false negatives) and fluorescent polymorphisms of autosomes exist that could produce false positives.

DNA sequences present on the X or, more usually, the Y chromosome can be used to distinguish between a male and a female conceptus without the need for dividing cells. DNA extracted from the test sample and hybridized to a Y chromosome-specific probe by Southern blot or dot blot hybridization provides a reliable method of identifying males (e.g. Gosden et al. 1984) and the introduction of the polymerase chain reaction for amplifying specific target DNA sequences makes this approach feasible with single-cell samples (e.g. Saiki et al. 1988; Handyside et al. 1989; discussed below). The presence of highly reiterated chromosome-specific DNA sequences provides a large target for hybridization and this means that it is also possible to use DNA-DNA in situ hybridization to identify the Y chromosome in interphase nuclei spread on a microscope slide. This offers a second feasible approach to sexing the pre-embryo when only a small number of cells are available.

A third approach makes use of the potential 2 : 1 difference in the amount of X chromosome-linked gene products before X chromosome inactivation occurs in the females. This approach is not useful for more conventional prenatal diagnosis because X chromosome inactivation is thought to occur around the time of implantation (as in the mouse) and would be completed well before cells are sampled, by chorionic villus biopsy or amniocentesis. With certain X-linked gene products, this approach provides a possible means of distinguishing male and female pre-embryos although there are considerable technical difficulties.

Three possible approaches to sexing the human pre-embryo (quantitative assays of X-linked gene products, in situ hybridization and polymerase chain reaction) are discussed below.

Sexing by Quantitative Biochemical Assays of X-linked Gene Products

In order for biochemical sexing to be feasible, the gene product must be assayed at a time when the residual oocyte-coded activity is insignificant compared to the embryo-coded activity but before X chromosome inactivation. This is not a trivial requirement and in order to judge whether this approach is feasible it is relevant to consider the theoretical problems and the experimental results with mouse embryos in some detail.

Figure 10.1 shows two hypothetical situations. In the first case (Fig. 10.1a) the oocyte-coded activity is low and the embryo-coded activity rises rapidly. By the morula and early blastocyst stage the expected activity in females (two X chromosomes active) is twice that in males (one X active) but by the late blastocyst stage this difference is reducd because X-inactivation in many cells of the female

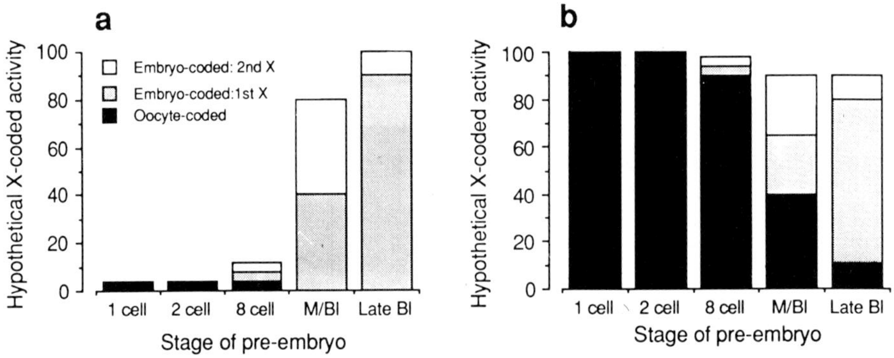

Fig. 10.1. Hypothetical changes in activity of an X-linked gene product during preimplantation development (M is morula and Bl is blastocyst). The shading distinguishes oocyte-coded activity and embryo-coded activity resulting from transcription of genes on both X chromosomes. The total activity expected in male pre-embryos (1 X chromosome) is shown by the black plus grey shading and the expected activity in females (2 X chromosomes) is shown by the total height of the bar (black plus grey plus white). **a** The oocyte-coded activity is low and the embryo-coded activity rises rapidly. By the morula and early blastocyst stage the expected activity in females (two X chromosomes active) is twice that in males (one X active) but by the late blastocyst this difference is reduced because X-inactivation in many cells of the female reduces the effective dose to a single X chromosome. **b** The oocyte-coded activity is high and persists for longer. In this case there is no time at which measurements of X-linked activity would provide a reliable prediction of the sex of a pre-embryo.

reduces the effective dose to a single X chromosome. (In reality, the situation is likely to be more complex because, for assays at the protein level, there will be a lag between transcription and a measurable increase in activity and also a lag between X-inactivation and a measurable decrease in activity per cell. Assay variation and variation in the rate of embryonic development may also cause problems.) In the second case (Fig. 10.1b) the oocyte-coded activity is high and persists for longer. The embryo-coded activity increases during preimplantation development but the expected activity in females is never twice that in males

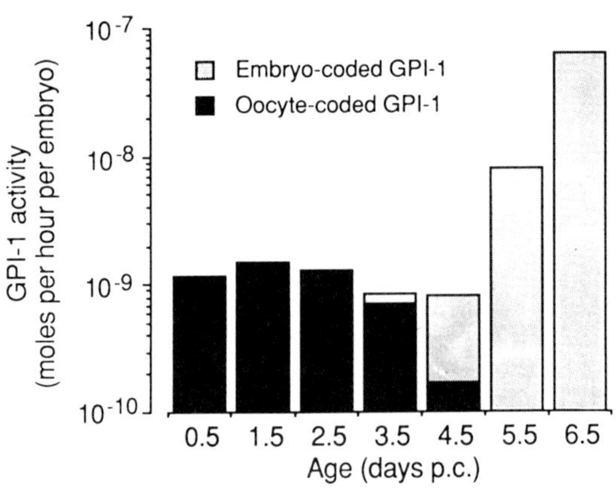

Fig. 10.2. Changes in oocyte-coded and embryo-coded activity of the autosomal-coded enzyme glucose phosphate isomerase during the preimplantation (0.5 to 4.5 days) and early postimplantation (5.5 and 6.5 days) stages of mouse development. (Redrawn from West et al. 1986.)

because significant levels of oocyte activity remain until X-inactivation reduces the 2 : 1 (female : male) activity ratio below a measurable difference. In this case there is no time at which measurements of X-coded activity would provide a reliable prediction of the sex of a pre-embryo.

For most enzymes we know little about the relative contributions of oocyte- and embryo-coded enzymes during preimplantation development but for some enzymes that have genetically determined electrophoretic variants (allozymes) something is known. Fig. 10.2 shows the relative activities of oocyte- and embryo-coded glucose phosphate isomerase (GPI-1) in mouse pre-embryos during the preimplantation (0.5–4.5 days) and early postimplantation (5.5 and 6.5 days) periods of development. This shows a situation with relatively high levels of oocyte-coded enzyme persisting to the blastocyst stage, rather similar to the hypothetical case shown in Fig. 10.1b. However, GPI-1 is encoded by an autosomal gene and we need to know about products of X-linked genes.

Several enzymes are known to be encoded by genes on the X chromosome in man, mouse and other mammals. Experimental studies of X-coded enzymes in mouse pre-embryos have laid the foundations to the development of methods that may be applicable to sexing the human pre-embryo. Fig. 10.3 shows the

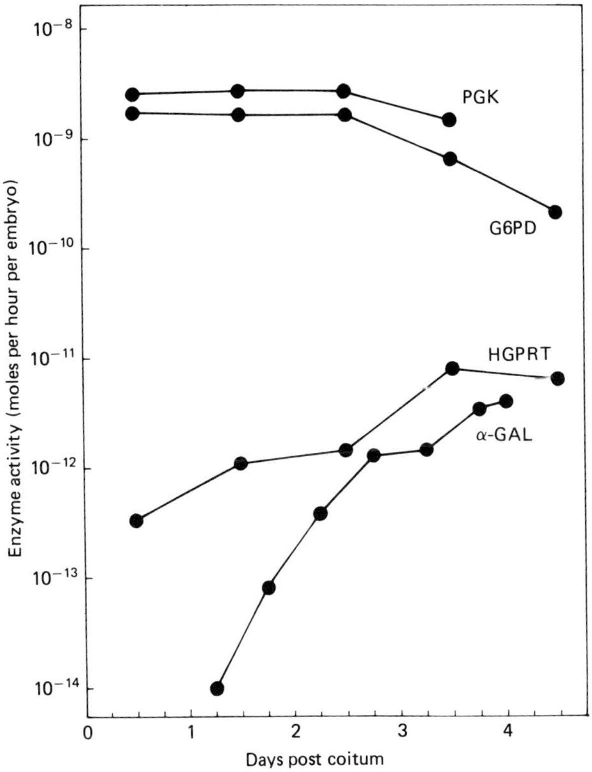

Fig. 10.3. The changes in total enzyme activity per pre-embryo for four X chromosome-coded enzymes during mouse preimplantation development (reproduced from West, 1982 with permission). PGK, phosphoglycerate kinase; G6PD, glucose-6-phosphate dehydrogenase; HGPRT, hypoxanthine guanine phosphoribosyltransferase; alpha-GAL alpha-galactosidase.

change in activity of four such enzymes during preimplantation mouse development. The activities of two of these enzymes (glucose-6-phosphate dehydrogenase (G6PD) and phosphoglycerate kinase (PGK)) are initially relatively high and remain stable or perhaps decline slightly during preimplantation development, in a pattern similar to the autosomal enzyme GPI-1 (Fig. 10.2).

The activities of the other two enzymes (alpha-galactosidase and hypoxanthine guanine phosphoribosyltransferase (HGPRT or HPRT)) are initially low but increase rapidly during preimplantation development. In addition, comparison of HGPRT activities between pre-embryos from XX and XO mothers has shown that by the 9–16 cell morula stage the HGPRT activity is embryo-coded (Epstein 1972; Monk and Harper 1978) but that significant levels of oocyte-coded HGPRT remain in 8-cell pre-embryos (Monk and Harper 1978). Although the relative contributions of oocyte- and embryo-coded activity is not known for alpha-galactosidase, alpha-galactosidase and HGPRT both increase rapidly during the preimplantation period (Fig. 10.3) and these two enzymes seem the most likely to provide a "developmental window" when the enzyme activity in female pre-embryos is close to double that in males (as in the hypothetical example shown in Fig. 10.1a).

In the 1970s a number of studies of X-linked enzymes were undertaken, in order to confirm that both X chromosomes were initially active in female mammalian pre-embryos and to try to determine when X chromosome inactivation occurs. The general approach was to assay the activity of an X-coded enzyme in a large number of pre-embryos and plot the distribution of activities at different stages of development. A bimodal distribution of enzyme activities was expected if both of the X chromosomes in the cells of female pre-embryos were active and the X-linked gene encoding the relevant enzyme was transcriptionally active. The two peaks of activity would represent male and female pre-embryos respectively.

No bimodal distributions were seen for G6PD in preimplantation mouse and rabbit pre-embryos (Brinster 1970) or for PGK in 4.5 day mouse pre-embryos (Kozak and Quinn 1975). However, these two enzymes do not increase in activity during preimplantation mouse development (Fig. 10.3) and it is likely that X chromosome inactivation begins before significant levels of embryo-coded activity are produced and perhaps before the relevant embryonic genes are activated. In contrast, bimodal distributions of alpha-galactosidase and HGPRT have been reported as discussed below.

Mouse Alpha-galactosidase and HGPRT

Bimodal distributions of alpha-galactosidase activity were found for groups of 8-cell and morula stage pre-embryos (Adler et al. 1977; Chapman et al. 1977, 1978) as shown in Fig. 10.4. Bimodal distributions were not usually seen at the 2-cell, 4-cell or blastocyst stage, nor were bimodal distributions seen at any stage of preimplantation development for the autosomally encoded enzymes ß-glucuronidase (Wudl and Chapman 1976; Wudl and Sherman 1976) and ß-galactosidase (Fig. 10.5) that also increase in activity during preimplantation development. The activity of alpha-galactosidase per cell increased to the morula stage and then declined between the morula and blastocyst stages. These results

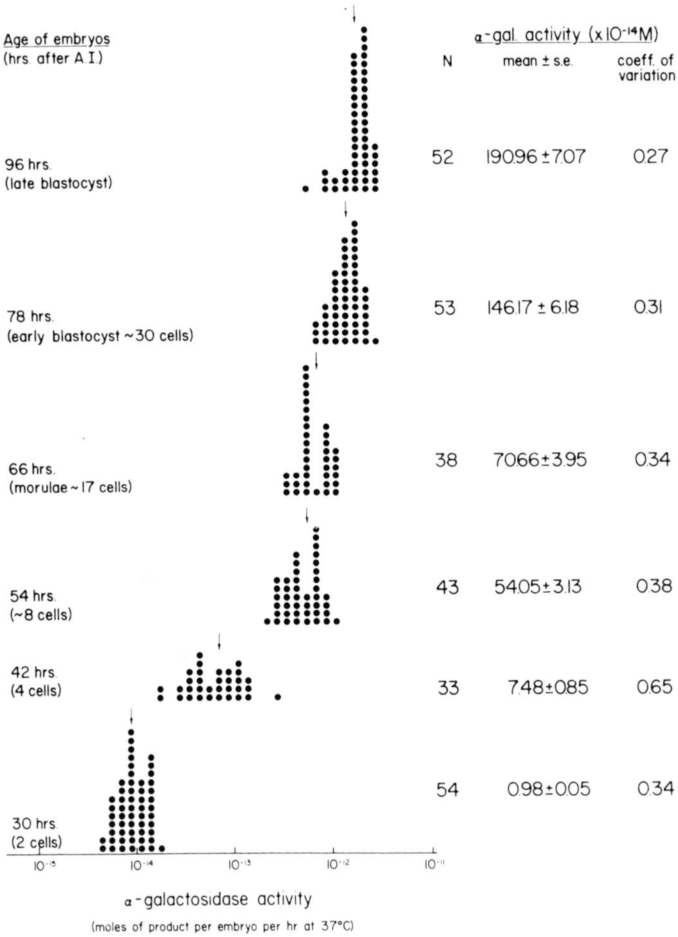

Fig. 10.4. Distributions of alpha-galactosidase activity per mouse pre-embryo from the 2-cell to blastocyst stage. Times shown are hours after artificial insemination and the stages of development are 2-cell (30 hrs), 4-cell (42 hrs), 8-cell (54 hrs), morula of about 17 cells (66 hrs), early blastocyst of about 30 cells (78 hrs) and late blastocyst of about 60 cells or more (96 hrs). Each symbol represents a single pre-embryo. Assay conditions were those given in Adler et al. (1977) except that the assay temperature was 37°C. (The data are from an experiment performed in 1976 by D.A. Adler, J.D. West and V.M. Chapman and are contemporaneous with experiments published by Adler et al. (1977) and Chapman et al. (1977, 1978). These data have not previously been published and are published with permission of Dr. V.M. Chapman.

suggested that both X-chromosomes were active in 8-cell and morula stage pre-embryos and that X-inactivation may have begun by the blastocyst stage. A large number of experiments were performed and although bimodal distributions were usually found at the 8-cell stage and morula stage, in some experiments the distributions were not clearly bimodal. This probably reflects the biological variation in the rate of preimplantation development.

Two laboratories reported similar experiments with mouse HGPRT. The first report (Monk and Kathuria 1977) focused on the 8-cell and blastocyst stages and

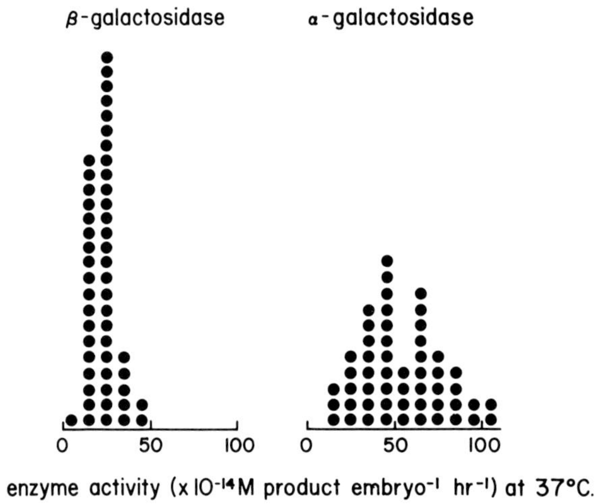

Fig. 10.5. Distributions of alpha-galactosidase and beta-galactosidase activity per 8-cell mouse pre-embryo (54 hours after artificial insemination). Pre-embryos were randomly allocated to either alpha-galactosidase or beta-galactosidase assays. (The data are from an experiment performed in 1976 by D.A. Adler, J.D. West and V.M. Chapman and are contemporaneous with experiments published by Adler et al [1977] and Chapman et al. [1977, 1978]. These data have not previously been published and are published with permission of Dr. V.M. Chapman.)

concluded that the results were not consistent with a bimodal distribution. Monk and Kathuria (1977) measured the autosomal enzyme adenosine phosphoribosyl transferase (APRT) and the X-coded enzyme HGPRT in the same embryos. Since both enzymes increase in activity at a similar rate during preimplantation development, the APRT activity was used to standardize for developmental variability and variability in extraction of the cytoplasmic content. This technical improvement allowed the results to be expressed as HGPRT activity and as the HGPRT : APRT ratio. However bimodality was not apparent for either HGPRT or the HGPRT : APRT ratio at the 8-cell or blastocyst stage.

Subsequent experiments by Monk and colleagues (Monk 1978a, b; Monk and Harper 1978) did reveal bimodal distributions at the morua stage (but not at the 8-cell or blastocyst stages). Kratzer and Gartler (1978a, b) carried out similar experiments and reported bimodal distributions of NGPRT at the 8-cell, morula and early to mid-blastocyst stages but not at the 4- to 8-cell stage or at the very late blastocyst stage. Although both groups found bimodal distributions there were some differences in the stages involved. Kratzer and Gartler found the distribution at the 8-cell and mid-blastocyst stages more convincingly bimodal than at the stages in between whereas Monk and her colleagues found the most convincing bimodal distributions at the morula stage.

Epstein et al. (1978a, b) took the analysis a stage further. They separated the two cells of 2-cell stage pre-embryos and cultured each half for 2.5 days to the blastocyst stage. (Both halves formed blastocysts in 71% of the pre-embryos.) For each pair of half-blastocysts, one half was frozen individually for later assay and the other half karyotyped to determine the sex of the pre-embryo. (Interpretable karyotypes were obtained from 47% of the half-blastocysts.) Groups of five half pre-embryos of the same sex were then pooled and assayed for HGPRT or APRT. The results (Fig. 10.6) demonstrated that females had

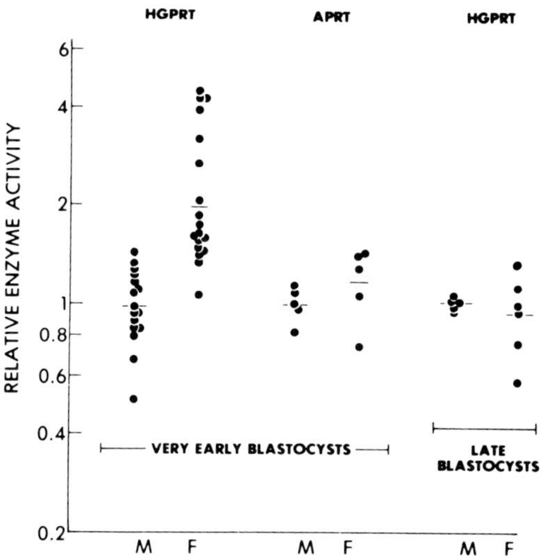

Fig. 10.6. HGPRT and APRT activities in very early and in late half-blastocysts of known sex. Each symbol represents the HGPRT or APRT activity in a group of 5 pooled half-blastocysts as described in the text. (Reproduced with permission from Epstein et al. [1978].)

approximately twice as much HGPRT as males at the very early blastocyst stage but the APRT activities were similar in both sexes. By the late blastocyst stage HGPRT levels were also similar in males and females. This confirmed the interpretation that the bimodal distributions of HGPRT (and presumably alpha-galactosidase) reflected a 2 : 1 enzyme activity difference between female and male pre-embryos.

More recently Monk and Handyside (1988) have tested whether HGPRT activity in a single cell removed from a mouse pre-embryo could accurately predict the morphological sex of the fetus. They isolated single blastomeres from zona-free 8-cell pre-embryos and cultured them for 12 hours. (In this time the sample would probably have divided to form two cells and the whole pre-embryo would have been equivalent to the 16-cell stage.) The biopsied cells were assayed for HGPRT and APRT and the sex of each pre-embryo (now at the blastocyst stage) was decided from the distribution of HGPRT : APRT activities in the biopsied samples for all of the pre-embryos in a litter of 40 (Fig. 10.7). Putative male and female pre-embryos were surgically transferred to separate recipient females and 15

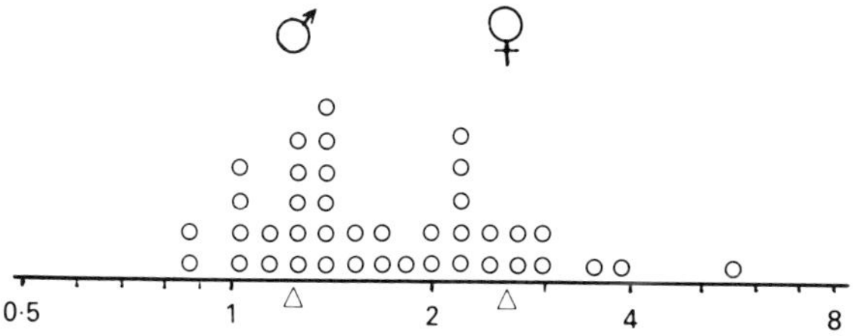

Fig. 10.7. Bimodal distribution of the HGPRT : APRT activity ratios in samples derived from biopsies of single blastomeres from mouse pre-embryos from a single litter. Each symbol represents the HGPRT : APRT ratio in a single biopsied sample. (Reproduced with permission from Monk and Handyside (1988).

fetuses were recovered on the 15th day of gestation and sexed by gonad morphology. The correct gonadal sex was predicted in 14 of the 15 fetuses examined.

This provided a possible model for preimplantation diagnosis of sex of human pre-embryos. If the developmental profile of HGPRT is similar in mouse and human pre-embryos, the biopsy could be performed at the 8-cell stage and the assay performed the following day. There would be no need for cryopreservation of the pre-embryos if transfers could be done at the blastocyst stage. However, present indications are that it may be preferable to transfer earlier stage pre-embryos (see p. 160) in which case cryopreservation would be needed.

Prospects for Sexing Human Pre-embryos with X-linked Gene Products

The above discussion of mouse pre-embryos shows that there is a "developmental window" between the 8-cell and blastocyst stages when female and male pre-embryos have different levels of HGPRT and probably also alpha-galactosidase. If a similar "developmental window" exists in human pre-embryos then it may also be possible to use biochemical assays of HGPRT or alpha-galactosidase to distinguish between male and female pre-embryos. However, there are inevitably some important differences between experimental studies with mouse pre-embryos and preimplantation diagnosis of sex of a human pre-embryo. First, the availability of inbred mice means that the mouse experiments can be designed to avoid genetic variability in enzyme activity that could confound the results. Second, in a clinical situation a patient will produce a relatively small number of pre-embryos, so that the results for each pre-embryo cannot be viewed against an overall distribution of a large number of contemporaneous samples. Several patients could be tested at the same time, particularly if the pre-embryos were stored frozen, but this might introduce another variable. If assay variability or developmental variation is significant it will be difficult to compare results obtained on different occasions and it will be difficult to sex a human pre-embryo that is one of a small group. Even for mouse pre-embryos, where large numbers can be obtained at a given stage of development to produce a bimodal distribution, there is an area of overlap and it is uncertain whether the pre-embryos that fall in the middle of the distribution are males or females. Bimodal distributions were not always demonstrated convincingly for mouse pre-embryos with either alpha-galactosidase or HGPRT (see above) and the difficulties in sexing human pre-embryos would be greater.

Is there a "developmental window" for human pre-embryos that would allow them to be sexed biochemically with X-linked gene products, such as alpha-galactosidase or HGPRT? Monk and Handyside (1988) cite their preliminary experiments that suggest that the developmental profiles of HGPRT and APRT activities in human pre-embryo are similar to those observed in the mouse. In other experiments, however, measurements of HGPRT activity in 75 unfertilized human oocytes and 51 human pre-embryos (between 1-cell and blastocyst stages) revealed no major increase in activity during the preimplantation period (Braude et al. 1988). The HGPRT activity level in human oocytes and pre-embryos, throughout the preimplantation period, was about 10 times the level found in mouse oocytes. It is therefore uncertain whether the HGPRT activity in human pre-embryos is oocyte- or embryo-coded, so a "developmental window" may not exist for the human pre-embryo.

Despite the encourging results with attempts to sex mouse pre-embryos (Monk and Handyside 1988), the present evidence forces us to conclude that there is little prospect of reliably sexing human pre-embryos biochemically with products of X-linked genes, such as alpha-galactosidase or HGPRT, in the near future. We are then left with molecular methods of sexing that rely on the identification of DNA sequences unique to the X or Y chromosome.

Sexing by In Situ Hybridization

DNA-DNA in situ hybridization involves the hybridization of a labelled DNA probe to a specific DNA sequence present in the target nuclei on a microscope slide. When the target DNA sequences are highly repeated on a single chromosome the numbers of copies of this chromosome can be determined in interphase nuclei ("interphase cytogenetics"). The DNA probe can be labelled in a variety of ways such as (1) incorporation of radioactive (e.g. tritiated) nucleotides, (2) the incorporation of nucleotides conjugated to either biotin or digoxygenin and (3) the chemical modification of the guanosine nucleotides with 2-acetylaminofluorene, AAF (Landegent et al. 1984). Radioactively labelled DNA can then be identified by autoradiography and DNA labelled in other ways can be identified by a variety of immunochemical or immunofluorescent methods as illustrated in Fig. 10.8

Sexing by DNA-DNA in situ hybridization requires a Y chromosome-specific DNA probe that detects a target sequence that is sufficiently repeated to give an unambiguous signal in both metaphase and interphase nuclei after hybridization. There are several such probes available (Table 10.1) and the choice

Table 10.1. Some DNA probes suitable for identification of the X or Y chromosome in interphase nuclei by in situ hybridization

Chromosome	Probe	Label[a]	References
Probes used for in situ hybridization with pre-embryos			
Y	pHY2.1	T, B	West et al. (1987, 1988)
Y	p102d	T	Jones et al. (1987)
Y	pHY2.1	B	Handyside et al. (1989), Penketh et al. (1989)
Probes used for in situ hybridization with other cells			
X	pXBR-1	T	Rappold et al. (1984)
X	pSV2X-5	B	Fantes et al. (1988)[b]
Y	CY1	T	Rappold et al. (1984)
Y	pHY2.1	B	Burns et al. (1985)
Y	pHY2.1	T	West et al. (1989a)
Y	pHY2.1	D	Fig. 10.8d, this Chapter
Y	pY3.4	T	Lau et al. (1985)
Y	pY3.4A	A	Pinkel et al. (1986a), Trask et al. (1988)
Y	pY431	B	Pinkel et al (1986b)
Y	pY431a	B	Guyot et al. (1988)
Y	Y190	B	Kozma and Adinolfi (1988)
Y	pDp105	T	Disteche et al. (1986)[b]

[a] A, AAF(2-acetylaminofluorine) modification of guanosine in DNA; B, biotin incorporation; D, digoxygenin incorporation; T, tritium incorporation.
[b] Not used with interphase nuclei.

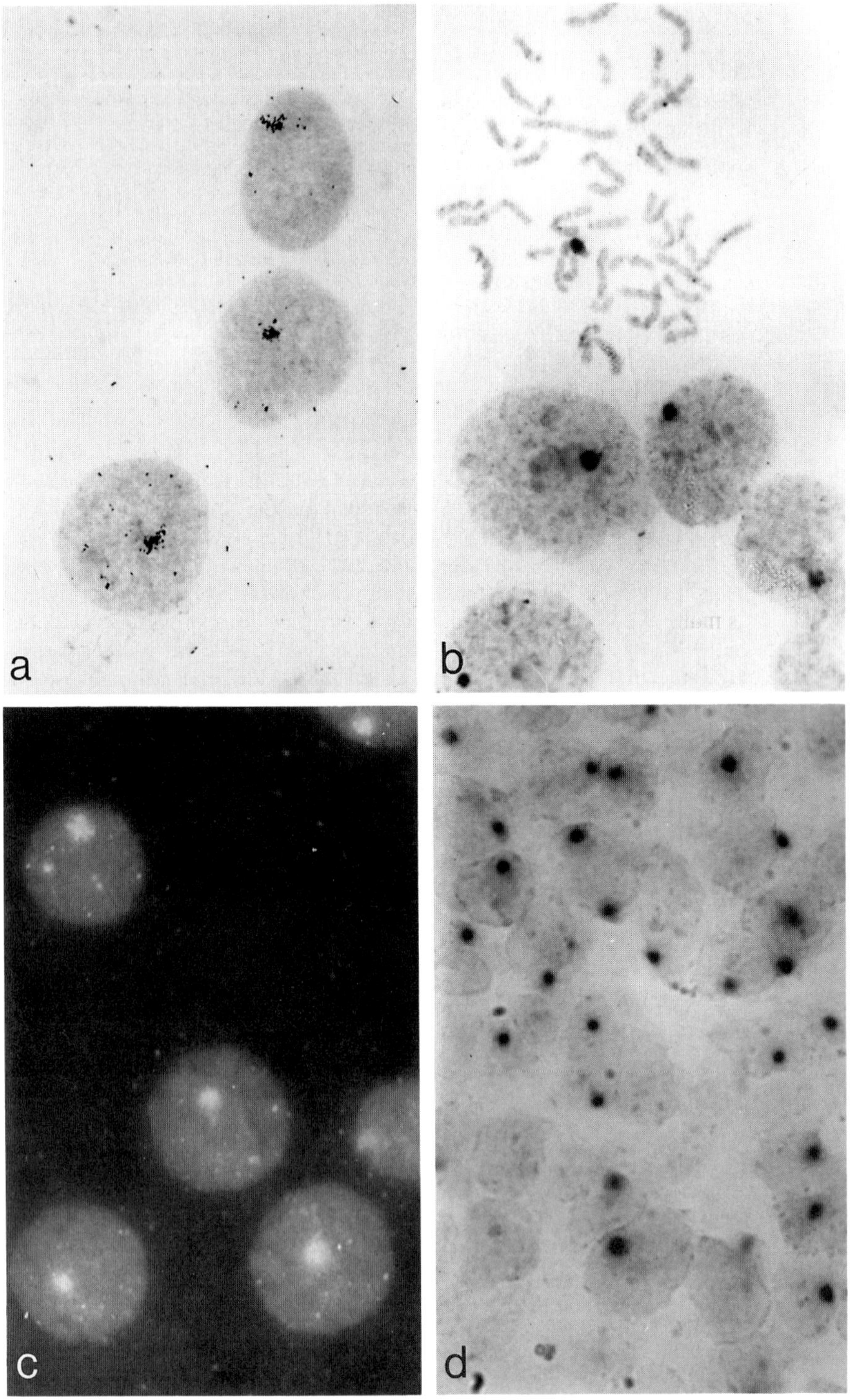
a
b
c
d

Fig. 10.8 a–d. Examples of four different detection systems for identifying the Y chromosome in interphase nuclei from males by DNA-DNA in situ hybridization. **a** Autoradiographic detection of tritiated Y probe hybridized to spreads of chorionic villus cells, counterstained with Giemsa. (From West et al. 1989.) **b** Immunochemical detection of biotinylated Y probe hybridized to spreads of adult lymphocytes. Visualized with goat anti-biotin anti-serum followed by horseradish peroxidase conjugated rabbit anti-goat anti-serum and diaminobenzidine staining to produce a brown coloured end-point; counterstained with Giemsa. (From West et al. 1988.) **c** Immunofluorescent detection of biotinylated Y probe hybridized to spreads of adult lymphocytes. Visualized with two rounds of FITC-conjugated avidin, each time followed by biotinylated goat anti-avidin (Vector Laboratories), mounted in Citifluor AF1 and viewed by ultraviolet microscopy (counterstained with propidium iodide). The nuclei appear orange and the Y chromosomes are bright yellow. (West and Keighren, unpublished.) **d** Immunochemical detection of digoxygenin-labelled Y probe hybridized to a histological section (brain) of a postimplantation human male conceptus at about 42 days. Visualized with alkaline phosphatase conjugated goat anti-digoxygenin anti-serum (from Boehringer) and nitroblue tetrazolium staining to produce a blue coloured end-point; no counterstain. (West and Keighren, unpublished.)

←

is determined by a variety of factors that include availability, number of copies of target DNA sequence on the Y chromosome, lack of significant cross-reacting autosomal target sequences and location of the target sequences on the human Y chromosome. In order to determine whether the individual is morphologically a male, probes close to the testis-determining factor gene (TDF) on the short arm (Page et al. 1987) would be most suitable. This would enable us to identify XX males as males if they retained a portion of the Y chromosome that included the target DNA as well as the TDF gene. However, for prenatal diagnosis we are usually more concerned with whether an individual has inherited an X chromosome from the father as well as from the mother because, in most cases at risk for X-linked diseases, the abnormal gene is passed from the Mother's X chromosome and only male offspring that are hemizygous for the defective gene are affected. In this case it is more useful to detect the presence of two X chromosomes and/or the absence of a Y chromosome. Although there are some X chromosome probes (Table 10.1), in practice it is easier to sex interphase nuclei by the presence or absence of a single Y hybridization site than to distinguish between 1 or 2 X chromosome hybridization sites. Ideally the Y probe should detect reiterated DNA sequences close to the centromere of the Y chromosome so that even Y chromosomes with small long arms are detected. However, prior hybridization to parental lymphocyte samples will forewarn of any inherited polymorphisms such as small Y chromosomes or Y/autosome translocations (Gosden et al. 1984; Ellis et al. 1990). Fortunately, the incidence of such polymorphisms arising de novo is low.

For our own studies we have used Y probe pHY2.1 (Cooke et al 1982) or the identical commercially-available probe, Amprobe RPN 1305X (Amersham). This probe recognizes a 2.12 kb sequence that is repeated 2000 times on the long arm of the Y chromosome. Most of these sequences are located on the distal fluorescent region of the Y chromosome but hybridization is still detectable to Y chromosomes that lack the fluorescent region (Gosden et al. 1984). An additional 100 copies of a related 2.00 kb sequence are located elsewhere in the genome but produce a much weaker signal after in situ hybridization than those on the Y chromosome. The Y chromosome is readily detected in metaphase or interphase nuclei where it is seen as strong hybridization site (hybridization body or Y body).

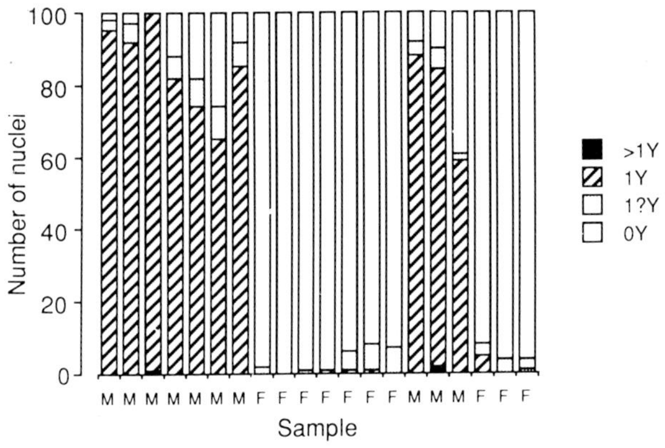

Fig. 10.9. Incidence of nuclei with 0, 1 equivocal, 1 or >1 Y-bodies from control slides hybridized to tritiated Y probe. (100 interphase nuclei scored per sample.) The first 14 samples were male (M) and female (F) lymphocyte cultures and the remaining 6 samples were lymphoblastoid cell lines. (Reproduced with permission from West et al. 1988.)

Most of our studies with human pre-embryos have been done with tritiated Y probe although a small number of pre-embryos were analysed with biotinylated Y probe and the Y chromosome visualized by diaminobenzidine staining of peroxidase-linked antibodies. Fig 10.9 shows the frequency of labelled nuclei from our male and female control preparations after hybridization with tritiated DNA probe (West et al. 1988). The proportion of unlabelled nuclei among the

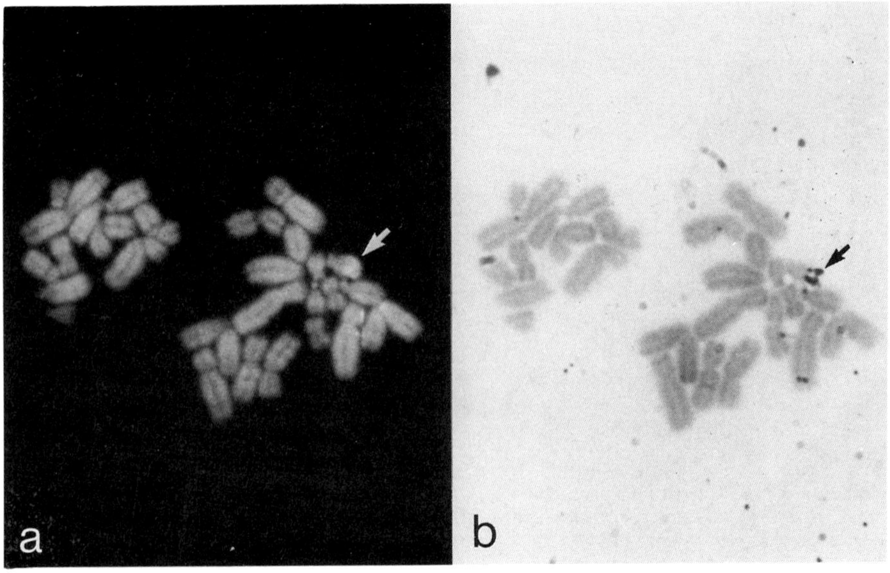

Fig. 10.10 a,b. Part of a metaphase spread from a control male lymphocyte culture; **a** pretreated with spermidine *bis*-acridine to reveal the fluorescent Y-chromosome then **b** hybridized to the tritiated Y probe to reveal specific hybridization to the Y chromosome. (Reproduced with permission from West et al. 1988.)

XY controls varied between experiments (typically 60%–100%) but the proportion of false positive nuclei among the XX controls was rarely more than a few percent. This provides excellent discrimination between preparations from males and females. Further confirmation that the clusters of grains identify the Y chromosome is shown in Fig. 10.10. This demonstrates that the Y proble labels the region of the Y chromosome that fluoresces after exposure to spermidine *bis*-acridine.

We have applied the same in situ hybridization technique to sex whole human pre-embryos after they had been treated with hypotonic, fixed and spread on a microscope slide. This work has established that it would be feasible to diagnose the sex of a pre-embryo by DNA-DNA in situ hybridization (West et al. 1987, 1988). Fourteen morphologically normal pre-embryos and nine that appeared abnormal were analysed by in situ hybridization to tritiated Y probe (Figs. 10.11

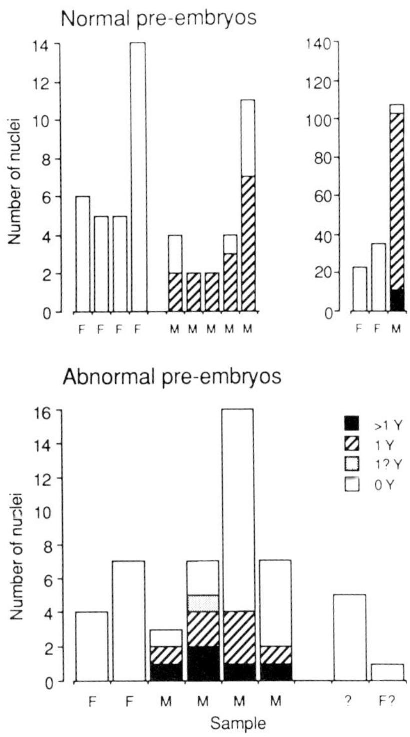

Fig. 10.11. Incidence of nuclei with 0, 1 equivocal, 1, or >1 Y hybridization bodies among 14 morphologically normal and 9 morphogically abnormal human pre-embryos. Based on the data of West et al. 1988. The assigned sex is shown as F (female) or M (male). One morphologically normal pre-embryo with one hybridization body in each of 2 of the 4 nuclei originally had 3 pronuclei and may have been an XXY triploid mosaic (West et al. 1987). Two of the abnormal pre-embryos were not sexed. In one case only one cell was recovered and, in the other, all five nuclei were negative but of abnormal morphology (probably fragmented). Small fragmented nuclei without hybridization bodies were also seen in some of the morphologically abnormal male pre-embryos. Pretreated pre-embryos (e.g. pre-embryos pretreated with spermidine *bis*-acridine for independent sexing by Fluorescent F-body analysis) are not included in this figure. (See West et al. [1987] for details.)

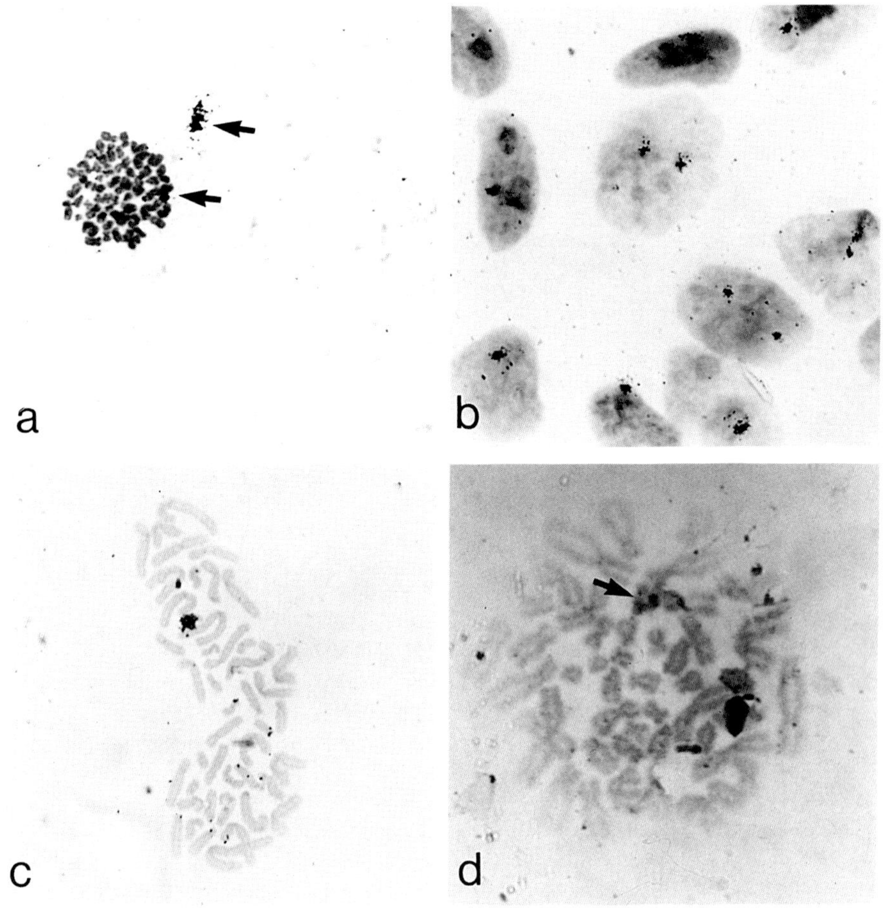

Fig. 10.12. Hybridization of tritiated (**a**, **b** and **c**) or biotinylated (**d**) Y probe to nuclei of human pre-embryos (Y hybridization bodies are arrowed). **a** Metaphase and part of a large interphase nucleus from a 6-cell pre-embryo. In the original preparation a Y body was clearly visible in both the metaphase spread and interphase nucleus. The chromatin in the interphase nucleus is very diffuse and fills the right half of the photograph. **b** interphase nuclei from a blastocyst showing presumptive polyploid nuclei with 2 Y bodies. **c** metaphase from a 2-cell pre-embryo. **d** metaphase from an 8-cell stage pre-embryo after hybridization with biotinylated Y probe and visualization with diaminobenzidine staning of peroxidase-linked antibodies. The brown precipitate (arrowed) shows both chromatids of the Y chromosome (the large dark mass is stain debris).

and 10.12). All 12 morphologically normal pre-embryos (ranging from the 2-cell stage to a blastocyst with 107 cells) were sexed with confidence (6 females and 6 males). Some of the morphologically abnormal pre-embryos had small (probably fragmenting) nuclei without hybridization bodies and two of these pre-embryos were not sexed. All 4 male morphologically abnormal, pre-embryos (4–8 cell stages) had one or more nucleus with multiple hybridization bodies and about 10% of nuclei in the morphologically normal blastocyst had two hybridization bodies. It seems likely that polyploidy occurs both during the

Table 10.2. Frequency of nuclei with Y bodies in 12 male pre-embryos after in situ hybridization with tritiated Y probe

	Pre-embryos	Metaphases	Interphase nuclei
Morphologically normal			
Cleavage stages	5	10/10	6/13 (46%)
Cleavage stages (pre-treated[a])	2	3/3	2/2 (100%)
Total cleavage stages			(54%)
Blastocysts	1	20/21	83/86 (97%)
Morphologically abnormal			
Cleavage stages	4	1/1	12/30 (40%)

Data from West et al. (1988)
[a] Pre-treated with spermidine *bis*-acridine or quinacrine dihydrochloride and UV light.

normal development of human blastocysts and in early cleavage stages of abnormally developing pre-embryos (Angell et al. 1987; West et al 1987, 1988). The polyploidy in the latter group may be a culture-induced phenomenon. In addition, some triploid pre-embryos are produced when two sperm fertilize a single egg (Angell et al. 1987) and two Y bodies are detectable by in situ hybridization in 69,XYY triploids (West et al. 1987, 1988).

Two other laboratories have also used DNA-DNA in situ hybridization to sex human pre-embryos. Jones et al (1987) illustrated three pre-embryos that were sexed with a different tritiated Y probe (p102d). Handyside et al. (1989) summarized the results of sexing 19 pre-embryos by in situ hybridization with biotinylated pHY2.1 and subsequent detection with streptavidin-linked alkaline phosphatase. (See Penketh et al. (1989) for full report.)

These studies show that it would be feasible to sex pre-embryos by DNA-DNA in situ hybridization but it is not clear how many cells would be required for a reliable sex determination. Early cleavage embryos had large nuclei with relatively diffuse hybridization bodies but were usually readily scored with the tritiated probe. Calculations based on the incidence of labelled nuclei in male and female lymphocytes suggest that it should normally be possible to sex morphologically normal pre-embryos with samples of three or more nuclei (West et al. 1988). The frequency of false negative interphase nuclei may be higher for early cleavage nuclei than for the control lymphocytes in which case more than three nuclei may be required for reliable sex determination. Table 10.2 summarizes the data given by West et al (1988) for 12 male pre-embryos. Although 97% of interphase nuclei from a large blastocyst had a Y hybridization body, the frequency was only 54% for the 15 nuclei from morphologically normal cleavage stage pre-embryos. If a Y body is detectable in only 50% of interphase nuclei then the probability of failing to observe any Y bodies is 12.5% (0.5^3) for a sample of 3 cells and 1.6% for 6 cells.

With tritiated DNA probe, sexing would take 4–8 days (allowing 3–7 days to expose the autoradiographs) but with DNA labelled with biotin (e.g. Burns et al. 1985; West et al. 1988; Handyside et al. 1989; Penketh et al. 1989) or digoxygenin (Fig 10.8d) this could be reduced to 2 days. Even so, it is unlikely that this would be fast enough to allow the identification of female pre-embryos in time for replacement in the same menstrual cycle.

If a Y probe is used clinically to sex pre-embryos by in situ hybridization to interphase nuclei, it would be important to test blood samples from both parents to screen for any abnormalities. For example, many interphase nuclei of male Y/autosome translocation carriers have two detectable Y bodies (Ellis et al. 1990) and so interphase nuclei from a female conceptus with a Y/autosome translocation would have a single hybridization body and thus, on this basis, be scored as a male, unless the parents are screened.

Sexing by Polymerase Chain Reaction

A technique known as the polymerase chain reaction (PCR) has been developed to amplify specific target DNA sequences (Mullis and Faloona 1987; Saiki et al. 1988; White et al. 1989). The PCR reaction requires two oligonucleotide primers that hybridize to opposite strands of the DNA, one either side of the target gene to be amplified with their 3' ends pointing towards each other. The procedure involves repeated cycles of heat denaturation of the DNA (e.g. 1 to 2 minutes at 90°C–96°C), annealing of the two flanking primer sequences (e.g. 2 minutes at 50°C–65°C), and extension of the hybridized primers across the target DNA sequence with thermostable DNA polymerase (e.g. 2 minutes at 65°C–72°C). The exact times and temperatures vary according to the sequence to be amplified. In theory each successive cycle doubles the number of copies of target DNA so that after 10 cycles there is a 2^{10}-fold amplification (1056-fold) of target DNA and after 20 cycles there is a 2^{20}-fold amplification (approximately 1 million-fold). This offers an enormously powerful means of amplifying specific DNA sequences to levels where they are readily detectable. Introduction of thermostable *Taq* DNA polymerase (Saiki et al. 1988) and the availability of specific apparatus to change the reaction temperature after defined intervals (programmable thermal cyclers) have simplified the procedure and PCR is now widely used.

In an impressive set of experiments, Handyside et al. (1989) have recently shown that it is feasible both to biopsy human pre-embryos and to sex them by amplification of target DNA, from a single blastomere, with the polymerase chain reaction. A single blastomere was removed from each of 38 human pre-embryos at the 6- to 10-cell stage via a micropipette inserted through a hole made in the zona pellucida (see Chapter 6) and PCR was used to sex the single blastomere. The whole procedure, from biopsy to sexing took only about 8 hours. The remaining portion of the pre-embryo was cultured to test its viability and to confirm the diagnosis of sex by in situ hybridization and/or fluorescent F-body staining with spermidine *bis* acridine. Ten of the 27 pre-embryos (37%) that were cultured developed into blastocysts which is similar to the proportion expected from cultured pre-embryos that are not biopsied.

PCR was used to amplify a 149 base pair DNA sequence that is repeated 800–1500 times on the Y chromosome. Sixty cycles of amplification were used and then the amplified DNA was stained with ethidium bromide and visualized under ultraviolet light. A cell was judged to be male if visualization under ultraviolet light revealed a strong band corresponding to the 149 base-pair Y chromosome-specific sequence. If the band was absent or very faint the cell was judged female.

Table 10.3. Sexing human pre-embryos by the polymerase chain reaction

Pre-embryos		Sexed by PCR	Other test resuts[a]		
			Agree	Disagree	Not done
Sexed pre-embryos with <2 pronuclei (parthenogenetic?)					
Male		0	–	–	–
Female		3	2	0	1
Sexed pre-embryos with 2 pronuclei (normal)					
Male		6	4	0	2
Female		12	11	0	1
Sexed pre-embryos with >2 pronuclei (polyspermic)					
Male		3	0	2	1
Female		1	0	0	1
Total	38	25	17	2	6

Data from Handyside et al. (1989).
[a] Sexed by in situ hybridization or fluorescent Y chromatin (F-body).

Of the single-cell biopsies from the 38 pre-embryos, 13 were lost because of technical problems and 25 were sexed by PCR (Table 10.3). Nineteen of these 25 pre-embryos were also sexed by an alternative method (in situ hybridization and/or F-body fluorescence on the remainder of the pre-embryo) and the sex was confirmed in 17 (90%) and contradicted in 2 (10%) cases. The two contradictory cases were both pre-embryos which had had three or more pronuclei after fertilization and were sexed as male by PCR but female by in situ hybridization. The authors suggest that this contradiction could be explained if the pre-embryo was a polyploid mosiac in which the Y chromosome segregated to only a proportion of the cells. This explanation requires that the single blastomere biopsied from both pre-embryos was the only one at the 6–10 cell stage that had a Y chromosome. Despite these two contradictory cases, this preliminary study is impressive and the prospects for sexing by PCR are encouraging.

One potential problem with amplifying DNA from a single blastomere is that contaminating DNA from sperm present in the medium, airborne skin cells or fragmented DNA, etc. could be amplified and produce spurious results. Handyside et al. (1989) observed stringent precautions to avoid contamination of the single-cell sample with foreign DNA that could have produced a false positive result. These precautions included washing the blastomere three times, the use of a class II containment cabinet throughout, filtration of buffers through a 0.2 μm filter and digestion of any contaminating target sequences present in the oligonucleotides and salmon sperm carrier DNA with restriction enzyme *EcoR1*. Negative controls were also run as a check on the effectiveness of the anti-contamination procedures. The authors commented that without these procedures they frequently produced false positive results from female samples or blank controls.

Conclusions and Future Prospects

In this chapter three possible methods of sexing human pre-embryos have been discussed. Although the attempts to sex mouse pre-embryos with assays of HGPRT activity (Monk and Handyside 1988) were encouraging it seems that this approach will be more difficult for human pre-embryos and may not be feasible. There would not be large "litters" of human pre-embryos and there may not be a "developmental window" when female pre-embryos have significantly more HGPRT activity than males (see p.150).

The other two approaches are both technically demanding but feasible. Further studies are needed to compare the success rate of sexing by in situ hybridization and DNA amplification by PCR. At present we have insufficient information to compare the success rates of the two techniques. Some information is summarized in Table 10.4 but figures for the two techniques are not comparable. The in situ hybridization data are for whole pre-embryos (from 2-cell to blastocyst) most of which were not sexed by another method. The PCR data are for individual blastomeres removed at the 8-cell stage, and, in most cases the remainder of the embryo was used to obtain an independent determination of sex.

In situ hybridization may not detect the Y chromosome in every interphase nucleus of a pre-embryo (Table 10.2) so more than one cell would be needed to avoid false negative test results (males scored as females). Although it may be possible to culture a single cell sample to routinely provide several cells for sexing by in situ hybridization, there is still a risk of some false negative results. If sexing was done to allow female pre-embryos to be selected for transfer to the uterus (in order to avoid conceiving a son affected by an X-linked genetic disease) false negative test results would pose a more serious clinical problem than false positives (females scored as males). PCR may be less likely to produce false negatives than in situ hybridization but may be more prone to false positives. It may be possible to avoid the occurrence of false positives with PCR by taking rigorous precautions against the possibility of contaminating the tiny sample with foreign DNA (Handyside et al 1989) but this requires further evaluation.

Table 10.4. Success rates for sexing human pre-embryos by in situ hybridization and PCR

Sexing by in situ hybridization with tritiated Y probe (West et al. 1988)	
Total pre-embryos[a]	27
Total sexed by in situ hybridization	20 (74%) 8 female : 12 male
	4/4 confirmed by other methods
Technical failures	7 (26%) 4 lost + 3 uncertain results
Sexing by polymerase chain reaction of Y chromosomal DNA (Handyside et al. 1989)	
Total pre-embryos	38
Total sexed by PCR	25 (66%) 16 female : 9 male
	17/19 (90%) confirmed by other methods
Technical failures	13 (34%) plus 2/19 (10%) results contradicted

[a] Excluding pre-embryos that failed to cleave and those mounted in DePeX before in situ hybridization or previously hybridized to biotinylated DNA probe but including morphologically abnormal pre-embryos and pre-embryos treated with spermidine *bis*-acridine or quinacrine dihydrochloride.

PCR has two other advantages over in situ hybridization. It requires only a single cell and so avoids the need for culturing the sample. It can be done more quickly and so avoids the need for cryopreservation, although cryopreservation could be used if this seemed appropriate.

At present, the success of blastocyst transfers in human IVF is low (Dawson et al. 1988) so that pre-embryos should be either transferred as soon after biopsy as possible or stored frozen and transferred at a later cycle. Although the first of these two options seems the most attractive at first sight, cryopreservation techniques are now successful. Several centres have achieved pregnancies in about 20% of patients receiving cryopreserved pre-embryos, which is similar to the success rates with fresh pre-embryos (e.g. Mohr et al. 1985; Fehilly et al. 1985; Testart et al. 1986). Also, it has been suggested that it may be beneficial to delay the transfer until a later menstrual cycle in order to improve the synchrony between the pre-embryo and the uterus and avoid exposing the pre-embryo to the abnormal endocrine environment of a stimulated IVF cycle (e.g. Fehilly et al. 1985; Frydman et al. 1988). In the context of preimplantation diagnosis, this would have the added advantage of removing the pressure on laboratory staff to produce a reliable diagnosis by a set deadline. Further studies are needed to evaluate the balance between the risk of damaging the pre-embryo by cryopreservation and the risk of transferring it to a suboptimal uterine environment.

Although in situ hybridization and PCR both appear to be feasible methods of sexing the pre-embryo, the results of the preliminary studies discussed here suggest that PCR may have several advantages. It requires only a single cell and does not require cryopreservation. If false positives can be routinely avoided by appropriate precautions against contamination, PCR may be a more efficient means of sexing pre-embryos than in situ hybridization.

Other types of preimplantation diagnosis are also likely to be feasible in the near future. In situ hybridization may be used for the identification of pre-embryos with specific numerical chromosome anomalies, such as specific trisomies, but the use of PCR to diagnose specific single gene defects is likely to have the biggest impact. Although 1500 copies of the target DNA were present in each nucleus that was sexed by PCR (Handyside et al 1989), PCR has also been used to detect a single copy sequence from one spermatozoa (Li et al. 1988) or human oocyte (Coutelle et al. 1989). This offers an enormous advance in the sensitivity of many molecular diagnosic tests and makes it feasible to use preimplantation diagnosis both to sex the pre-embryo and to diagnose specific genetic disorders.

Preimplantation diagnosis is likely to benefit couples who are at high risk for sex-linked disorders or autosomal single-gene defects and anxious to avoid the need for a therapeutic abortion. Preimplantation diagnosis may be used less frequently for couples at lower risk for genetic disorders, such as many of the spontaneous chromosomal aberrations, where the risk of therapeutic termination is correspondingly lower. For couples at risk, the risk of conceiving an affected conceptus is typically 25% for an autosomal recessive, 50% for an autosomal or X-linked dominant and 25% (50% of the males) for an X-linked recessive trait. In contrast, the frequency of the most common chromosomal disorder (trisomy 21) is ony 2.42% at term for mothers over the age of 40 and lower still for younger mothers (e.g. Brock 1982).

Finally, in situ hybridization can also be used to distinguish between X-bearing and Y-bearing spermatozoa (West et al. 1989b). This provides a means of evaluating the various methods that purport to separate X- and Y-bearing spermoatozoa. If a woman who is heterozygous for an X-linked genetic disease could be inseminated with only X-bearing spermatozoa, she would avoid the risk of conceiving an affected son without the need for prenatal or preimplantation diagnosis.

Acknowledgements. I am grateful to many scientific, clinical and technical collaborators. These include J.R. Gosden, R.R. Angell, C.M. Gosden, K.M. West, M. Keighren, L. Harkness, S.S. Thatcher, A.F. Glasier, M.W. Rodger, D.T. Baird, N. Hastie and H.J. Evans. I also thank T. McFetters and E. Pinner for preparing the illustrations, M. Keighren for reading the manuscript, V.M. Chapman, C.J. Epstein, M. Monk and A.H. Handyside for permission to reproduce illustrations and the Wellcome Trust for financial support.

References

Adler DA, West JD, Chapman VM (1977) Expression of alpha-galactosidase in preimplantation mouse embryos. Nature 267: 838–839

Angell RR, Sumner AT, West JD, Thatcher SS, Glasier AF, Baird DT (1987) Post fertilization polyploidy in human preimplantation embryos fertilized in vitro. Hum Reprod 2: 721-727

Angell RR, Hillier SG, West JD, Glasier AF, Rodger MW, Baird DT (1988) Chromosome anomalies in early human embryos. J Reprod Fertil Suppl 36: 73–81

Braude PR, Monk M, Pickering S, Johnson MH, Cant A (1988) Preimplantation diagnosis of genetic activity in genetic disease: measurements of HPRT activity in human oocytes and preimplantation embryos grown in vitro. In: Human Reproduction: abstracts from the fourth meeting of the European Society of Human Reproduction and Embryology. IRL Press, Oxford, p 44 (abstr 143)

Brinster RL (1970) Glucose-6-phosphate dehydrogenase activity in the early rabbit and mouse embryo. Biochem Genet 4: 669–676

Brock DJH (1982) Early diagnosis of fetal defects. Churchill Livingstone, Edinburgh

Burns J, Chan VTW, Jonasson JA, Fleming KA, Taylor S, McGee JOD (1985). Sensitive system for visualising biotinylated DNA probes hybridised in situ: rapid sex determination of intact cells. J Clin Pathol 38: 1085–1092

Buster JE, Bustillo M, Rodi IA, et al. (1985) Biologic and morphologic development of donated human ova recovered by nonsurgical uterine lavage. Am J Obstet Gynec 153: 211–217

Chapman VM, West JD, Adler DA (1977) Genetics of early mammalian embryogenesis. In: Sherman MI (ed) Concepts in early mammalian development. MIT Press, Cambridge, Massachusetts, pp 95–135

Chapman VM, West JD, Adler DA (1978) Bimodal distribution of alpha-galactosidase activities in mouse embryos. In: Russell LB (ed) Genetic mosaics and chimeras in mammals. Plenum Press, New York, pp 227–237

Cooke HJ, Schmidtke J, Gosden JR (1982) Characterisation of a human Y chromosome repeated sequence and related sequences in higher primates. Chromosoma 87: 491–502

Coutelle C, Williams C, Handyside A, Hardy K, Winston R (1989) Genetic analysis of DNA from single human oocytes: a model for preimplantation diagnosis of cystic fibrosis. Br Med J 299: 22–24

Dawson KJ, Rutherford AJ, Winston NJ, Subak-Sharpe R, Winston RML (1988) Human blastocyst transfer, is it a feasible proposition? In: Human Reproduction: abstracts from the fourth meeting of the European Society of Human Reproduction and Embryology. IRL Press, Oxford, pp 44–45 (abstr 145)

Disteche CM, Brown L, Saal H, et al. (1986) Molecular detection of a translocation (Y;15) in a 45X male. Hum Genet 74: 372–377

Ellis PM, West JD, West KM, Murray RS, Coyle MC (1990) Relevance to prenatal diagnosis of the identification of a human Y/autosome translocation by Y chromosome specific in situ hybridization. Mol Reprod Dev Incorp Gamete Res 25: 37–41

Epstein CJ (1972) Expression of the mammalian X chromosome before and after fertilization. Science 175: 1467–1468

Epstein CJ, Travis B, Tucker G, Smith S (1978a) The direct demonstration of an X-chromosome dosage effect prior to inactivation. In: Russell LB (ed) Genetic mosaics and chimeras in mammals. Plenum Press, New York, pp 261–267

Epstein CJ, Smith S, Travis B, Tucker G (1978b) Both X chromosomes function before visible X chromosome inactivation in female mouse embryos. Nature 274: 500–503

Fantes J, Gosden JR, Piper J (1988) Use of an alphoid satellite sequence to automatically locate the X chromosome, with particular reference to the identification of the fragile X. Cytogenet Cell Genet 48: 142–147

Fehilly CB, Cohen J, Simons RF, Fishel SB, Edwards RG (1985) Cryopreservation of cleaving embryos and expanded blastocysts in the human: a comparative study. Fertil Steril 44: 638–644

Frydman R, Forman RG, Belaisch-Allart J, Hazout A, Testart J (1988) An assessment of alternative policies for embryo transfer in an in vitro fertilization-embryo transfer program. Fertil Steril 50: 466–470

Gosden JR, Gosden CM, Christie S, Cooke HJ, Morsman JM, Rodeck CH (1984) The use of cloned Y-chromosome-specific DNA probes for fetal sex determination in first trimester prenatal diagnosis. Hum Genet 66: 347–351

Guyot B, Bazin A, Sole Y, Julien C, Daffos F, Forestier F (1988) Prenatal diagnosis with biotinylated chromosome specific probes. Prenatal Diagn 8: 485–493

Handyside AH, Pattinson JK, Penketh RJA, Delhanty JDA, Winston RML, Tuddenham EGD (1989) Biopsy of human preimplantation embryos and sexing by DNA amplification. Lancet ii: 347–349

Jones KW, Singh L, Edwards RG (1987) The use of probes for the Y chromosome in preimplantation embryo cells. Hum Reprod 2: 439–445

Kozak LP, Quinn PJ (1975) Evidence for dosage compensation of an X-linked gene in the 6 day embryo of the mouse. Dev Biol 45: 65–73

Kozma R, Adinolfi M (1988) In situ fluorescence hybridisation of Y translocations: cytogenetic analysis using probes Y190 and Y431. Clin Genet 33: 156–161

Kratzer PG, Gartler SM (1978a) HGPRT activity changes in preimplantation mouse embryos. Nature 274: 503–504

Kratzer PG, Gartler SM (1978b) Hypoxanthine guanine phosphoribosyl transferase expression in early mouse development. In: Russell LB (ed) Genetic mosaics and chimeras in mammals. Plenum Press, New York, pp 247–260

Landegent JE, Jansen In De Wal N, Baan RA, Hoeijmakers JHJ, Van Der Ploeg M (1984) 2-Acetylaminofluorene-modified probes for the indirect hybridocytochemical detection of specific nucleic acid sequences. Exp Cell Res 153: 61–72

Lau YF, Ying KL, Donnell GN (1985) Identification of a case of Y:18 translocation using a Y-specific repetitive DNA probe. Hum Genet 69: 102–105

Li A, Gyllensten UB, Cui X, Saiki RK, Erlich HA, Arnheim N (1988) Amplification and analysis of DNA sequencies in single human sperm and diploid cells. Nature 335: 414–419

McLaren A (1985) Prenatal diagnosis before implantation: opportunities and problems. Prenatal Diagn 5: 85–90

McLaren A (1986) Prelude to embryogenesis. In: Human embryo research. Yes or no? Ciba Foundation. Tavistock Publications, London pp 5–23

Mohr LR, Trounson A, Freeman L (1985) Deep-freezing and transfer of human embryos. J In Vitro Fertil Embryo Transf 2: 1–10

Monk M (1978a) Biochemical studies of X-chromosome activity in preimplantation mouse embryos. In: Russell LB (ed) Genetic mosaics and chimeras in mammals. Plenum Press, New York, pp 239–246

Monk M (1978b) Biochemical studies on mammalian X-chromosome activity. In: Johnson MH (ed) Development in mammals vol 3, pp 189–223. North-Holland Publishing Co, Amsterdam

Monk M (1988) Preimplantation diagnosis. BioEssays 8: 184–189

Monk M, Handyside AH (1988) Sexing of preimplantation mouse embryos by measurement of X-linked gene dosage in a single blastomere. J Reprod Fertil 82: 365–368

Monk M, Harper M (1978) X chromosome activity in preimplantation mouse embryos from XX and XO mothers. J. Embryol Exp Morphol 46: 53–64

Monk M, Kathuria H (1977) Dosage compensation for an X-linked gene in preimplantation mouse embryos. Nature 270: 599–601
Mullis KB, Faloona FA (1987) Specific synthesis of DNA in vitro via a polymerase-catalysed chain reaction. Methods Enzymol 155: 335–350
Page DC, Mosher R, Simpson EM, et al. (1987) The sex-determining region of the human Y chromsome encodes a finger protein. Cell 51: 1091–1104
Papaioannou VE (1986) Microsurgery and micromanipulation of early mouse embryos. In: Techniques in cellular physiology– part 1. Elsevier/North-Holland, Amsterdam, pp 1–27
Penketh R, McLaren A (1987) Prospects for prenatal diagnosis during preimplantation human development. In: Fetal diagnosis of genetic defects. Baillière's international clinical obstetrics and gynaecology, volume 1, pp 747–764
Penketh RJA, Delhanty JDA, Van den Berghe JA, et al. (1989) Rapid sexing of human embryos by non-radioactive in situ hybridization: potential for preimplantation diagnosis of X-linked disorders. Prenatal Diagn 9: 489–500
Pinkel D, Gray JW, Trask B, Van den Engh G, Fuscoe J, Van Dekken H (1986a) Cytogenetic analysis by in situ hybridization with fluorescently labeled nucleic acid probes. Cold Spring Harbor Symposia on Quantitative Biology 51: 151–157
Pinkel D, Straume T, Gray JW (1986b) Cytogenetic analysis using quantitative high sensitivity, fluorescence hybridization. Proc Natl Acad Sci USA 83: 2934–2938
Rappold GA, Cremer T, Hager HD, Davis KE, Muller CR, Yang T (1984) Sex chromosome positions in human interphase nuclei as studied by in situ hybridization with chromosome specific DNA probes. Hum Genet 67: 317–325
Saiki RK, Gelfand DH, Stoffel S, et al. (1988) Primer-directed enzymatic amplification of DNA with a thermostable DNA polymerase. Science 239: 487–491
Summers PM, Campbell JM, Miller MW (1988) Normal in vivo development of marmoset monkey embryos after trophectoderm biopsy. Hum Reprod 3: 389–393
Testart J, Lassalle B, Belaisch-Allart J, et al. (1986) High pregnancy rate after human embryo freezing. Fertil Steril 46: 268–272
Trask B, Van den Engh G, Pinkel D, et al. (1988) Fluorescence in situ hybridization to interphase cell nuclei in suspension allows flow cytometric analysis of chromosome content and microscopic analysis of nuclear organization. Hum Genet 78: 251–259
West JD (1989) The use of DNA probes in preimplantation and prenatal diagnosis. Mol Reprod Dev 1: 138–145
West JD, Gosden JR, Angell RR, et al. (1987) Sexing the human pre-embryo by DNA-DNA in situ hybridization. Lancet i: 1345–1347
West JD, Gosden JR, Angell RR et al (1988) Sexing whole human pre-embryos by in situ hybridization to a Y-chromosome specific DNA probe. Hum Reprod 3: 1010–1019
West JD, Gosden CM, Gosden JR, et al. (1989a) Sexing the human fetus and identification of polyploid nuclei by DNA-DNA in situ hybridization in interphase nuclei. Mol Reprod Dev 1: 129–137
West JD, West KM, Aitken RJ (1989b) Detection of Y-bearing spermatozoa by DNA-DNA in situ hybridization. Mol Reprod Dev 1: 201–207
White TJ, Arnheim N, Erlich HA (1989) The polymerase chain reaction. Trends Genet 5: 185–189
Wudl LR, Chapman VM (1976) The expression of ß-glucuronidase during preimplantation development of mouse embryos. Dev Biol 48: 104–109
Wudl LR, Sherman MI (1976) In vitro studies of mouse embryos bearing mutations at the T locus t^{w5} and t^{12}. Cell 9: 523–532

11. Embryonic Development: The Origin of Neural Tube Defects

A.J. Copp

Introduction

The early postimplantation period is a critical time in mammalian development when the major processes of organogenesis are proceeding. This period encompasses the third to eighth weeks of human embryonic development and the seventh to thirteenth days in the mouse. Among the organ-forming events to occur during this period are the formation of the central nervous system primordium, the development of a four-chambered heart, the establishment of the gland and duct systems of many gastrointestinal organs and the patterning of the limb bud cartilaginous elements. Disturbance of these and other early organogenetic events can lead to the appearance of major congenital malformations. Thus, it is essential to subject early postimplantation embryos to detailed study if we are to understand the mechanisms underlying these embryonic events and, ultimately, to develop rational approaches for preventing birth defects.

Unfortunately, early postimplantation mammalian embryos are not easily accessible for observation, due to their small size and intimate relationship with the uterus. This has meant that relatively few human embryos of this age have been described in detail. Current hypotheses about the developmental mechanisms operating during this period derive almost entirely from studies of mouse and rat embryos. Even rodent embryos are not easily manipulated in utero and making repeated observations on single embryos, for instance to determine the effects of a surgical intervention, is not straightforward. A great advance came in the 1960s and 1970s when Denis New and his colleagues described a culture system (New et al. 1973) in which intact postimplantation rat and mouse embryos can develop in vitro, for limited periods, in a manner closely similar to that in utero. Fig. 11.1 shows that many organogenetic events are in progress during the period when whole rodent embryos can be cultured, making these embryonic events readily accessible for experimental analysis.

The purpose of this chapter is to illustrate the use of rodent embryos, developing both in utero and in whole embryo culture, as a means of analysing

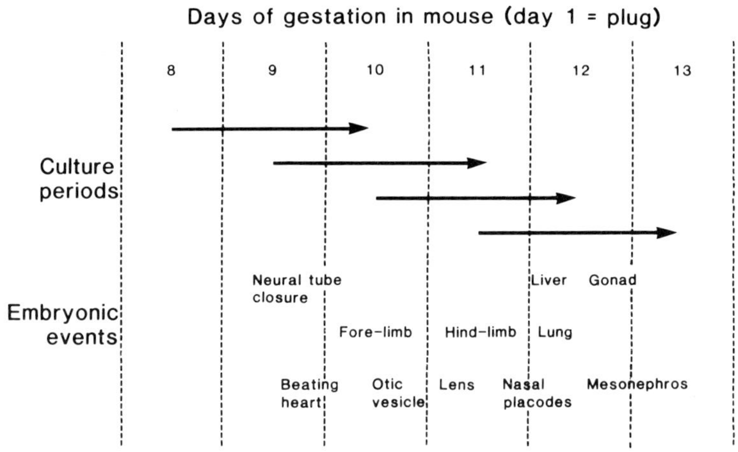

Fig. 11.1. *Top:* The four main periods of development (arrows) during which mouse embryos may be grown in the whole-embryo culture system of New et al. (1973). Forty-eight hours is the usual maximum period that mouse embryos are cultured since, beyond this time, rates of growth and development in vitro fall behind those in utero. *Bottom:* The approximate time in mouse development at which particular organs are first established. It can be seen that a wide range of organogenetic events may be studied in cultured embryos.

postimplantation developmental mechanisms and the pathogenesis of congenital malformations. As an example, recent advances in our understanding of the process of neurulation and the origin of congenital malformations affecting the central nervous system will be described.

Neurulation and Neural Tube Defects

The process of neurulation in which the primordium of the central nervous system, the neural tube, forms is one of the earliest organogenetic events to occur in embryonic development. Abnormalities of neurulation lead to a variety of congenital malformations, referred to collectively as neural tube defects (NTD), among which anencephaly and spina bifida are the best known. NTD are the second commonest cause of perinatal death in the UK due to congenital malformation (after congenital heart defects, see Office of Population Censuses and Surveys. Series DH3 no. 1, 1985). Nevertheless, many cases of spina bifida are compatible with postnatal life, producing multiple handicap in childhood. These malformations present a major challenge both to the paediatrician and to the handicapped person and his/her family.

Normal Neurulation: An Overview

Neurulation can be divided into primary and secondary phases. Primary neurulation occurs during the third and fourth weeks of human development (fertilization occurs at the start of the first week) and between days 9 and 11 in the mouse (fertilization occurs at approximately 1.00 a.m. on day 1). In primary neurulation, the neural plate ectoderm which covers the dorsal midline of the embryo (and which was induced to form earlier in development by interaction with underlying chordomesodermal structures) undergoes dorsal folding, transforming via a deepening groove to form a closed tube which sinks beneath the surface of the embryo. Primary neurulation is responsible, in both humans and rodents, for the formation of the entire brain and of the rostral portion of the spinal cord, down to the level of the sacrum. Neural tube formation at more caudal levels of the spine occurs following completion of primary neurulation by an entirely different process, secondary neurulation, in which there is direct canalization of a solid cord of cells, the medullary cord, without involvement of neural folds. In rodents, secondary neurulation is responsible for forming the caudal half of the neural tube, which is incorporated into the tail. In humans,

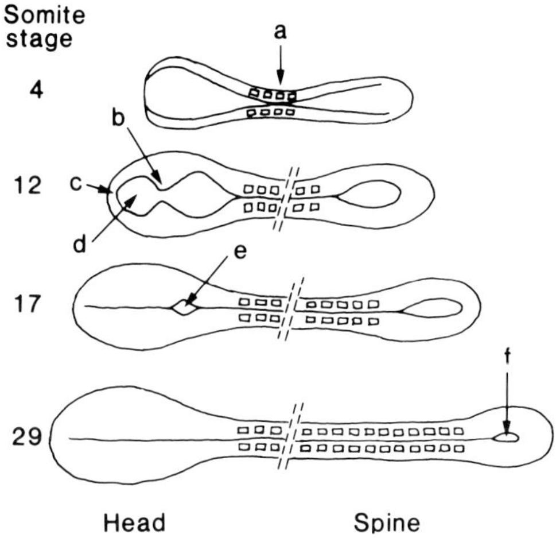

Fig. 11.2. The sequence of events comprising primary neurulation in the mouse embryo. At the 4 somite stage, neural fold closure is initiated in the future cervical region (a). Closure spreads from this point in both rostal and caudal directions. At the 12 somite stage, a second site of closure is initiated at the forebrain/midbrain junction (b), and soon afterwards closure is also initiated at the extreme anterior end of the axis (c). Closure spreads forward from point (b) and backwards from (c) leading to complete closure of the forebrain neural tube, at the anterior neuropore (d). Closure also spreads backwards from (b) so that, around the 17 somite stage, the hindbrain neural tube will become completely closed (e). From the 4 somite stage onwards, closure spreads caudally along the future spine and this process is completed at the 29 somite stage with closure of the posterior neuropore (f). Thereafter, neural tube formation continues in the tail region by a different process, secondary neurulation, which involves canalization of a solid cord of cells, the medullary cord. Dashed lines indicate that part of the embryonic axis has been omitted, for the sake of clarity, from the 12, 17 and 29 somite stage embryos.

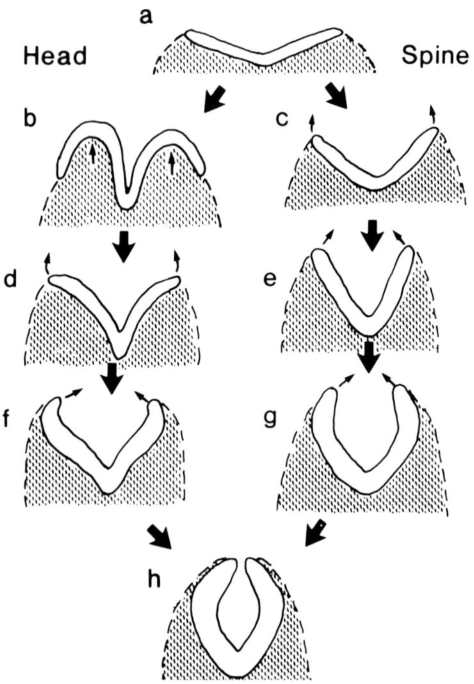

Fig. 11.3. Schematic transverse sections through the hindbrain (left) and lower spine (right) of mouse embryos to demonstrate the region-specific morphology of neurulation movements. In both cases the neural plate (a) is transformed into a neural tube (h). However, in the hindbrain region, the process involves two steps: initially, the neural plate becomes biconvex (b) and subsequently the apices of the neural folds bend medially (d and f) and approach one another in the dorsal midline. By contrast, in the spine, neurulation is an apparently simple process in which the neural groove deepens with the apices of the neural folds elevating and converging medially (c, e and g). Key to tissue layers: white, neuroepithelium; stippled, mesoderm and notochord; dashed line, surface ectoderm. Small arrows show the predominant direction of neural plate deformation. For a detailed morphological account of cranial neurulation, see Morriss-Kay (1981).

a short caudal region forms by secondary neurulation, and subsequently degenerates leaving only the coccyx (Lemire 1969).

Even within the portion of the neural tube that arises by primary neurulation, there is marked regionalization with respect to both timing and morphology

Timing

Neural tube formation begins in the cervical region of the embryo and then spreads in both rostral and caudal directions (Fig. 11.2). In the mouse a second site of initiation of neural tube closure arises later at the midbrain/forebrain boundary (Geelen and Langman 1977). It is not yet clear whether a similar closure event occurs in human embryos. Completion of closure in the mouse occurs, therefore, at three sites: within the forebrain (the anterior neuropore), within the hindbrain and at the caudal end of the embryo (Fig. 11.2). Primary neurulation in the spine continues for some time after completion of cranial neural tube closure, ceasing with closure of the posterior neuropore in the sacral region.

Morphology

Neurulation in the cranial region is a two-step process (Morriss-Kay 1981) in which the neural folds form initially as biconvex structures (Fig. 11.3a and b) and then undergo a marked change in morphology as the apices bend medially towards each other until they contact and fuse (Fig. 11.3d, f and h). By contrast, spinal neurulation appears to be a simpler process, morphologically, with the neural folds becoming elevated to form a v-shaped neural groove with gradual progressive convergence of the apices of the folds in the midline (Fig. 11.3 a, c, e, g and h).

Animal Models of NTD

Animal models of NTD fall into two broad categories with respect to their aetiology: genetic and environmental. A number of specific genetic loci are known in the mouse at which mutations cause NTD (Table 11.1). These mutations produce distinct patterns of NTD distribution which may indicate that different functional aspects of the neurulation process are disturbed in each case. Apart from these specific loci, trisomy for particular chromosomes can also lead to the appearance of NTD (Table 11.1). In addition, "non-mutant" inbred strains of mice differ in their propensity to develop NTD in response to teratogens such as hyperthermia (Finnell et al. 1986) and valproic acid (Naruse et al. 1988). Thus, genetic control of neurulation may involve both major all-or-nothing genes and minor quantitative genes.

A variety of environmental factors have been identified which produce NTD in non-mutalt rodent strains (Kalter 1968). These teratogens often appear non-specific in their effects, NTD being one of a number of congenital anomalies occurring in treated embryos.

In order to investigate the sequence of steps that underlies the process of neurulation, it seems most appropriate to analyse genetic mutant models of NTD pathogenesis. At least in the case of point mutations, it may be assumed that the defective production of a single protein species is responsible for the development of NTD. By contrast, the specificity of teratogen action in producing NTD cannot be assumed. Nevertheless, as I hope to demonstrate in the following sections, studying the interaction of mutants with environmental influences is often a most instructive method of analysis.

Table 11.1. Mouse mutants and trisomies producing neural tube defects

Mutant or trisomy	Linkage	NTD		Lethality	Reference[c]
		Cranial	Spinal		
Bn, Bent-tail	X	Exenc[a]	Sp bif[b]	All homozygotes	1
crn, Cranio-schisis	–	Exenc	None	Exenc only	2
Cd, Crooked	6	Exenc	None	Exenc only	3
ct, Curly tail	–	Exenc	Sp bif	Exenc only	4
xn, Exencephaly	–	Exenc	None	All homozygotes	5
Lp, Loop tail	1	Cranio-rachischisis		All homozygotes	6
Rf, Rib fusion	–	Exenc	None	Exenc only	3
SELH/Bc strain	–	Exenc	None	Exenc only	7
Sp, Splotch	1	Exenc	Sp bif	All homozygotes	8
Sp^d, Delayed splotch	1	Exenc	Sp bif	Survive to term	2
vl, Vacuolated lens	1	None	Sp bif	None	9
Trisomy 12	–	Exenc	None	Exenc only	10
Trisomy 14	–	Exenc	None	Exenc only	10

[a]Exenc: Exencephaly.
[b]Sp bif: Spina bifida.
[c]References: (1) Johnson 1976; (2) Kalter 1985; (3) Cole and Trasler 1980; (4) Seller and Adinolfi 1981; (5) Wallace et al. 1978; (6) Stein and Rudin 1953; (7) MacDonald et al. 1989; (8) Auerbach 1954; (9) Wilson and Wyatt 1986; (10) Putz and Morriss-Kay 1981.

The Curly Tail Mouse Mutant as a Model of Human NTD

Work in this author's laboratory has been concerned with the development of lower spinal NTD in mouse embryos carrying the incompletely penetrant mutation curly tail (*ct*, see Table 11.1). Sixty percent of *ct*/*ct* embryos develop lumbosacral NTD comprising either spina bifida (in which the spinal neural tube remains open throughout development; Fig. 11.4a) or tail flexion defects (the tail exhibits a curl or kink; Fig. 11.4b) whereas the remaining 40% of *ct*/*ct* embryos are developmentally normal (Fig 11.4c). An additional small number (2%–5%) of *ct*/*ct* embryos develop cranial NTD, namely exencephaly, in which the cranial neural tube remains open. Exencephaly is the embryonic forerunner of the birth defect anencephaly, in which the cranial vault and brain are partially or completely absent. Curly tail embryos develop NTD in a manner closely resembling the human embryo, making curly tail the best animal model of human NTD available (Seller and Adinolfi 1981). The main similarities between NTD in *ct* mice and in humans are summarized in Table 11.2.

Our studies of the *ct* mutant model system are designed to elucidate the sequence of events at the molecular, cell and organ level, that links the expression

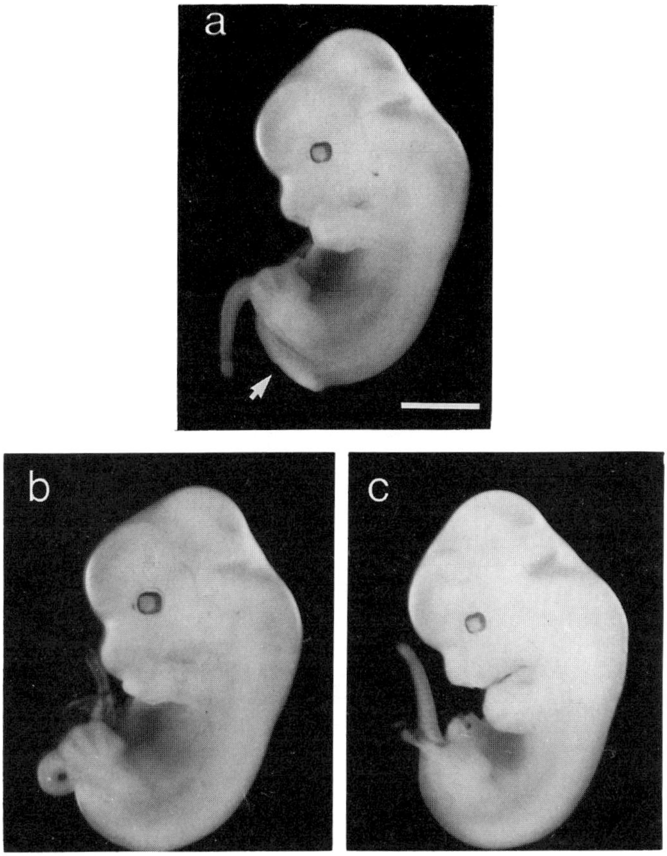

Fig. 11.4. Homozygous mutant curly tail embryos of day 13 gestation to illustrate the range of phenotypes seen in the lower spine. **a** Lumbosacral spina bifida (arrow) with tail flexion; **b** tail flexion with otherwise normal morphology; **c** normal lower spine and tail. Scale bar = 2 mm.

of the defective gene to the development of NTD in homozygous embryos. To date, our studies have concentrated on the pathogenesis of lower spinal NTD and we have attempted to answer the following specific questions:

1. Does lumbosacral spina bifida arise from faulty neural folding or defective canalization (i.e. primary or secondary neurulation)?
2. What is the basic cellular defect that gives rise to lumbosacral NTD?
3. Can this defect be corrected experimentally, as a means of preventing the development of NTD?
4. How does the cellular defect become manifest as a failure of neurulation?
5. What is the molecular basis of the cellular defect?

Table 11.2. Comparison between NTD in curly tail mice and humans

	Curly tail	Humans
Site		
Cranial	Exencephaly[a]	Anencephaly[a]
Spinal	Spina bifida and tail defects	Spina bifida
Inheritance	Recessive gene with penetrance under polygenic control	Polygenic
Prenatal lethality	Exencephaly only	Anencephaly mainly
Sex ratio		
Cranial	Female excess	Female excess
Low spinal	Male excess	Male excess
Amniotic fluid alpha-fetoprotein	Elevated in open defects	Elevated

[a]Exencephaly and anencephaly represent different developmental stages of cranial NTD. Exencephaly is present during the embryonic period and is the main cranial NTD observed in curly tail mice, whereas anencephaly is the main cranial NTD seen in human fetuses, either at birth or following abortion.

Lumbosacral Spina Bifida Arises by Defective Neural Folding

A long-standing controversy centres on whether NTD arise by failure of primary neural fold closure or by reopening of a previously closed neural tube (Gardner 1973; Marin-Padilla 1978). It is now generally assumed that the majority of spontaneous NTD result from defective primary closure. Nevertheless, a re-examination of this question was prompted by a recent study of aborted human fetuses with NTD (Seller 1987) in which it was found that NTD involving the head and upper spine affect mostly females, whereas lower spinal NTD affect mainly males. This finding was interpreted as indicating that female embryos may be especially susceptible to disturbance of primary neurulation, whereas males may be more susceptible to abnormalities of the secondary neurulation process. Since neural tube formation in secondary neurulation occurs entirely without the presence of open neural folds, the implication was that low spinal NTD must arise by pathological opening of the lumbosacral neural tube.

We tested this hypothesis in the mouse embryo as follows (Copp and Brook 1989). The precise axial level of lumbosacral spina bifida was determined in curly tail embryos and the rostral limit of the NTD was found to lie between somites 27 and 32 in over 90% of embryos examined (n=34). India ink marking experiments using non-mutant embryos developing in the whole-embryo culture system showed that primary neurulation is completed, with closure of the posterior neuropore, at the level of somites 32 to 34. Since neurulation in mammals progresses in a rostrocaudal sequence, without overlap between regions of primary and secondary neurulation (Schoenwolf 1984), we concluded that spina bifida in *ct*/*ct* embryos must arise initially as a defect of primary neurulation. The position of posterior neuropore closure in human embryos is estimated to lie at the level of the future second sacral segment (Muller and O'Rahilly 1987) indicating that in humans, as in the *ct* mouse, lumbosacral spina bifida usually arises as a defect of posterior neuropore close. There is no reason to believe, therefore, that disruptive opening of the neural tube in the lower spine is a major factor in the pathogenesis of spina bifida.

Hans Gruneberg, in his original description of the curly tail mutant (Gruneberg 1954), noted that the posterior neuropores of a proportion of *ct/ct* embryos were larger than normal indicating delayed neural fold closure. We confirmed this observation in a study of embryos undergoing completion of primary neurulation (closure of the posterior neuropore, see Fig. 11.2) both in utero and in whole-embryo culture (Copp et al. 1982). Delayed neuropore closure was found to correlate with development of spinal NTD and, moreover, to occur independently of the maternal environment, in vitro.

We asked whether there is a cause-and-effect relationship between delayed neuropore closure and the later development of spina bifida and/or tail defect. Homozygous *ct/ct* embryos were explanted from pregnant females on day 11 of gestation (when they had between 25 and 29 somites), scored for neuropore size as a measure of neuropore closure delay and then cultured for 36 h until the presence or absence of an NTD could be clearly determined. Embryos with little or no closure delay at the start of culture developed normally in most cases, those with moderate delay developed tail defects and those with severe delay developed spina bifida and/or tail defects (Copp, 1985). These findings established two things. First, that spina bifida and tail defects, although morphologically distinct malformations, in fact result from a single embryonic abnormality, delay of neuropore closure; the severity of the closure defect determines the final phenotype. Second, *ct/ct* embryos destined to develop NTD can be recognized early in development, prior to the completion of normal neuropore closure, by virtue of their large neuropores. This morphological marker of abnormal embryo fate has formed the basis of a number of subsequent studies on the cellular and molecular basis of NTD development in the curly tail mutant (see Fig. 11.5).

The Basic Cellular Defect in *ct/ct* Embryos

Neurulation takes place at the time of intense embryonic growth, raising the possibility that disturbance of cell proliferation may play an important role in the pathogenesis of NTD. Indeed, one of the earliest findings in relation to the development of human NTD was of an apparent "overgrowth" of neuroepithelial cells in the region of spina bifida (Patten 1953). Later studies of mouse embryos showed that, in fact, there is a reduction in the rate of proliferation of neuroepithelial cells following defective neural closure (Wilson 1980). The appearance of neuroepithelial overgrowth in these embryos derives from the lateral projection of the bifid neural folds and the arrest of neuroepithelial cells in mitosis, producing an artefactually high mitotic index value.

Notwithstanding these studies of fully formed NTD, there have been few investigations of cell proliferation rates during the early stages of abnormal neural fold closure. We performed such a study (Copp et al. 1988a), measuring rates of cell proliferation in the five resident cell types within the posterior neuropore

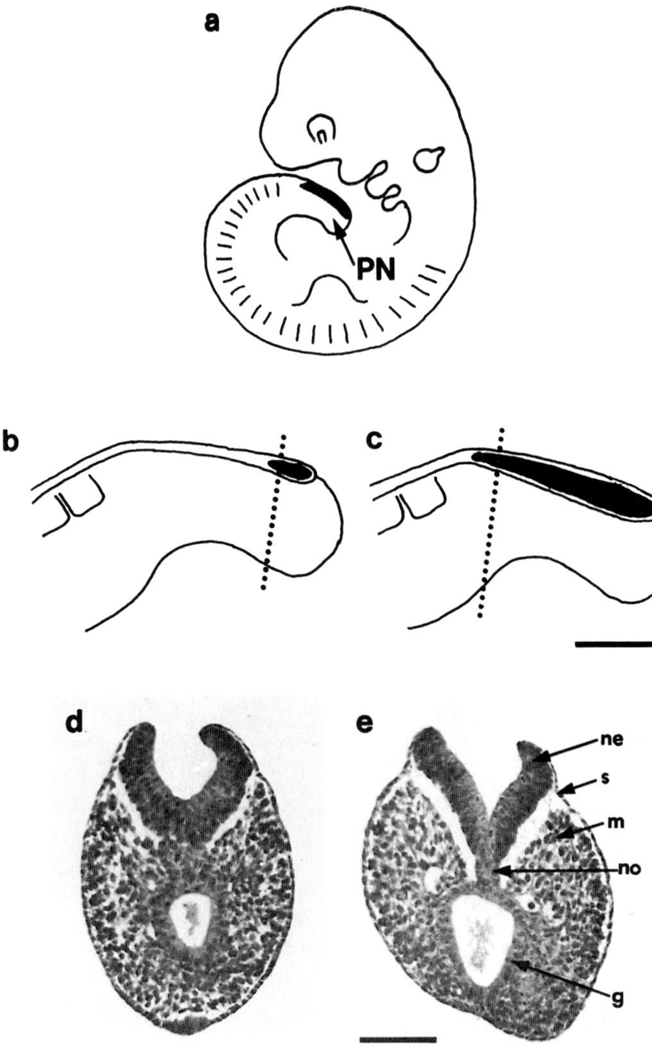

Fig. 11.5. Diagrams and histological sections of embryos to illustrate the enlarged posterior neuropore as seen in affected *ct/ct* embryos and the cell types analysed in the cell proliferation analysis. **a** Embryo on day 11 gestation with approximately 27 somites. The posterior neuropore (PN) is the only embryonic region still undergoing primary neurulation. **b** and **c** Enlarged views of the posterior neuropore regions of unaffected (b) and affected (c) *ct/ct* embryos. Note that the neuropore of the affected embryo (c) occupies almost the entire length of the presomitic mesdermal region. **d** and **e** Transverse histological sections, stained with haemalum and eosin, through the posterior neuropore regions of unaffected (d) and affected (e) *ct/ct* embryos. Planes of section are indicated by dotted lines in (b) and (c). Cell types studied in the cell proliferation analysis: ne, neuropithelium; s, surface ectoderm; m, mesoderm; no, notochord; g, hindgut endoderm. Scale bars: (b) and (c), 0.3 mm; (d) and (e), 0.1mm.

Table 11.3. Length of the cell cycle in various cell types within the posterior neuropore region of normal and affected *ct/ct* embryos

Cell type	Length of cell cycle (h)[a]	
	Normal	Affected
Neuroepithelium	10.2	9.1
Surface ectoderm	16.5	18.2
Mesoderm	13.9	12.8
Notochord	12.4	17.3
Hindgut endoderm	8.3	11.2

[a]Length of cell cycle calculated from the formula $t_g = \ln 2 \times t_m/\text{MI}$, where t_g is the cell cycle length, t_m is the length of mitosis (assumed to be 0.5 h) and MI is the mean mitotic index.

region of *ct/ct* embryos. A comparison was made between embryos with normal-sized neuropores at the 27–29 somite stage (normal controls) and those with abnormally enlarged neuropores (presumptive abnormal). The study measured mitotic index values, length of S-phase of the cell cycle, and the rate of appearance of unlabelled cells in a [^{3}H] thymidine pulse-chase experiment. All three of these independent measures yielded the same, unexpected, result: the neuroepithelium proliferated in an identical manner in normal and abnormal embryos, as did the underlying mesoderm and the surface ectoderm (the presumptive epidermis). On the other hand, the hindgut endoderm and notochord proliferated significantly more slowly in abnormal embryos than in normal controls (Table 11.3). Thus, a cell proliferation defect is present in affected *ct/ct* embryos within tissues subjacent to the neural plate but not within the neuroepithelium itself.

Spinal NTD are Prevented by Correcting the Cell Proliferation Imbalance

Following the discovery of the hindgut/notochord cell proliferation defect, we considered the hypothesis that spinal NTD may arise in *ct/ct* embryos as a result of an imbalance in growth rates between these affected tissues and the unaffected neuroepithelium. One way of testing this hypothesis was to retard embryonic growth experimentally which, by analogy with cytotoxic cancer chemotherapy, should have the greatest effect on the most rapidly growing cells in the embryo. In the case of *ct/ct* embryos, proliferation of the neuroepithelium should be reduced to a greater extent than proliferation of the hindgut or notochord, thereby re-establishing a balance of cell proliferation rates, and preventing the development of spinal NTD.

Embryos were growth-retarded in utero by depriving pregnant females of food for 24 h or 48 h. Growth retardation for 48 h, before closure of the posterior neuropore, significantly reduced the overall incidence of spinal NTD and prevented spina bifida almost completely (Table 11.4), whereas growth retardation for the same length of time following neuropore closure (and for 24 h at any time) had no effect on the incidence of NTD (Copp et al. 1988b). In

Table 11.4. Effect of growth retardation in utero on development of curly tail embryos

Period of food deprivation				Developmental outcome				Measurements of development and growth	
				No. embryos showing					
Hours	Days gestation	No. embryos	% resorption	Normal spine	Curly tail	Spina bifida	% NTD	No. somites	Protein content (mg)
0	–	36	18.2	14	14	8	61.1	53.7 ± 0.5	3.5 ± 0.4
24	9–10	33	23.3	17	15	1	48.5	54.1 ± 0.5	3.2 ± 0.4
	10–11	36	5.3	12	16	8	66.6	53.5 ± 0.4	3.4 ± 0.2
	11–12	46	8.0	16	22	8	65.2	53.5 ± 0.3	2.7 ± 0.2
48	8–10	37	17.4	25	12	0	32.4	50.9 ± 0.3	2.9 ± 0.1
	9–11	59	10.4	42	16	1	28.8	49.4 ± 0.4	1.6 ± 0.2
	10–12	52	8.8	26	24	2	50.0	52.5 ± 0.3	3.5 ± 0.2

Data from Copp et al. (1988b).

a separate experiment, embryos were growth-retarded in vitro by culture at 40.5°C rather than the usual 38°C; culture at 40.5°C has previously been shown to induce growth retardation in rat embryos without producing NTD (Cockroft and New 1978). In vitro growth retardation reduced the proportion of embryos undergoing delayed neuropore closure, showing that growth retardation acts to prevent NTD by normalizing the primary spinal neurulation process. In order to determine the effects of growth retardation on cell proliferation rates, embryos were labelled for 1 h with [^{3}H] thymidine in vitro and then subjected to autoradiographic analysis. This experiment showed that, as expected, cell proliferation had been inhibited by culture at 40.5°C primarily in the neuroepithelium and to a lesser extent in other cell types (Copp et al. 1988b). Thus, growth retardation re-establishes a balance between the proliferation rates of hindgut/notochord and neuroepithelium, and leads to normal spinal neurulation.

A Mechanical Link Between the Cell Proliferation Defect and Spinal NTD

Having established that the hindgut/notochord cell proliferation defect is directly responsible for the appearance of spinal NTD in *ct*/*ct* embryos we asked the question: by what mechanism does the cell proliferation imbalance lead to defective neural fold closure? Previous studies by Jacobson and his colleagues had provided evidence for a role of axial elongation in amphibian (Jacobson and Gordon 1976) and chick (Jacobson 1984) neural tube closure. Moreover, in the mouse embryo, there is circumstantial evidence that ventral curvature of the embryonic axis may retard neurulation, specifically in the midbrain region (Jacobson and Tam 1982). We therefore examined the hypothesis that the cell proliferation imbalance leads to delay of posterior neuropore closure either by reducing axial elongation, or by increasing ventral curvature, in the caudal embryonic region. Measurements were made on camera lucida drawings of embryos in profile view and these revealed that whereas axial length is not reduced in affected *ct*/*ct* embryos, compared with unaffected controls, ventral curvature of the caudal embryonic region is abnormally increased in embryos undergoing delayed neuropore closure (F.A. Brook and A. J. Copp, unpublished). In another experiment, surgical enlargement of the neuropore failed to produce increased ventral curvature, suggesting that the excessive curvature in affected *ct*/*ct* embryos is a cause, and not a result, of delayed neural fold closure (F.A. Brook and A. J. Copp, unpublished).

Clues to the Molecular Basis of the NTD in *ct/ct* Embryos

A group of macromolecules that may play a role in neurulation are the glycosaminoglycans (GAGs), which are constituents of the interstitial extracellular matrix and basement membranes of both embryonic and adult tissues. Previous studies of rat (Solursh and Morriss 1977) and mouse (Copp and Bernfield 1988b) embryos, undergoing cranial and spinal neurulation respectively, revealed a spatial and temporal correlation between the neurulation process and accumulation of a particular GAG, hyaluronate. In order to determine whether hyaluronate, or other GAG species, may play a role in the development of spinal NTD, we studied the accumulation of these macromolecules in *ct*/*ct* embryos.

Glucosamine is a useful precursor for such studies since it is converted by mammalian cells to N-acetyl-glucosamine, which is then incorporated into a wide range of carbohydrates including GAGs. Embryos were metabolically labelled by culture in medium containing [^{3}H] glucosamine, and the relative amounts of radioactivity in the various GAG species was determined for specific regions of the labelled embryos. Curly tail embryos with delayed neuropore closure accumulated significantly less hyaluronate in the posterior neuropore region than unaffected *ct*/*ct* embryos (Copp and Bernfield 1988a). This difference was specific: normal and abnormal embryos were closely similar with respect to their accumulation of non-hyaluronate GAGs at the neuropore site, and also to their accumulation of hyaluronate in regions where neurulation had already been completed (e.g. the hindbrain).

Sections of labelled embryos were subjected to autoradiographic analysis with or without prior treatment with *Streptomyces* hyaluronidase, an enzyme that specifically digests hyaluronate. A heavy localization of newly synthesized hyaluronate was seen in unaffected *ct*/*ct* embryos at the site of developing basement membranes, beneath the neuroepithelium and around the notochord. Hyaluronate accumulation at this site was markedly reduced in *ct*/*ct* embryos with delayed neuropore closure (Copp and Bernfield 1988a).

These findings may provide a clue to the molecular basis of the cellular defect in *ct* embryos. Hyaluronate has been implicated in the promotion of proliferation of cultured fibroblasts (Tomida et al. 1975; Cohn et al. 1976; Matuoka et al. 1987), thus raising the possibility that normal proliferation of hindgut and notochordal cells is stimulated by close proximity to extracellular matrix hyaluronate. In this case, subnormal accumulation of hyaluronate in affected *ct*/*ct* embryos may be the cause of the observed cell proliferation defect. On the other hand, the possibility that reduced hyaluronate accumulation is actually a result of defective hindgut and notochordal cell proliferation, rather than a cause, cannot be ruled out.

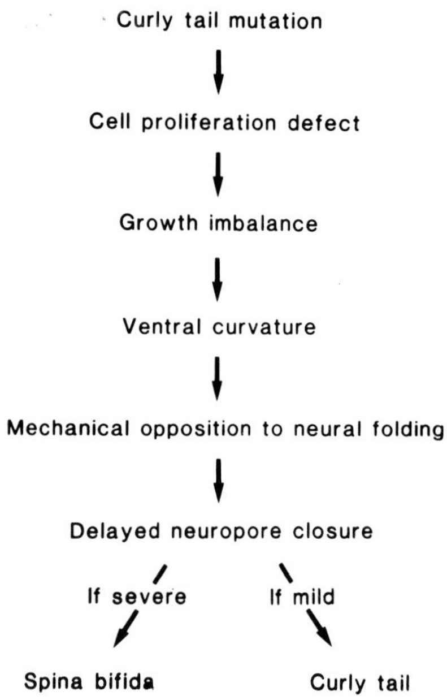

Fig. 11.6. Flow diagram showing the sequence of events in the development of spinal NTD in *ct/ct* embryos. The earliest cellular defect identified to date is a reduced rate of proliferation of hindgut endoderm and notochord cells in the posterior neuropore region. This cell proliferation defect produces a growth imbalance within the embryo which leads to ventral curvature of the caudal extremity. Ventral curvature opposes dorsally-directed neurulation movements and so leads to delayed neuropore closure. If the closure delay is mild, only a tail flexion results whereas, if it is severe, neural tube closure fails to be completed and a spina bifida results, usually in conjunction with a curly tail.

Discussion and Conclusions

The previous sections have outlined the experimental evidence on which is based our current understanding of the cellular and morphogenetic basis of spinal NTD development in *ct/ct* embryos. The presumed sequence of events is presented in the form of a flow-diagram in Fig. 11.6. The next step in our research will be to investigate in greater detail the molecular basis of the hindgut/notochord cell proliferation defect in *ct/ct* embryos. Although our findings with regard to hyaluronate accumulation are interesting, it is not yet possible to draw firm conclusions about the role of extracellular matrix defects in the pathogenesis of the *ct* phenotype.

The finding of a cell proliferation defect in *ct/ct* embryos that affects cell types other than the neuroepithelium is unexpected in the light of results obtained with other mouse mutants. For instance, hindbrain NTD in embryos homozygous for splotch (*Sp*) and looptail (*Lp*) are both associated with a reduction in the rate of neuroepithelial cell proliferation (Wilson 1974; Wilson and Center 1974). It seems possible, therefore, that the different mutations disrupt different cellular functions, each of which is essential for normal completion of neurulation. This raises the exciting possibility of using comparative studies of the various mutations (Table 11.1), to "dissect" the normal neurulation process into a series of functional steps each of which, when disrupted, leads to development of NTD.

The finding that embryonic growth retardation leads to normalization of spinal neurulation in *ct/ct* embryos is in sharp contrast to the often-stated maxim that intrauterine growth retardation is a predisposing factor for congenital malformations (Spiers 1982). Our result is not without precedent. Seller and colleagues were able to reduce the incidence of spinal NTD in *ct* mice by maternal administration of the DNA synthesis inhibitors hydroxyurea (Seller and Perkins

1983) and mitomycin C (Seller and Perkins 1986). Thus, it would appear likely that any influence which retards embryonic growth, if acting at the appropriate stage of gestation, will redress the balance of cell proliferation rates in the embryo and prevent the development of spinal NTD. It should be noted, however, that growth retardation is not effective in preventing cranial NTD: hydroxyurea and mitomycin C act as potent teratogens, increasing the incidence of exencephaly in *ct* mice (Seller and Perkins 1983; Seller and Perkins, 1986). Thus, the pathogenetic mechanism underlying exencephaly must differ fundamentally from that responsible for lumbosacral spina bifida in *ct/ct* embryos. This conclusion fits well with the observed difference in sex ratio in the two types of NTD (Carter 1974) and suggests that it is misleading to classify NTD as a single group of malformations. Rather, cranial and lower spinal NTD should be seen as distinct malformations with quite different pathogenetic origins.

*Acknowledgements.*rI am most grateful to Dr. Karen Downs for commenting on the manuscript and to the Imperial Cancer Research Fund for financial support.

References

Auerbach R (1954) Analysis of the developmental effects of a lethal mutation in the house mouse. J Exp Zool 127: 305–329

Carter CO (1974) Clues to the aetiology of neural tube malformations. Dev Med Child Neurol 16, suppl 32: 3–15

Cockroft DL, New DAT (1978) Abnormalities induced in cultured rat embryos by hyperthermia. Teratology 17: 277–284

Cohn RH, Cassiman J-J, Bernfield M (1976) Relationship of transformation, cell density, and growth control to the cellular distribution of newly synthesized glycosaminoglycan. J Cell Biol 71: 280–294

Cole WA, Trasler DG (1980) Gene-teratogen interaction in insulin-induced mouse exencephaly. Teratology 22: 125–139

Copp AJ (1985) Relationship between timing of posterior neuropore closure and development of spinal neural tube defects in mutant (curly tail) and normal mouse embryos in culture. J Embryol Exp Morphol 88: 39–54

Copp AJ, Bernfield M (1988a) Accumulation of basement membrane-associated hyaluronate is reduced in the posterior neuropore region of mutant (curly tail) mouse embryos developing spinal neural tube defects. Dev Biol 130: 583–590

Copp AJ, Bernfield M (1988b) Glycosaminoglycans vary in accumulation along the neuraxis during spinal neurulation in the mouse embryo. Dev Biol 130: 573–582

Copp AJ, Brook FA (1989) Does lumbosacral spina bifida arise by failure of neural folding or by defective canalisation? J Med Genet 26: 160–166

Copp AJ, Seller MJ, Polani PE (1982) Neural tube development in mutant (curly tail) and normal mouse embryos: the timing of posterior neuropore closure in vivo and in vitro. J Embryol Exp Morphol 69: 151–167

Copp AJ, Brook FA, Roberts HJ (1988a) A cell-type-specific abnormality of cell proliferation in mutant (curly tail) mouse embryos developing spinal neural tube defects. Development 104: 285–295

Copp AJ, Crolla JA, Brook FA (1988b) Prevention of spinal neural tube defects in the mouse embryo by growth retardation during neurulation. Development 104: 297–303

Finnell RH, Moon SP, Abbott LC, Golden JA, Chernoff GF (1986) Strain differences in heat-induced neural tube defects in mice. Teratology 33: 247–252

Gardner WJ (1973) The dysraphic states. From syringomyelia to anencephaly. Excerpta Medica, Amsterdam

Geelen JA, Langman J (1977) Closure of the neural tube in the cephalic region of the mouse embryo. Anat Rec 189: 625–640

Gruneberg H (1954) Genetical studies on the skeleton of the mouse. VIII. Curly tail. J Genet 52: 52–67
Jacobson AG (1984) Further evidence that formation of the neural tube requires elongation of the nervous system. J Exp Zool 230: 23–28
Jacobson AG, Gordon R (1976) Changes in the shape of the developing vertebrate nervous system analysed experimentally, mathematically and by computer simulation. J Exp Zool 197: 191–246
Jacobson AG, Tam PPL (1982) Cephalic neurulation in the mouse embryo analysed by SEM and morphometry. Anat Rec 203: 375–396
Johnson DR (1976) The interfrontal bone and mutant genes in the mouse. J Anat 121: 507–513
Kalter H (1968) Teratology of the central nervous system. University of Chicago Press, Chicago
Kalter H (1985) Experimental teratological studies with the mouse CNS mutations cranioschisis and delayed splotch. J Craniofac Genet Dev Biol Suppl 1: 339–342
Lemire RJ (1969) Variations in development of the caudal neural tube in human embryos (Horizons XIV–XXI). Teratology 2: 361–370
MacDonald KB, Juriloff DM, Harris MJ (1989) Developmental study of neural-tube closure in a mouse stock with a high-incidence of exencephaly. Teratology 39: 195–213
Marin-Padilla M (1978) Clinical and experimental rachischisis. In: Vinken PJ, Bruyn GW, Myrianthopoulos NC (eds) Handbook of clinical neurology, no 32. Congenital malformations of the spine and spinal cord. Elsevier/North-Holland Medical Press, Amsterdam, pp 159–191
Matuoka K, Namba M, Mitsui Y (1987) Hyaluronate synthetase inhibition by normal and transformed human fibroblasts during growth reduction. J Cell Biol 104: 1105–1115
Morriss-Kay GM (1981) Growth and development of pattern in the cranial neural epithelium of rat embryos during neurulation. J Embryol Exp Morphol 65 (suppl): 225–241
Muller F, O'Rahilly R (1987) The development of the human brain, the closure of the caudal neuropore, and the beginning of secondary neurulation at stage 12. Anat Embryol 176: 413–430
Naruse I, Collins MD, Scott WJ (1988) Strain differences in the teratogenicity induced by sodium valproate in cultured mouse embryos. Teratology 38: 87–96
New DAT, Coppola PT, Terry S (1973) Culture of explanted rat embryos in rotating tubes. J Reprod Fertil 35: 135–138
Office of Population Censuses and Surveys, Series DH3 no18 (1985) Mortality statistics. Her Majesty's Stationery Office, London
Patten BM (1953) Embryological stages in the establishing of myeloschisis with spina bifida. Am J Anat 93: 365–395
Putz B, Morriss-Kay GM (1981) Abnormal neural fold development in trisomy 12 and trisomy 14 mouse embryos. I. Scanning electron microscopy. J Embryol Exp Morphol 66: 141–158
Schoenwolf GC (1984) Histological and ultrastructural studies of secondary neurulation of mouse embryos. Am J Anat 169: 361–374
Seller MJ (1987) Neural tube defects and sex ratios. Am J Med Genet 26: 699–707
Seller MJ, Adinolfi M (1981) The curly-tail mouse: an experimental model for human neural tube defects. Life Sci 29: 1607–1615
Seller MJ, Perkins KJ (1983) Effect of hydroxyurea on neural tube defects in the curly-tail mouse. J Craniofac Genet Dev Biol 3: 11–17
Seller MJ, Perkins KJ (1986) Effect of mitomycin C on the neural tube defects of the curly-tail mouse. Teratology 33: 305–309
Solursh M, Morriss GM (1977) Glycosaminoglycan synthesis in rat embryos during the formation of the primary mesenchyme and neural folds. Dev Biol 57: 75–86
Spiers PS (1982) Does growth retardation predispose the fetus to congenital malformation? Lancet i: 312–314
Stein KF, Rudin IA (1953) Development of mice homozygous for the gene for loop-tail. J Hered 44: 59–69
Tomida M, Koyama H, Ono T (1975) Induction of hyaluronic acid synthetase activity in rat fibroblasts by medium change of confluent cultures. J Cell Physiol 86: 121–130
Wallace ME, Knights PJ, Anderson JR (1978) Inheritance and morphology of exencephaly, a neonatal recessive with partial penetrance, in the house mouse. Genet Res 32: 135–149
Wilson DB (1974) Proliferation in the neural tube of the splotch (Sp) mutant mouse. J Comp Neurol 154: 249–256
Wilson DB (1980) Cellular proliferation in the exencephalic brain of the mouse embryo. Brain Res 195: 139–148
Wilson DB, Center EM (1974) Neural cell cycle in the Looptail mutant of the mouse (Lp). J Embryol Exp Morphol 32: 697–705
Wilson DB, Wytt DP (1986) Pathogenesis of neural dysraphism in the mouse mutant vacuolated lens (*vl*). J Neuropathol Exp Neurol 45: 43–55

12. Ultrasound and Biochemical Assessment of First Trimester Pregnancy

B. Brambati, A. Lanzani and L. Tului

Introduction

Within the last two decades new investigative tools have become available for timing of fertilization and implantation, for detection of genetic anomalies, and for predicting pregnancy outcome in the first trimester. A close interaction between the conceptus and the mother has been defined and embryonic signals have been identified which may lead to local, regional and general maternal responses (Table 12.1). The first detectable change in the maternal circulation is the appearance of early pregnancy factor (EPF) within 24 hours of conception; this could be a gestational signal to the corpus luteum and endometrium (Morton et al. 1977). In addition, a mild maternal thrombocytopenia has been observed in the first week as a result of production of the embryo-derived platelet activating factor (ED-PAF) which has been found in the supernatants of mouse and human embryo cultures (O'Neill 1985). The development of sensitive and specific radioimmunoassays for human chorionic gonadotrophin (hCG), together with in vitro fertilization and embryo transfer, has permitted determination of the mean and confidence limits for the first appearance of hCG. Serial serum determinations from the time of implantation may predict pregnancy failure before clinical signs are apparent (Lenton et al. 1982).

Almost three-quarters of conceptuses do not survive to livebirth. Most pregnancies fail in the first 14 days after fertilization (Edwards 1986; Kline et al. 1986) and about 15% of recognized clinical pregnancies are lost in the first trimester (Brambati and Lanzani 1987). There is no consensus about the role of environmental factors, or of unfavourable endocrine (Macdonald 1989) or immunological (Adinolfi 1986; Sargent et al. 1988) conditions. Spontaneous or induced gene mutations are possible causes, and gene sequences with specific regulatory functions in the embryo have been demonstrated in the human (Boncinelli et al. 1988). However, chromosome anomalies are probably the major cause of reproductive loss in early pregnancy and have been detected in about 80% of missed abortions between 6 and 11 weeks (Guerneri et al. 1987).

Table 12.1. Biophysical and biochemical markers for determining fertilization and implantation, and post-implantation embryo development

Marker	First detection	
	Days post-conception	Days post-LMP
EPF	1	15
ED-PAF (maternal thrombocytopenia)	1	15
hCG	8–11	22–25
(Subjective symptoms)	14–21	28–35
Gestational sac	16–20	30–34
SP1	18–23	32–37
Heart activity	24–26	38–40
PAPP-A	28–33	42–37

Investigation of early gestation has in general been very disappointing. Several biochemical markers have been used to predict the evolution of early pregnancy, but in many cases abnormal levels are not observed until weeks after embryo death when heart activity is no longer evident by ultrasound. Inappropriate use of ultrasound to detect fetal viability at the time of maternal blood sampling and the clinical heterogeneity of the population investigated may explain the discordant results of different authors. Some well-designed studies addressed only selected cases with both a living fetus and a clinical diagnosis of threatened abortion (Ho and Jones 1980; Mantoni 1985; Westergaard et al. 1985; Stabile et al. 1989).

The aim of the present study was to assess the utility of a number of biophysical and biochemical parameters as prognostic indicators in clinically normal first-trimester pregnancies. Moreover, because serial evaluation is often impractical, and would anyway delay diagnosis and treatment, the value of single measurements in detecting viability of the conceptus and predicting pregnancy progress has been explored.

Prognostic Indicators of Early Pregnancy Failure

The patients in this study were women referred to our prenatal clinic in the early first trimester (6 to 9 weeks amenorrhoea) for genetic counselling. Maternal blood was taken and ultrasound examination performed using a 5 MHz abdominal sector scan and, when required, a 6.5 MHz vaginal probe. Serum specimens were stored at −20°C until assayed and all biochemical analysis was performed in the Departments of Obstetrics, Gynaecology and Reproductive Physiology (Prof. J.G. Grudzinskas and Prof. T. Chard), The London Hospital. The normal limits of ultrasonic and biochemical parameters were determined from a population of women with regular menstrual cycles, a reliable menstrual history, and normal pregnancy outcome. In no case were clinical signs of threatened abortion present, and the fetal heart beat was observed in all cases.

Alpha-fetoprotein (AFP), human chorionic gonadotrophin (hCG), Schwangerschafts protein 1 (SP1), pregnancy-associated plasma protein A (PAPP-A) and progesterone (P) were measured by radioimmunoassay methods (Westergaard et al. 1985). All viable pregnancies underwent chorionic villus sampling (CVS) for fetal karyotyping; 44 out of 91 cases (48%) ending in spontaneous abortion before CVS were karyotyped by a direct method after surgical evacuation of the uterus (Guerneri et al. 1987). An abnormal karyotype was found in 36 cases (81.9%). The time interval between the scan showing a live embryo and miscarriage ranged from 2 days to 3 weeks. Pregnancy failure was diagnosed by the absence of a fetal heart beat (87 cases) or by spontaneous expulsion of the conceptus (4 cases).

Ultrasound Investigation

The length of the embryo (CRL) and the gestational sac (GS) volume were determined in 2317 normal pregnancies between 6 and 12 weeks using the standard procedures devised by Robinson and Fleming (1975) and Robinson

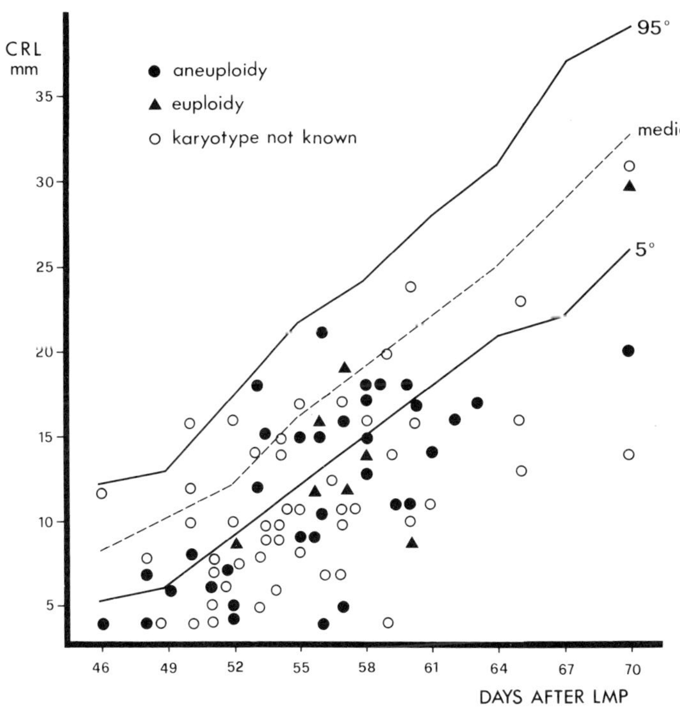

Fig. 12.1. CRL values of 91 cases, ending later in spontaneous abortion, are superimposed on the normal range (median, 5th and 95th centiles). In 33, 8 and 50 cases chorionic villi karyotype was abnormal, normal, and not known, respectively.

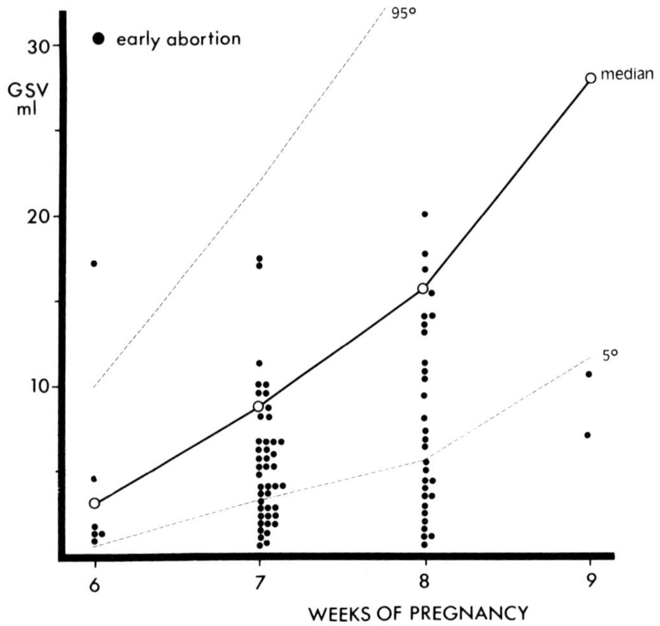

Fig. 12.2. GS volume values of 82 cases, ending later on in spontaneous abortion, are superimposed on the normal range (median, 5th and 95th centiles).

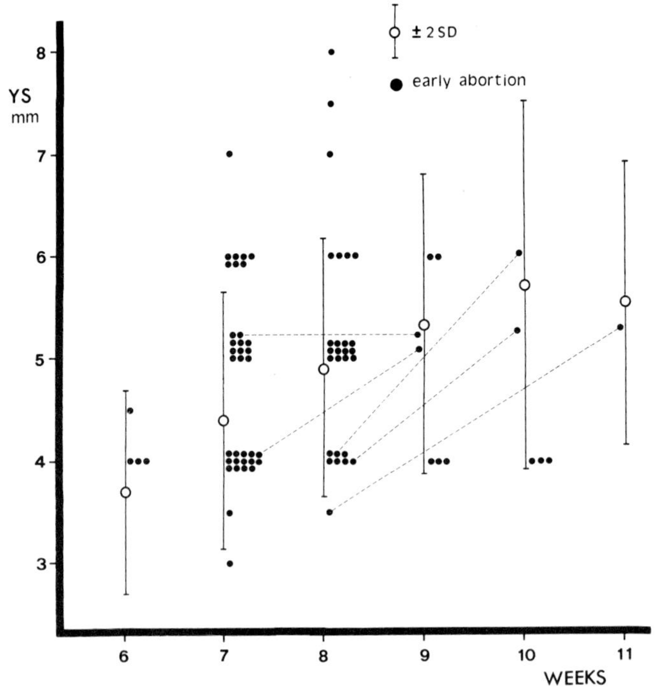

Fig. 12.3. YS diameter values of 73 cases, ending later in spontaneous abortion, are superimposed on the normal range (mean ± 2SD).

Table 12.2. Sensitivity, specificity, predictive value and efficiency of a single CRL, GS volume and YS diameter measurement in predicting imminent pregnancy failure (cut off level: the 5th centile of normal range)

	CRL (≤5°)	GS volume (≤5°)	YS diameter (≤5° ≥95°)
Sensitivity	61.5%	41.3%	38.2%
Specificity	95.0%	95.0%	90.0%
Predictive value of (+) test	33.5%	24.8%	10.2%
Predictive value of (−) test	98.3%	97.6%	95.0%
Efficiency	94 %	93 %	74 %

(1985). Yolk sac (YS) diameter was also calculated as the mean of two orthogonal diameters. CRL, GS volume and YS diameter values of 91 cases ending in spontaneous abortion were compared with normals.

CRL and GS volumes (Figs 12.1 and 12.2) in case of subsequent pregnancy failure were within the lower end of the normal range (61.5% [CRL] and 51.3% [GS] being less than the 5th percentile). The tendency towards reduced yolk sac size, as previously described (Brambati and Lanzani 1987), was not confirmed in the present study; instead there was an excess of values both in the highest and the lowest range (Fig. 12.3). Table 12.2 shows the predictive value analysis for CRL, GS volume and YS diameter. These results suggest a close association between early growth delay and pregnancy failure in the first trimester. Sonographic evidence of growth delay between 6 and 9 gestation weeks suggests an increased risk of embryo death. In cases of miscarriage the embryos were an average of 6 days smaller than would be expected from the period of amenorrhoea.

Many factors might influence fetal growth (Vorherr 1982). Genetic constitution is believed to be the major factor affecting growth of the conceptus in the first months of intrauterine life. This is further supported in our study by the fact that in 63.8% of the pregnancies in which an abnormal karyotype was reported, CRL values were below normal limits. However, low CRL values were also present in 62.5% of chromosomally normal cases, and this would indicate that other genetic and/or environmental factors may cause early growth delay.

Biochemical Markers

AFP, hCG, SP1, PAPP-A and P were assayed at 6 to 9 weeks in 240 uncomplicated pregnancies with a normal outcome, and in 47 viable pregnancies in which fetal death was observed days or weeks later. Because this was not a complete population study the predictive value of the biochemical determinations could not be estimated. The relation between the abnormal and normal populations were evaluated using the 5th percentile as a cutoff.

All biochemical indices showed depressed values. In 77%, 85%, 90%, 77% and 85% of cases respectively maternal levels of hCG, PAPP-A, SP1, AFP and P were lower than the median. A clear-cut discrimination between normal and abnormal was only possible with the placental proteins. Around half of cases of pregnancy failure had hCG, SP1 and PAPP-A below the 5th percentile

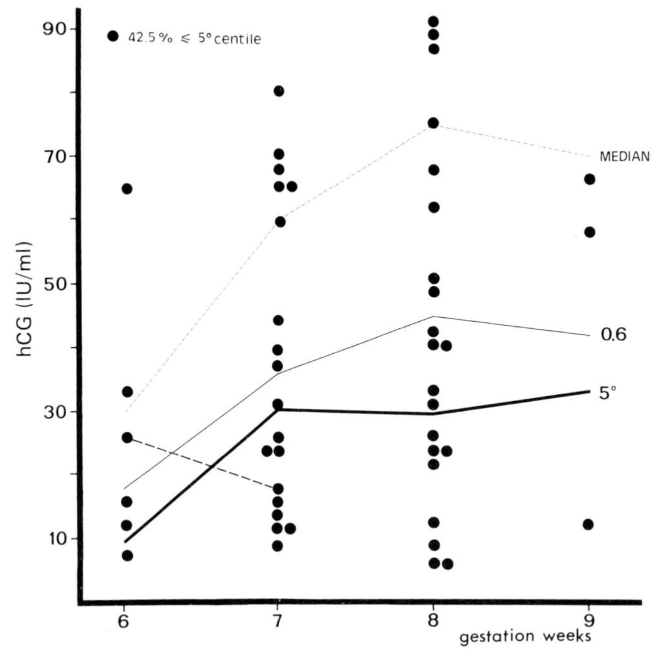

Fig. 12.4. Maternal serum level of human chorionic gonadotrophin (hCG) in 48 cases ending later in spontaneous abortion; the heavy line represents the 5th centile.

(Figs. 12.4–12.6), whereas AFP and P (Fig. 12.7) were low in only one-quarter of the abnormal population (Table 12.3). Although the proportion of cases with a normal fetal chromosome constitution was small (18.1%), karyotype does not seem to affect the efficiency of the tests: abnormal values of at least one of the biochemical (100%) or ultrasonic (71%) parameters were found in cases with normal chromosomes. The fact that several fetal and placental markers are affected by early pregnancy failure suggests that fetal demise is the end-result of a complex and general disturbance of the feto-placental unit.

The present investigation permits evaluation of the potential value of single sonographic and biochemical tests in the prediction of an abnormal outcome of an apparently normal first-trimester pregnancy. The sensitivity of biochemical testing is further enhanced (to 95%) by combining at least three tests (hCG, PAPP-A and SP1). This, together with sonographic examination, is a promising rapid test screen at 6 to 9 weeks gestation.

Table 12.3. Sensitivity of a single P, AFP, hCG, PAPP-A and SP1 maternal blood measurement between 6 and 9 weeks for detecting imminent pregnancy failure (cut off level: the 5th centile of normal range)

	P	AFP	hCG	PAPP-A	SP1	hCG+PAPP−A+SP1
Sensitivity (TP/TP+FN ×100%)	21	28	42	51	52	95

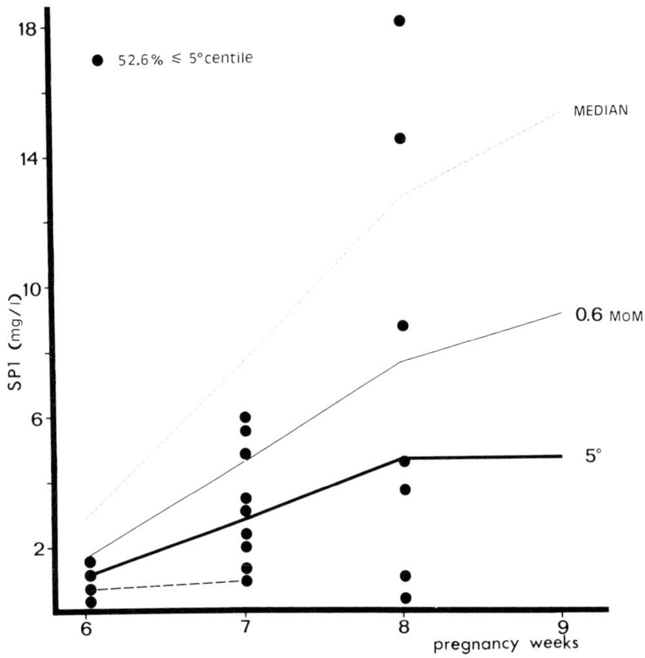

Fig. 12.5. Maternal serum level of Schwangerschaftsprotein 1 (SP1) in 19 cases ending later in spontaneous abortion; the heavy line represents the 5th centile.

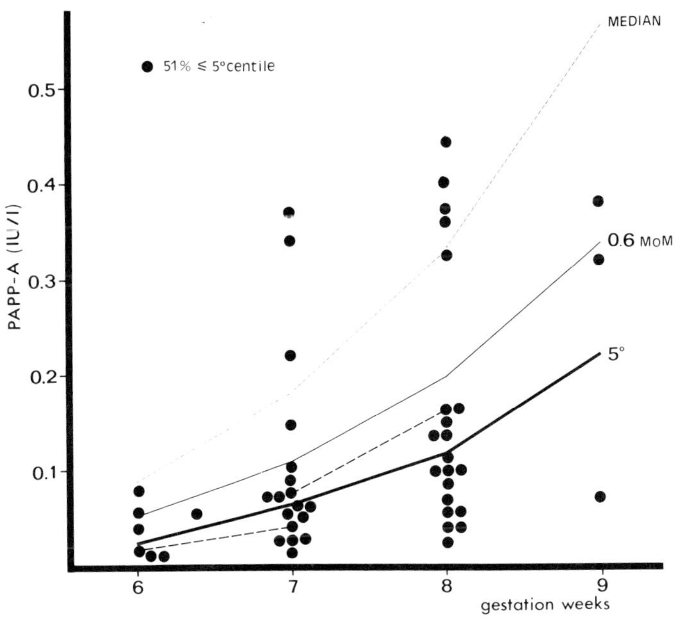

Fig. 12.6. Maternal serum level of pregnancy associated plasma protein-A (PAPP-A) in 47 cases ending later in spontaneous abortion; the heavy line represents the 5th centile.

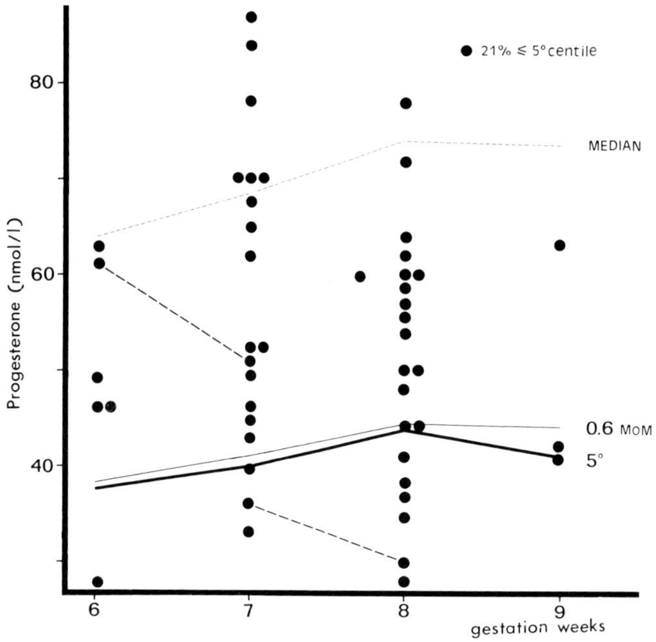

Fig. 12.7. Maternal serum level of progesterone (P) in 48 cases ending later in spontaneous abortion; the heavy line represents the 5th centile.

Assessment of Genetic Diseases and Developmental Anomalies

The last two decades have witnessed rapid growth of prenatal diagnosis methods (amniocentesis, cordocentesis and CVS) as routine components of genetic counselling and obstetric management. The low risk and high efficiency of these methods in preventing the birth of severely affected fetuses have been confirmed, and at the present time more than 100 different genetic abnormalities can be diagnosed in the first or second trimester (Weaver 1989). CVS has been introduced as a routine clinical procedure in recent years (Fig. 12.8) and offers the psychological and medical advantages of very early diagnosis. Moreover the high yield of DNA from chorionic tissue allows rapid molecular diagnosis of a growing number of hereditary diseases.

First-trimester genetic diagnosis by CVS is now performed throughout the world and analysis of the WHO-CVS Registry data (Jackson 1989) shows a 50% annual increase; around 50 000 CVS procedures will be carried out in 1990 in Europe alone.

Trials have been conducted at 11 Canadian and 7 American clinics on a comparison between CVS and amniocentesis (Canadian Collaborative CVS-Amniocentesis Trial Group 1989; Rhoads et al. 1989). In both studies transcervical aspiration was the only CVS method used, and no significant difference in fetal loss rate between CVS and amniocentesis was found.

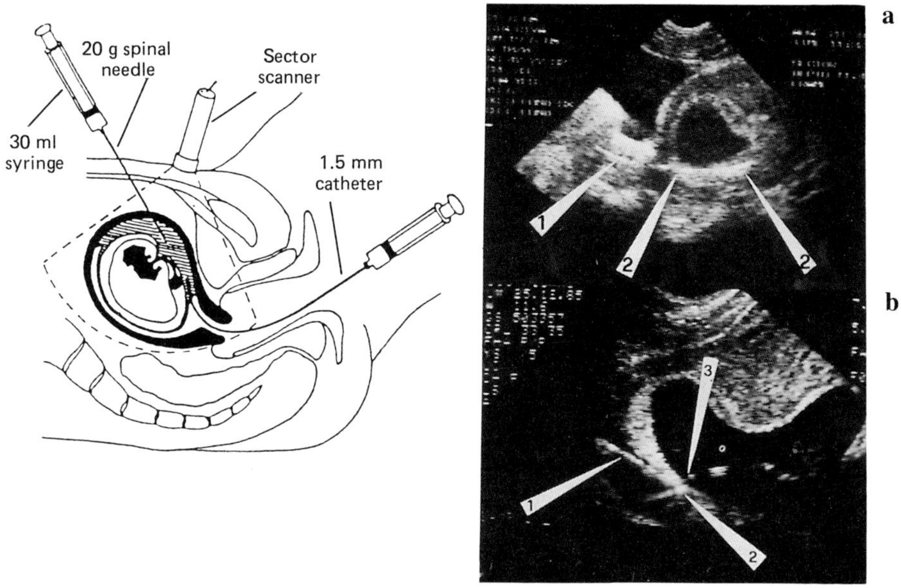

Fig. 12.8. Schematic and sonographic representation of transcervical (**a**) and transabdominal (**b**) chorionic villus sampling methods. Arrows: sampling devices introduced in the placenta.

Extrapolating from the Danish randomized trial on amniocentesis (Tabor et al 1986), the expected fetal loss rate resulting from CVS would be about 1%. The risk of transcervical and transabdominal sampling have been compared in our randomized trial of 1156 patients between 8 and 12 weeks (Brambati et al. 1988b; Brambati et al. 1989, unpublished). Although fetal loss rate did not differ between the two techniques, there was a higher success rate at the first insertion for transabdominal needling, a smaller number of early complications, a shorter learning time and reduced procedure time. Finally, the transabdominal approach permits CVS as early as the 6th and 7th gestation weeks (Brambati ct al. 1988a); results can be obtained in a few days by dircct karyotyping and DNA analysis by the polymerase chain reaction. If abortion is required, biochemical interruption of pregnancy by antiprogestins and prostaglandins is possible (WHO Task Force on Post-Ovulatory Methods for Fertility Regulation 1989).

High-resolution ultrasound permits detection of more than 200 fetal defects in the second and third trimesters (Weaver 1989), but only a small number of

Table 12.4. Abnormalities of the conceptus diagnosed by ultrasound in the second and third month of pregnancy

Abnormality	Detection time (gestation weeks)	Ultrasound method
Conjoined twins	7–11	Abdominal 5 MHz Vaginal 6.5 MHz
Anencephaly and spina bifida	9	Vaginal 6.5 MHz
Encephalocele	12	Abdominal 5 MHz
Cystic nuchal hygroma (with/without generalized oedema)	9–11	Abdominal 5 MHz Vaginal 6.5 MHz
Omphalocele	12	Abdominal 5 MHz

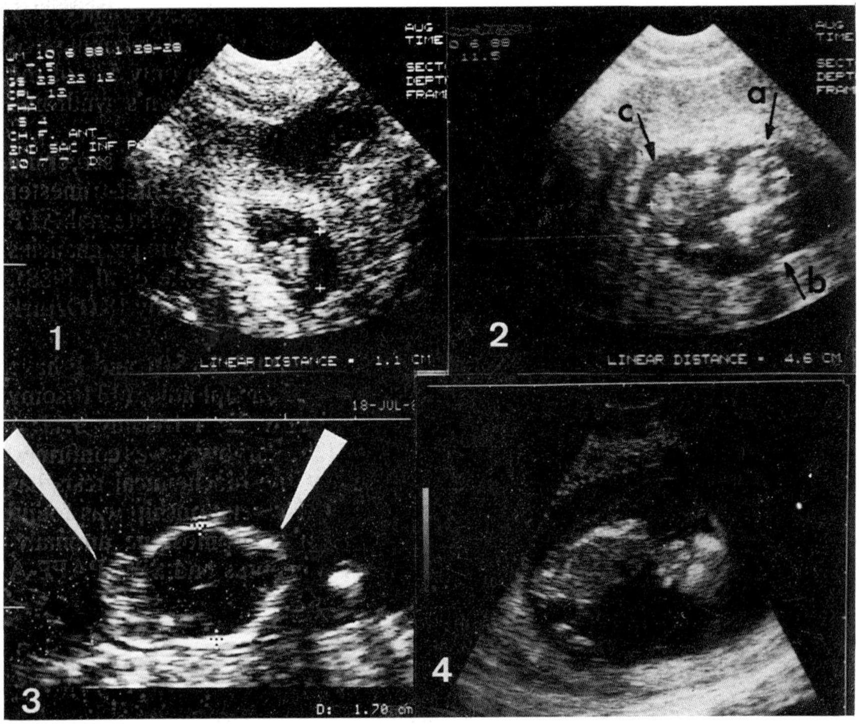

Fig. 12.9. Sonographic evidence of: conjoined twins (thoraco-omphalopagus) at 7 (1) and 11 (2) gestation weeks, arrows indicating cephalic poles (a and b) and common omphalocele (c); encephalocele (3) at 12 weeks; cystic nuchal hygroma with generalized oedema (4) at 10 weeks in a trisomy 18 fetus.

anomalies can be recognized in the first trimester (Table 12.4 and Fig 12.9). Our prospective study of 3157 pregnancies between 6 and 12 weeks by abdominal scanning with a 5 MHz probe yielded a detection rate of about 3 per thousand. The potential of early gestation sonography has recently been increased by the use of high-frequency 6.5–7.5 MHz probes specially designed for intravaginal use (Rottem et al. 1989). Transvaginal sonography permits detailed examination of the appearance of embryonic structures (Rottem 1989, personal communication). This new approach should increase the possibility of screening for some gross embryo abnormalities in the first trimester.

Screening for Fetal Chromosome Anomaly

The risk of fetal aneuploidy due to an extra chromosome increases with maternal age, but since some 90% of births are from women under 35, maternal age criteria for prenatal diagnosis has little impact on the incidence of chromosome anomalies at birth. Moreover, because of limited cytogenetic laboratory facilities, it is not possible to extend prenatal tests to all pregnant women. There is, therefore, a need for screening tests other than age to identify higher-risk pregnancies. It is now clear that measurement of hCG, AFP and unconjugated oestriol (uE3) between 15 and 20 weeks, and amniocentesis on only 5% of the pregnant population, will identify over 60% of fetuses with Down's syndrome (Schoenfeld et al. 1987; Wald et al. 1988).

However, the prevention of Down's syndrome by second-trimester screening programmes and late terminations is not entirely satisfactory and a first-trimester screening test togehter with CVS should be of obvious benefit. Maternal AFP and uE3 levels between 8 and 12 weeks are lower than the median in pregnancies in which the fetus has aneuploidy (Brambati et al. 1986; Cuckle et al. 1988), and a low hCG alpha/beta free subunit ratio seems specific to trisomy 18 (Ozturk et al. 1989, unpublished work).

In the present investigation maternal hCG, AFP, PAPP-A, SP1 and P have been evaluated between 6 and 9 weeks of gestation in 25 aneuploidies (13 trisomy 21; 6 trisomy 18, 2 triploidies; 1 trisomy 13; 2 trisomy 22; 1 trisomy 5,11; 1 trisomy 11, 18). All the patients underwent CVS and the karyotype was confirmed on fetal tissues after termination. The sensitivity of the biochemical tests has been evaluated using the 5th percentile lower limit. No relationship was found between maternal P and hCG levels and embryonic chromosome anomaly, whereas some 50% of patients with an abnormal conceptus had SP1, PAPP-A

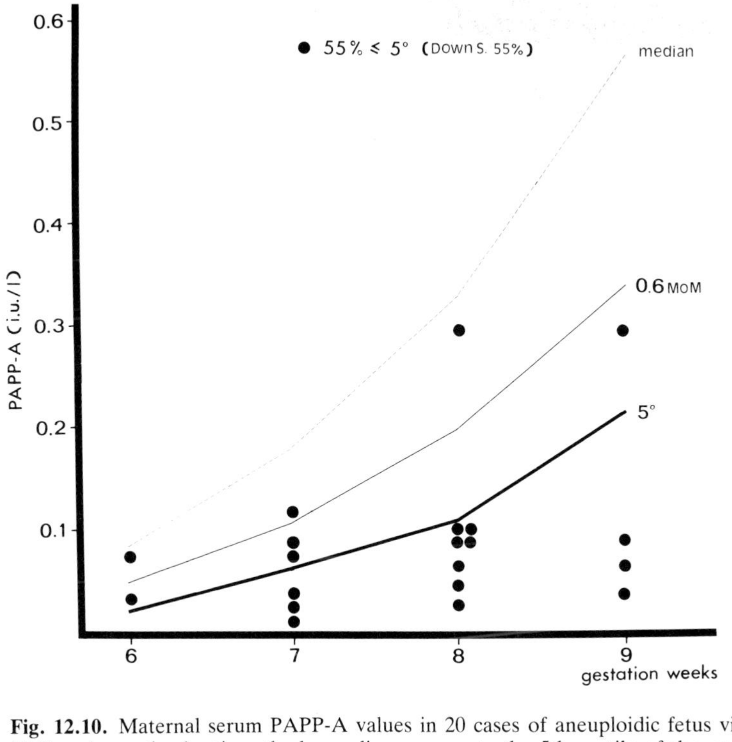

Fig. 12.10. Maternal serum PAPP-A values in 20 cases of aneuploidic fetus viable at the time of CVS and genetic abortion; the heavy line represents the 5th centile of the normal range.

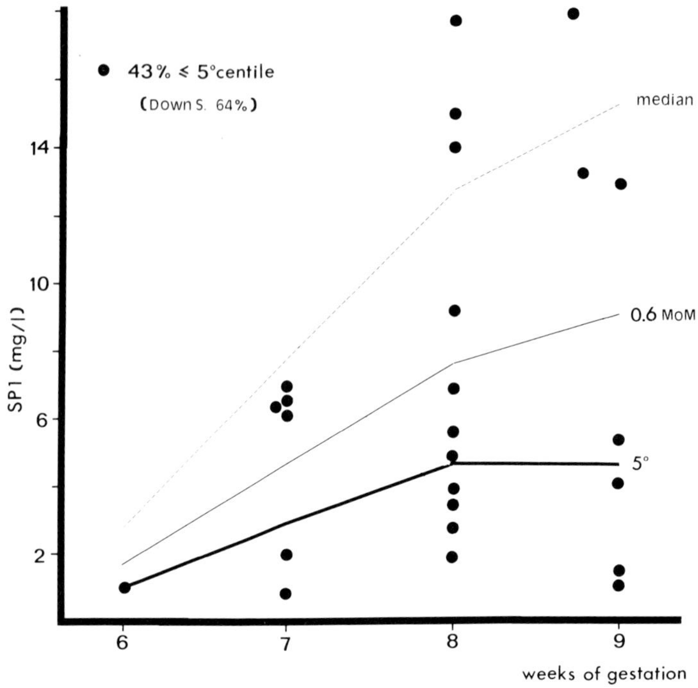

Fig. 12.11. Maternal serum SP1 values in 25 cases of aneuploidic fetus viable at the time of CVS and genetic abortion; the heavy line represents the 5th centile of the normal range.

and AFP values below the 5th percentile (Figs. 12.10 and 12.11); the sensitivity of AFP and SP1 was higher for Down's syndrome than for other chromosome defects. Furthermore, the simultaneous determination of SP1, PAPP-A and AFP would permit detection of up to 85% of conceptuses with a chromosome aberration.

Our data confirm previous observations that AFP concentrations in the first trimester are low in pregnancies with Down's syndrome as well as with other aneuploidies and suggest for the first time the association with low PAPP-A and SP1 levels. The steady increase of AFP, PAPP-A and SP1 during the first trimester may explain the reduced levels in chromosomally abnormal pregnancies. Cuckle and colleagues (1988) have put forward the hypothesis of "genetic" immaturity of the conceptus and its placenta, with reduced synthesis of fetal and placental proteins. However, this hypothesis does not explain the biochemical findings in the second trimester when placental products are elevated (see Chapter 14).

Conclusions

Until recently, early pregnancy management consisted of pregnancy tests and evaluation of uterine size. The only clinically recognizable conditions were ectopics and threatened or spontaneous abortions. Now, the new procedures of embryonic tissue sampling and advances in cytogenetic and molecular analysis can clearly reveal the genetic constitution of the conceptus.

The results reported here confirm the efficiency of sonographic biometry of the embryo and placental protein evaluation in maternal serum in determining prognosis of early gestation. Indeed, a single CRL measurement and serum hCG, PAPP-A and SP1 estimation at 6 to 9 weeks can predict impending abortion of a live embryo days or weeks before the event. Moreover, the results of single maternal PAPP-A, SP1 and AFP determinations suggest the possibility of identifying women at an increased risk to whom CVS should be offered.

References

Adinolfi M (1986) Recurrent habitual abortion. HLA sharing and deliberate immunization with partner's cells: a controversial topic. Hum Reprod 1: 45–48

Boncinelli E, Somma R, Acampora D, et al. (1988) Organization of human homeobox genes. Hum Reprod 3: 880–886

Brambati B, Lanzani A (1987) A clinical look at early post-implantation pregnancy failure. Hum Reprod 2: 401–405

Brambati B, Simoni G, Bonacchi I, Piceni L (1986) Fetal chromosomal aneuploidies and maternal serum alpha-fetoprotein levels in first trimester. Lancet ii: 165–166

Brambati B, Tului L, Simoni G, Travi M (1988a) Prenatal diagnosis at 6 weeks. Lancet ii: 397

Brambati B, Oldrini A, Lanzani A, Terzian E and Tognoni G (1988b) Transabdominal versus transcervical chorionic villus sampling: a randomized trial. Hum Reprod 3: 911–813

Canadian Collaborative CVS-Amniocentesis Clinical Trial Group (1989) Multicentre randomized clinical trial of chorionic villus sampling and amniocentesis. Lancet i: 1–6

Cuckle HS, Wald NJ, Barkai G, et al. (1988) First-trimester biochemical screening for Down's syndrome. Lancet ii: 851–852

Edwards RG (1986) Causes of early embryonic loss in human pregnancy. Hum Reprod 1: 185–198

Guerneri S, Bettio D, Simoni G, Brambati B, Lanzani A, Fraccaro M (1987) Prevalence and distribution of chromosome abnormalities in a sample of first trimester internal abortion. Hum Reprod 2: 735–739

Ho PC, Jones WR (1980) Pregnancy-specific beta-1-glycoprotein as a prognostic indicator in complications of early pregnancy. Am J Obstet Gynecol 138: 253–256

Kline J, Stein Z, Susser M (1986) Very early pregnancy: fertilization and implantation frequency and cause of loss. In: Porter IH, Hatcher NH, Willey AM (eds) Perinatal genetics: diagnosis and treatment. Academic Press, Orlando, San Diego, New York, London, Toronto, pp 3–22

Jackson LG (1989) CVS Newsletter, 30 Setpember, Philadelphia

Lenton EA, Neal LM, Sulaiman R (1982) Plasma concentrations of human chorionic gonadotropin from the time of implantation until the second week of pregnancy. Fertil Steril 37: 773–778

Macdonald RR (1989) Does treatment with progesterone prevent miscarriage? Br J Obstet Gynaecol 96: 257–264

Mantoni M (1985) Ultrasound signs in threatened abortion and their prognostic significance. Obstet Gynecol 65: 471–475

Morton H, Rolfe B, Clunie GJA, Anderson MJ, Morrison J (1977) An early pregnancy factor detected in human serum by the rosette inhibition test. Lancet i: 394–397

O'Neill C (1985) Examination of the causes of early pregnancy associated thrombocytopenia. J Reprod Fertil 73: 567–577

Rhoads GG, Jackson LG, Schlesselman SE, et al. (1989) The safety and efficacy of chorionic villus sampling for early prenatal diagnosis of cytogenetic abnormalities. N Engl J Med 320: 609–617

Robinson HP (1975) Gestation sac volumes as determined by sonar in the first trimester of pregnancy. Br J Obstet Gynaecol 82: 100–107

Robinson HP, Fleming JEE (1975) A critical evaluation of sonar crown-rump length measurements. Br J Obstet Gynaecol 82: 702–710

Rottem S, Bronshtein M, Thaler I, Brandes JM (1989) First trimester transvaginal sonographic diagnosis of fetal anomalies. Lancet i: 444–445

Sargent IL, Wilkins T, Redman CWG (1988) Maternal immune responses to the fetus in early pregnancy and recurrent miscarriage. Lancet ii: 1099–1104

Schoenfeld M, DiMaio M, Baumgarten A, Greenstein RM, Saal HM, Mahoney MJ (1987) Screening for fetal Down's syndrome in pregnancy by measuring maternal serum alpha-fetoprotein levels. N Engl J Med 317:342–346

Stabile I, Campbell S, Grudzinskas JG (1989) Ultrasound and circulating placental protein measurements in complications of early pregnancy. Br J Obstet Gynaecol 96: 1182–1191

Tabor A, Madsen M, Obel EB, Philip J, Bang J, Norgaard-Pedersen B (1986) Randomized controlled trial of genetic amniocentesis in 4606 low-risk women. Lancet i: 1287–1293

Worherr H (1982) Factors influencing fetal growth. Am J Obstet Gynecol 142: 577–588

Wald NJ, Cuckle HS, Densem JW, et al. (1988) Maternal serum screening for Down's syndrome in early pregnancy. Br Med J 297: 883–887

Weaver DD (1989) Catalog of prenatally diagnosed conditions. The John Hopkins Univerity Press, Baltimore and London

Westergaard JG, Teisner B, Sinosich MJ, Madsen LT, Grudzinskas JG (1985) Does ultrasound examination render biochemical tests obsolete in the prediction of early pregnancy failure? Br J Obstet Gynaecol 92: 77–83

WHO Task Force on post-ovulatory methods for fertility regulation (1989) Termination of early human pregnancy with RU 486 (mifepristone) and the prostaglandin analogue sulprostone: a multi-centre, randomized comparison between two treatment regimens. Hum Reprod 4: 718–725

13. Endocrinology and Metabolism in Early Pregnancy

J.G. Grudzinskas and T. Chard

Introduction

The synthesis and secretion of human chorionic gonadotrophin (hCG) by the conceptus at implantation is the first in a series of endocrine and metabolic events which are involved in maternal adaptation to the pregnant state. These changes can be exploited clinically by the measurement of hormones and proteins in peripheral blood, urine or amniotic fluid. thus the detection of hCG in maternal blood or urine is the standard method of early pregnancy diagnosis. Examination of the fetus and related tissues has also revealed a number of other proteins which may be used in the diagnosis of early pregnancy and its failure (Table 13.1). For example, measurements of Schwangerschaftsprotein 1 (SP-1) can be used in the biochemical diagnosis of pregnancy (Grudzinskas et al. 1977) and consistently depressed levels of pregnancy-associated plasma protein A (PAPP-A)

Table 13.1. Major fetal, trophoblast and decidual proteins identified in early pregnancy

Fetal
Alpha-fetoprotein (AFP)
Fetal antigen 1 (FA-1)
Fetal antigen 2 (FA-2)
Trophoblast
Human chorionic gonadotrophin (hCG)
Schwangerschaftsprotein 1 (SP1)
Human placental lactogen (hPL)
Pregnancy-associated plasma protein A (PAPP-A)
Placental protein 5 (PP5)
Decidual/endometrial
Insulin-like growth factor binding protein (IGF-bp: a_1PEG, PP12, a_1 PAMG)
Progestogen-dependent endometrial protein (PEP: a_2PEG, PP14, a_2CMG, a_2PAMG, AUP)

have been shown in early pregnancy failure (Westergaard et al. 1985). Elevated maternal serum alpha-fetoprotein (AFP) levels may indicate fetal spina bifida; and reduced AFP levels are associated with an increased risk of trisomy 21 (Wald et al. 1988). The recent identification of specific secretory proteins of endometrial and decidual origin holds the promise of the first non-invasive indices of the function of these tissues. This chapter deals with recent developments in measurement of hormones and proteins of fetal, maternal and placental origin in normal and abnormal early pregnancy.

Diagnosis of Pregnancy

The early diagnosis of pregnancy depends on the detection of hCG in maternal urine, or 1–2 days earlier in blood. Current assay technology has solved most of the problems of non-specific results. However, highly sensitive assays have shown hCG at low concentrations (<5 iu/l), may be present in normal subjects and in clinical practice a single estimation of hCG should only be considered indicative of pregnancy if it is greater than 25 iu/l or if a lower level of hCG is seen to increase twofold at an interval of three days (Jones et al. 1983). If hCG has been given therapeutically, estimations should be delayed until clearance of the exogenous hCG has occurred, possibly delaying the diagnosis by up to 14 days. In these circumstances, assays for placental proteins such as SP1 may be appropriate. Other pregnancy-associated proteins, such as human placental lactogen (hPL), pregnancy-associated plasma protein A (PAPP-A) and placental protein 5 (PP5), are not candidates for early diagnosis since they cannot be detected in maternal blood until after six weeks of amenorrhoea. Even hCG results should be interpreted with care immediately after implantation; the sooner the diagnosis is made, the less likely is the outcome to be normal (Table 13.2) given the very high rate of spontaneous pregnancy failure in the peri-implantation period (see below.)

Table 13.2. Pregnancy outcome in relation to time of diagnosis

Time of diagnosis	Likelihood of normal outcome (%)
Preimplantation	25–30
Postimplantation	43–60
Six weeks' amenorrhoea	85–90
Second trimester	95
Third trimester	98

Endocrinology and Metabolism of Normal Early Pregnancy

The stimulus for the initial production of placental products, hCG, hPL, SP1 and PAPP-A, is unknown. The secretion of hPL, SP1, PAPP-A, PP5 and progesterone into the maternal circulation appears to parallel the growth of functioning trophoblast (Grudzinskas et al. 1977; Lenton et al. 1981; Ahmed and Klopper 1985; Fig. 13.1). In normal pregnancy this pattern contrasts with that of hCG. The synthesis of SP1, at least for the initial weeks of pregnancy, seems to be independent of the presence of an embryo or fetus as seen in women with hydatidiform mole, and also of the site of implantation, as seen in women with ectopic gestation. In normal pregnancy the doubling times for hCG and SP1 are very similar, 2–3 days in the first 6 weeks of pregnancy (Lenton et al. 1981).

The disappearance rates (40–60 h) of these molecules after removal of the placenta are also equivalent. Curiously, there is not an extensive literature on hPL in early pregnancy, and this hormone is not considered to be useful as a pregnancy test (Letchworth 1976). Blood levels of hPL increase as pregnancy advances, and are related to functioning trophoblast mass. Circulating PAPP-A can be detected in the maternal circulation 28 days after conception; the relatively late appearance precludes its use as an early diagnostic test for pregnancy (Chemnitz et al. 1986; Fig 13.2). PAPP-A levels increase throughout gestation with a main doubling time of 4.9 days during the first trimester; the disappearance rate after removal of the placenta is 4–7 days (Sinosich 1985).

The main source of oestradiol and progresterone shifts from the corpus luteum to the fetoplacental unit in the middle of the first trimester (Klopper 1985). The synthesis of AFP by embryonal endodermal tissues is reflected by an increase in circulating levels during the first trimester; substantial amounts of AFP are detected consistently after 10 weeks' gestation (Kunz and Keller 1976; Olajide et al. 1989). Synthesis of the secretory proteins of the endometrium parallel the morphological changes which this tissue undergoes (Bell 1986). Progesterone-

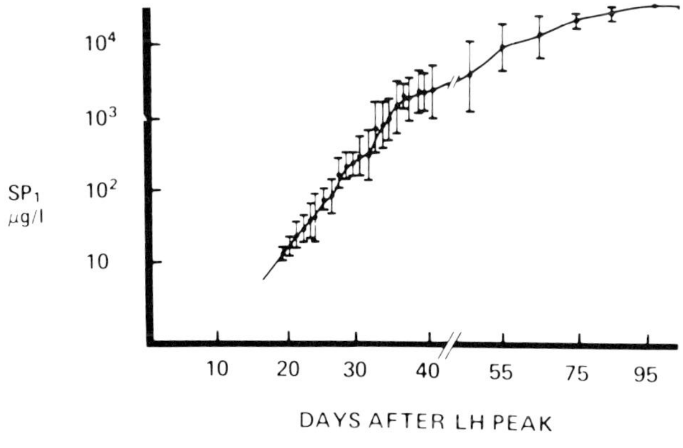

Fig. 13.1. Mean serum SP1 levels in nine women in the first trimester of normal pregnancy. (From Lenton et al. [1981], by permission of *Acta Obstetricia et Gynecologica Scandinavia.*)

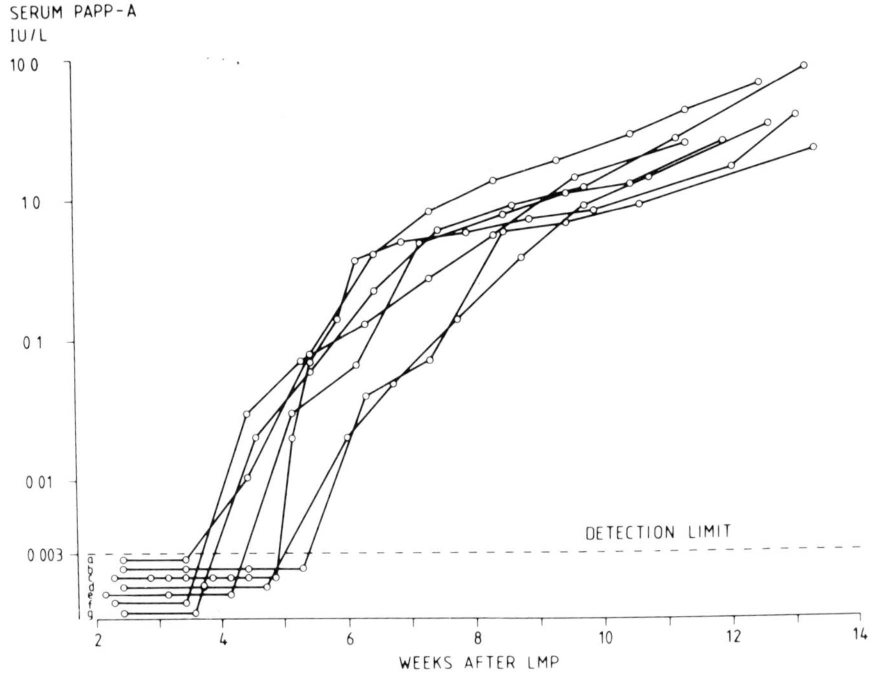

Fig. 13.2. Serum PAPP-A levels in seven women in the first trimester of normal pregnancy. (From Chemnitz et al. [1986], by permission of *British Journal of Obstetrics and Gynaecology*.)

dependent endometrial protein (PEP; also known as PP14 – see Table 13.1), which is derived from the glandular epithelium of the endometrium, shows a pattern of blood levels almost identical to those of hCG. By contrast, the insulin-like growth factor binding protein (IGF-bp; also known as PP12) which is derived from the stromal cells of the gestational endometrium has peak levels in mid pregnancy (Bell 1989).

Control of Synthesis and Secretion

The mechanisms which control the synthesis of trophoblast proteins are poorly understood; uteroplacental perfusion probably plays a major role, influencing synthesis and secretion according to the law of mass action (Chard and Grudzinskas 1985). The ovary, the embryo and the endometrium may all contribute. Firstly, with no ovarian function in women who are pregnant as a result of embryo donation, pregnancy is dependent on synthetic oestrogens and progestagens adminstered only for the first 8–9 weeks (Lutjen et al. 1984). Secondy, depressed levels of trophoblast proteins are seen when complications of early pregnancy become evident clinically, but the initiation of secretion appears to be unrelated to the presence of the embryo, as evidenced by the apparently normal blood levels seen in blighted ovum and hydatidiform mole.

Circulating placental hormones and proteins are consistently present in ectopic gestation, but the abnormalities in synthesis have varied widely, the earliest and greatest difference being seen in low levels of progesterone PAPP-A and PEP, and the least for hCG (Sinosich et al. 1985). Finally, with the possible exception of PAPP-A in association with Cornelia de Lange syndrome, fetal congenital abnormalities are not related to changes in circulating levels of trophoblast proteins (Westergaard et al. 1983), as pregnancy outcome is normal in the apparent absence of hPL asnd SP1. Gross elevations of hCG and SP1 in amniotic fluid have been reported in pregnancies complicated by Meckel's syndrome, but these changes are not reflected in the maternal circulation (Heikinheimo et al. 1982). By contrast, the dramatic changes in ovarian hormones observed in early pregnancy are part of the maternal response to pregnancy rather than a primary phenomenon. The information on endometrial and decidual proteins is less extensive (see reviews by Bell, 1988; 1989; Huhtala et al. 1988), but it is likely that both PEP and IGF-bp synthesis is modulated by progesterone.

Complications of Early Pregnancy

Early Pregnancy Failure

The chances of pregnancy leading to a viable offspring in any one ovarian cycle is approximately 25%. Detailed studies using sensitive biochemical tests confirm that failure rate of pregnancy is similar whether ovulation and pregnancy have occurred spontaneously, or as a result of in-vitro fertilization-embryo transfer (IVF-ET) programme (Table 13.2). The incidence of clinically obvious miscarriage is 10%–15%. Estimates of the incidence of the failure of subclinical and clinical pregnancy vary from 8% to 55%. (For review, see Grudzinskas et al. 1986). Differences in clinical study design, assay technology, and study groups account for the discordance in the literature. A major issue is the specificity of the substances measured as an index of trophoblastic activity. In this respect, hCG estimations must still be considered superior to those of SP1 (unless hCG has been given therapeutically). By contrast, ultrasonic findings such as uterine distension or a gestational sac cannot be considered as specific signs of pregnancy (Stabile et al. 1988a).

Threatened and Spontaneous Miscarriage

Circulating levels of hormones and proteins of fetal trophoblastic and maternal origin have been used to predict the outcome in women with vaginal bleeding in early pregnancy (Niven et al. 1972; Nygren et al. 1973; Garoff and Seppala 1975; Kunz and Keller 1976; Braunstein et al. 1978; Damber et al. 1978; Jovanovic et al. 1978; Schultz-Larsen and Hertz 1978; Jouppila et al. 1979; Masson et al. 1983a, b; Salem et al. 1984). As ultrasound examination has now revolutionized this practice, these tests are probably obsolete if fetal life can be demonstrated by ultrasound (Jouppila et al. 1980a, b; Hertz et al. 1980; Stabile et al. 1987). Nevertheless, a proportion of patients in whom fetal heart action has been demonstrated will spontaneously miscarry. We have described serum levels of hPL, SP1, PAPP-A, progesterone, oestradiol, AFP and pregnancy-zone protein (PZP) in the latter situation. In the 108 patients in whom the history and clinical findings were diagnostic of threatened miscarriage (Westergaard et al. 1985) ultrasound revealed a fetal heart action in 77 women, and no clearcut evidence of fetal life in the remaining 31 patients. Spontaneous miscarriage occurred in 42 pregnancies, 31 of which showed no sign of fetal heart action on repeated scan examination. In the remaining 11 patients, the fetal heart action was observed repeatedly until miscarriage occurred. The sensitivity, predictive values and relative risk of normal and abnormal levels of the biochemical indices measured in the first sample, and in all samples in relation to the scan findings in the women who aborted, revealed that the predictive value of an abnormal level in the sample obtained at presentation was greatest for PAPP-A, particularly if there was scan evidence of fetal life (54%). When all abnormal results were considered, the predictive value was highest for AFP and PAPP-A.

The differences between the indices, both in single and serial samples, were less if the ultrasound findings were not included. However, when ultrasound demonstrated a live fetus, the predictive value of a normal test i.e. PV negative, was highest (99%) for PAPP-A estimations. The relative risk of miscarriage was highest for depressed levels of PAPP-A, being three times greater than the other biochemical indices if the fetus was alive, and five to ten times greater if examined independent of the ultrasound findings. All the 11 women who had evidence of a live fetus but subsequently miscarried had depressed PAPP-A levels, levels being abnormal at least 4 weeks before miscarriage in 4 patients and in every sample obtained in the other 7.

By contrast, the levels of the other substances measured generally remained within the normal range – the only exception being AFP. A similar study showed that if the fetal heart action was not evident ultrasonically after 7 weeks gestation, or if the gestational sac volume is greater than 3 ml, then measurements of hCG, hPL, SP1, PAPP-A and oestradiol, were of no clinical value (Grudzinskas et al. 1988). Further, spontaneous miscarriage after the observation of a heart beat is extremely uncommon; in this small group the levels of hormones and proteins were in the normal range, the possible exception being PAPP-A.

Finally, recent studies in women with apparently normal pregnancies at 6–10 weeks' gestation have shown reduced levels of AFP, PAPP-A and hCG within 2–3 weeks of spontaneous miscarriage (Brambati, Grudzinskas and Chard, unpublished observations). Most of these fetuses had or were likely to have an abnormal karyotype, so measurement of hormones and proteins in the first trimester may identify this group as do hCG, AFP and oestriol measurement in the second trimester.

Anembryonic Pregnancy

Early arrest of embryonic development permits an examination of the contribution of the conceptus to the control of hormone and protein synthesis by the trophoblast. Stabile and colleagues (1989) have described the ultrasonic diagnosis of this condition.

If a heart beat cannot be seen in a sac of greater than 3 ml, the diagnosis can be confidently made. Prior to this time, measurements of serum hCG and SP1 have a specificity in excess of 90% in the exclusion of this condition. Serum AFP levels are normal in many of these women suggesting that an embryo was present at an earlier stage and that the term anembryonic pregnancy is a misnomer (Stabile et al. 1989).

Circulating hCG is also reduced at 4 weeks' gestation in a group of women studied with this condition at a subfertility clinic; mean levels of maternal PAPP-A, oestradiol and progesterone fell some 3 weeks later (Yovich et al. 1986). These findings confirm that a failure in the normal rise of hCG is suggestive of failed pregnancy at a time before ultrasound can provide useful information (i.e. in the absence of fetal heart action).

Ectopic Pregnancy

The use of quantitative hCG tests in this condition has been reviewed elsewhere (Kadar 1983) confirming the value of assays capable of detecting the very low levels of hCG present in this condition. A positive hCG tests alerts the clinician to the possibility of a pregnancy-related disorder and a negative result (i.e. $<$ 25 iu/l) virtually excludes the diagnosis. (Seppälä et al. 1980).

Stabile and colleagues (1988a) have reported a sensitivity of 100% for a combination of hCG and ultrasound. Quantitative estimations of hCG may also be of value, since depressed levels are commonly seen in ectopic gestation. In conjunction with ultrasonic examination this can often distinguish between normal or failed intrauterine pregnancy and ectopic gestation. The use of discriminatory zone for hCG in conjunction with ultrasound can also be helpful. If levels of hCG are greater than 6500 iu/l, ultrasound examination should reveal the presence of a live embryo in utero; if this is not the case, failed pregnancy, in particular ectopic gestation, should be suspected (Kadar 1983; Rottem and Timor-Tritsch 1988).

The data on SP1 are similar to that on hCG, while the findings with PAPP-A levels suggest that secretion is more severely compromised in ectopic pregnancy (Chemnitz et al. 1984; Sinosich et al. 1985). A preliminary report has shown that PAPP-A levels were depressed or absent in all of 17 women with ectopic gestation (Sinosich et al. 1985). In our study of 60 women with ectopic pregnancy, circulating PAPP-A was detected in only 30 and levels were depressed in 24 women (Fig. 13.3) (Stabile et al. 1988a). Thus the synthesis of PAPP-A appears to be more severely compromised than that of other placental products in ectopic gestation.

Westergaard and colleagues (1988) examined serum levels of oestradiol-17ß, progesterone, and the major secretory protein of the gestational endometrium (PP14 – see Table 13.1) in ectopic pregnancy. They noted depressed levels, especially of progesterone and PP14. They concluded that it was not possible to distinguish beteen failed intrauterine pregnancy and ectopic gestation by the measurement of hormones and proteins in serum, but that it could be possible to exclude ectopic pregnancy by these measurements. At first presentation, the presence of hCG would alert the clinician to the possibility of a pregnancy-related

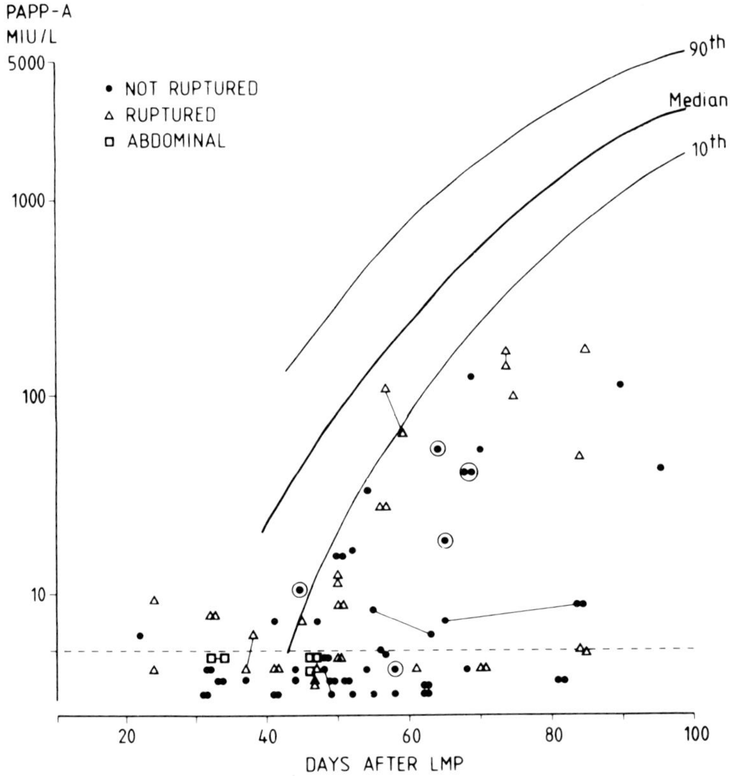

Fig. 13.3. Circulating PAPP-A levels in 60 women with ectopic gestation in relation to the normal range. The encircled symbols indicate that fetal tissue was identified. (From Stabile et al. [1988b], by permission of Springer-Verlag.)

disorder: normal levels of progesterone, PAPP-A, or PP14 would indicate a normal intrauterine pregnancy, and that ectopic pregnancy is unlikely (Stabile et al. 1988b).

Trophoblastic Disease

Trophoblastic tissue in hydatidiform mole maintains its ability to synthesize hormones and proteins, and although this capacity is reduced for hPL and steroids, it is usually greater for hCG.

The risk of choriocarcinoma is higher in women with the highest levels of hCG (Newlands 1983). We have evaluated measurements of other trophoblast proteins (e.g. SP1, PP5 and PAPP-A)- in this context. In untreated hydatidiform mole reduced levels of PAPP-A for gestational age have been observed in women prior to treatment and elevated levels of circulating SP1 and PP5 (Fig 13.4) (Tsakok et al. 1983). High SP1 levels were characteristic of women who

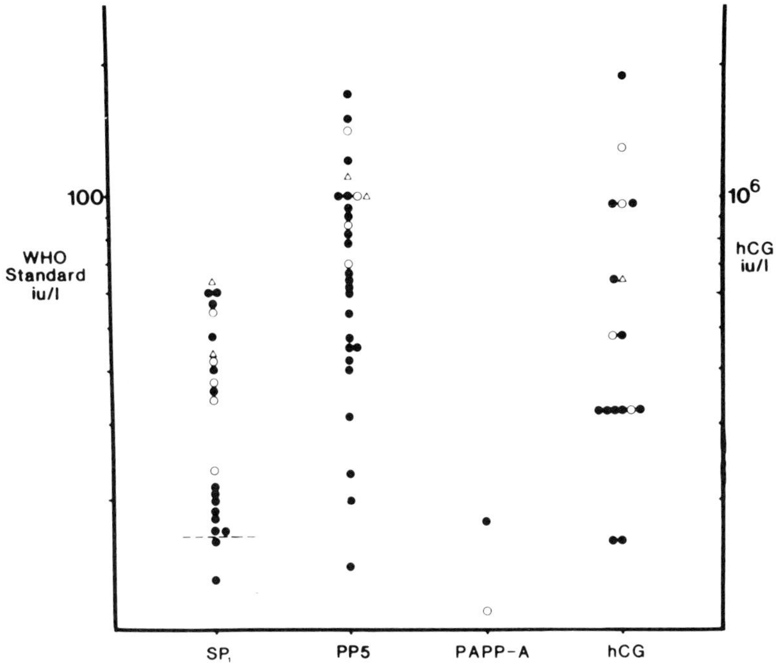

Fig. 13.4. Serum SP1, PP5, PAPP-A and hCG levels in 31 women with gestational trophoblastic disease before treatment: ●, hydatidiform mole; ○ chorioncarcinoma; △, lung metastases, ..., 16.5 IU/l (WHO standard 78/610). Levels of SP1, PP5 or PAPP-A <IU/l, or hCG <100 000 IU/l, are not shown. (From Tsakok et al. [1983], by permission of the *British Journal of Obstetrics and Gynaecology*.)

developed subsequent malignant disease. Than and his colleagues (1988) observed high serum concentrations of PP14 in women prior to treatment for hydatidiform mole which fell rapidly after evacuation. PP14 was not found in women with choriocarcinoma. In patients with choriocarcinoma, serum SP1 levels are usually lower than in benign disease and circulating PP5 cannot be detected (Seppälä et al. 1979; Soma et al. 1981; Lee et al. 1981, 1982). Although the place of hCG estimation in the monitoring of women with this disease is firmly established, estimations of endometrial or trophoblast-specific proteins may give further insight into the biology and clinical management of this condition.

Prenatal Diagnosis: Chorionic Villus Sampling

Miscarriage occurring in women scheduled for chorionic villus sampling (CVS) has been examined to determine whether the pregnancies which failed were destined to miscarry or whether the miscarriage was a direct result of the surgical procedure.

Some women with an apparently normal live fetus will miscarry spontaneously before a scheduled CVS. Reduced levels of AFP, PAPP-A and hCG have been observed in most of these subjects, (Brambati, Chard, Grudzinskas, unpublished observations) together with an abnormal karyotype. Wald and colleagues (1988) have also reported reduced AFP and oestriol levels in women carrying a fetus affected by Down's syndrome (see Chapter 17).

Ward and colleagues (1985) examined serum levels of AFP, hCG, SP1 and PAPP-A before and 6 h after chorionic villus sampling. AFP levels usually rose after sampling. Depressed or elevated preoperative levels of AFP, hCG and PAPP-A were associated with fetal anomalies and pregnancy loss in 7 of the 11 pregnancies which did not progress. All pregnancies but one (a missed abortion) were apparently normal when assessed by ultrasound, and the two highest levels of hCG were seen in the pregnancies in which the fetus was homozygous for alpha- and beta-thalassaemia. Similar observations have been made for hPL and SP1 in pregnancies complicated by hydrops fetalis in late pregnancy (Bellman et al. 1980).

We have subsequently confirmed that serum AFP levels usually rise within 30 mins of CVS (Knott et al. 1988) but that there are no consistent fluctuations in proteins and hormones of trophoblastic origin (Stabile et al. 1988c).

Conclusion

Ultrasound has made a major contribution to assessment of early pregnancy. Nevertheless, hCG estimations are still the mainstay of the diagnosis of early pregnancy and, when used in conjunction with ultrasound, provide valuable clinical information on the wellbeing of the pregnancy prior to 6 weeks' gestation.

Once a fetal heart beat has been detected at 6 weeks' gestation, spontaneous miscarriage is very uncommon. However, some apparently normal women who will subsequently miscarry display reduced levels of AFP, hCG and PAPP-A. It is still unclear whether this information can be exploited by the clinician. In women presenting with vaginal bleeding arter 7 weeks' gestation, and in whom a fetal heart beat is seen, measurement of PAPP-A but not other trophoblast proteins, may predict the small group who will subsequently miscarry. Furthermore, a systematic examination of these phenomena in relation to fetal karyotype is required to establish whether these measurements indicate women at increased risk of fetal chromosomal abnormality.

In women with suspected ectopic gestation, whereas the detection of hCG confirms the pregnancy, high levels of progesterone or PEP may exclude this condition while reduced levels of PAPP-A may confirm it.

The identification of specific endometrial and decidual proteins (IGF-bp and PEP) suggests that these may be active rather than passive participants in the reproductive process. Indeed, it is now possible to consider the endometrium/decidua as an endocrine organ (Grudzinskas 1987; Bell 1988; Fay et al. 1990a, b). The ability to measure these substances, in particular IGF-Bp and PEP, may provide both a non-invasive test of endometrial function for the assessment of fertility, and an index of endometrial/decidual function in the earliest days and weeks of pregnancy.

References

Ahmed AG, Klopper A (1985) Concomitant secretion of Schwangershaftsprotein and human chorionic gonadotrophin following conception. Clin Endocrinol 23: 677–681

Bell SC (1986) Secretory endometrial and decidual proteins: studies on clinical significance of a maternally derived group of pregnancy associated serum proteins. Hum Reprod 1: 129–143

Bell SC (1988) Synthesis and secretion of proteins by the endometrium and decidua. In: Chapman MG, Grudzinskas JG, Chard T (eds) Implantation. Springer-Verlag, London, pp 95–118

Bell SC (1989) Decidualisation and insulin-like growth factor (IGF) binding protein: implications for its role in stromal cell differentiation and the decidual cell in haemochorial placentation. Hum Reprod 4: 125–130

Bellman O, Tebbe, J, Lang N, Baur MP (1980) Determination of SP1 and hPL for predicting perinatal asphyxia. In: Klopper A, Genazzani A, Crosignani PG (eds) The human placenta: proteins and hormones. Academic Press, London, pp 99–108

Braunstein GD, Karow WG, Gentry WC, Rasor I, Wade MM (1978) First trimester chorionic gonadotrophin measurements as an aid in the diagnosis of early pregnancy disorders. Am J Obstet Gynecol 143: 25–32

Chard T, Grudzinskas JG (1985) Placental and pregnancy-associated proteins: control mechanisms and clinical application. In: Bischof P, Klopper A (eds) Proteins of the placenta. Karger, Basel, pp 104–113

Chemnitz J, Tornehave D, Teisner B, Poulsen HK, Westergaard JG (1984) The localisation of pregnancy proteins (hPL, SP1 and PAPP-A) in intra- and extrauterine pregnancies. Placenta 5: 489–494

Chemnitz J, Folkersen J, Teisner B et al. (1986) Comparison of different antibody preparations against pregnancy-associated plasma protein A (PAPP-A) for use in localisation and immunoassay studies. Br J Obstet Gynaecol 93: 111–18

Damber MG, von Schoultz B, Solheim F, Stigbrand T, Carlstrom K (1978) Prognostic value of the pregnancy zone protein during early pregnancy in spontaneous abortion. Obstet Gynaecol 51: 677–681

Fay TN, Lindenberg S, Teisner B, Westergaard LG, Westergaard JG, Grudzinskas JG (1990a) De novo synthesis of placental protein-14 (PP14) and not PP12 by monolayer cultures of glandular epithelium of gestational endometrium. J Clin Endocrinol Metab 70: 515–518

Fay TN, Jacobs IJ, Teisner B, Westergaard JG, Grudzinskas JG (1990b) A biochemical test for the direct assessment of endometrial function: measurement of the major secretory endometrial protein PP14 in serum during menstruation in relation to ovulation and luteal function. Hum Reprod 5: 382–386

Garoff L, Seppala M (1975) Prediction of fetal outcome in threatened abortion by maternal serum placental lactogen and alphafetoprotein. Am J Obstet Gynecol 121: 257–261

Grudzinskas JG (1987) Secretory proteins of the endometrium. Tokyo Med Coll J 45: 170–175

Grudzinskas JG, Gordon YB, Jeffrey D, Chard T (1977) Specific and sensitive determination of pregnancy specific beta-1 glycoprotein by radioimmunoassay. Lancet i: 333–335

Grudzinskas JG, Westergaard JG, Teisner B (1986) Biochemical assessment of placental function: early pregnancy. Clin Obstet Gynaecol 13: 553–5469

Grudzinskas JG, Stabile I, Campbell S (1988) Early pregnancy failure: biochemical and biophysical assessment. In: Beard RW, Sharp F (eds) Early pregnancy loss mechanisms and treatment. Royal College of Obstetricians and Gynaecologists/Springer-Verlag, London, pp 183–190

Heikinheimo M, Wahlstrom T, Aula P, Seppala M (1982) Pregnancy specific beta-1 glycoprotein in amniotic fluid. In: Grudzinskas JG, Teisner B, Seppala M (eds) Pregnancy proteins: biology, chemistry and clinical application. Academic Press, Sydney, pp 215–221

Hertz JB, Mantoni M, Svenstrup B (1980) Threatened abortion studies by estradiol-17-beta in serum and ultrasound. Obstet Gynecol 55: 324–328

Huhtala ML, Seppala M, Julkenen M, Koistinen R (1988) Characterisation, biological action and clinical studies of endometrial proteins. In: Chapman MG, Grudzinskas JG, Chard T (eds) Implantation. Springer-Verlag, London, pp 119–134

Jones HW, Acosta AA, Andrews MC et al. (1983) What is pregnancy? A question for in vitro fertilisation. Fertil Steril 40: 728–733

Jouppila P, Tapanainen J, Huhtaniemi I (1979) Plasma hCG levels in patients with bleeding in the first and second trimesters of pregnancy. Br J Obstet Gynaecol 86: 343–349

Jouppila P, Seppala M, Chard T (1980a) Pregnancy-specific beta-1 glycoprotein in complications of early pregnancy. Lancet i: 667–668

Jouppila P, Huhtaniemi I, Tapanainen J (1980b) Early pregnancy failure: study by ultrasonic and hormonal methods. Obstet Gynecol 55: 42–47

Jovanovic L, Dawood MY, Landesmann R, Saxena BB (1978) Hormonal profile as a prognostic index of early threatened abortion. Am J Obstet Gynecol 130: 274–278

Kadar N (1983) Ectopic pregnancy. In: Studd J (ed) Progress in obstetrics and gynaecology, vol 3. Churchill Livingstone, Edinburgh, pp 305–323

Klopper A (1985) Steroids in pregnancy. In: Shearman RP (ed) Clinical reproductive endocrinology. Churchill Livingstone, Edinburgh, pp 209–223

Knott PD, Chan, B, Ward RHT et al. (1988) Changes in circulating alphafetoprotein and human chorionic gonadotrophin following chorionic villus sampling. Eur J Obstet Gynaecol Reprod Biol 27: 277–281

Kunz J, Keller PJ (1976) hPL, oestradiol, progesterone and AFP in patients with threatened abortion. Br J Obstet Gynaecol 83: 640–644

Lee JN, Salem HT, Al-Ani ATM et al. (1981) Circulating concentrations of specific placental proteins (human chorionic gonadotrophin, pregnancy-specific beta-1 glycoprotein and placental protein 5) in untreated gestational trophoblastic tumours. Am J Obstet Gynecol 39: 702–704

Lee JN, Salem HT, Chard T, Huang SC, Ouyang PC (1982) Circulating placental proteins (hCG SP1 and PP5) in trophoblastic disease. Br J Obstet Gynaecol 89: 69–72

Lenton EA, Grudzinskas JG, Gordon YB, Chard T, Cooke ID (1981) Pregnancy specific beta-1 glycoprotein and chorionic gonadotrophin in early pregnancy. Acta Obstet Gynecol Scand 60: 489–492

Letchworth AT (1976) Human placental lactogen assay as a guide to fetal wellbeing. In: Klopper A (ed) Plasma hormone assays in evaluation of fetal wellbeing. Churchill Livingstone, Edinburgh, pp 147–173

Lutjen C, Trounson A, Leeton J, Findlay J, Wood C, Renou P (1984) The establishment and maintenance of pregnancy using in-vitro fertilisation and embryo donation in a patient with primary ovarian failure. Nature 307: 174–175

Masson GM, Anthony F, Wilson MS, Lindsay K (1983a) Comparison of serum and urine hCG levels with SP1 and PAPP-A levels in patients with first-trimester vaginal bleeding. Obstet Gynecol 61: 223–226

Masson GM, Anthony F, Wilson MS (1983b) Value of Schwangerschaftprotein 1 (SP1) and pregnancy associated plasma protein (PAPP-A) in the clinical management of threatened abortion. Br J Obstet Gynaecol 90: 146–149

Newlands ES (1983) Treatment of trophoblastic disease. In: Studd J (ed) Progress in obstetrics and gynaecology, vol 3. Churchill Livingstone, Edinburgh, pp 158–174

Niven PAR, Landon J, Chard T (1972) Placental lactogen levels as a guide to outcome of threatened abortion. Br Med J iii: 799–801

Nygren KG, Johansson EDG, Wide L (1973) Evaluation of the prognosis of threatened abortion from the peripheral levels of plasma progesterone, oestradiol and human chorionic gonadotrophin. Am J Obstet Gynecol 116: 916–922

Olajide F, Kitau MJ, Chard T (1989) Maternal serum AFP levels in the first trimester of pregnancy. Eur J Obstet, Gynecol Reprod Biol 30: 123–1238

Rottem S, Timor-Tritsch IE (1988) In: Timor-Tritsch IE, Rottem S (eds) Transvaginal ultrasonography. Heinemann Medical Books, London, pp 125–142

Salem HT, Ghaneimah SA, Shabaan MM, Chard T (1984) Prognostic value of biochemical tests in the assessment of fetal outcome in threatened abortion. Br J Obstet Gynaecol 91: 382–385

Schultz-Larsen P, Hertz JB (1978) The predictive value of pregnancy specific beta-1 glycoprotein in threatened abortion. Eur J Obstet Gynecol Reprod Biol 8: 253–257

Seppälä M, Wahlstrom T, Bohn H (1979) Circulating levels and tissue localisation of placental protein 5 (PP5) in pregnancy and trophoblastic disease: absence of PP5 expression in the malignant trophoblast. Int J Cancer 24: 6–10

Seppälä M, Tontti K, Ranta T, Stenman UH, Chard T (1980) Use of a rapid hCG beta sub-unit radioimmunoassay in acute gynaecological emergencies. Lancet i: 165–166

Sinosich MJ (1985) Biological role of pregnancy-associated plasma protein A in human reproduction. In: Bischof P, Klopper A (eds) Proteins of the placenta. Karger, Basel, 158–184.

Sinosich MJ, Ferrier A, Teisner B et al. (1985) Circulating pregnancy-associated plasma and its tissue concentration in tubal ectopic gestation. J Clin Reprod Fertil 3: 311–317

Soma H, Kikuchi M, Takayama M et al. (1981) Concentrations of SP1 and beta-hCG in serum and cerebrospinal fluid and concentrations of hCG in urine in patients with trophoblastic tumour. Arch Gynecol 230: 321–327

Stabile I, Grudzinskas JG, Campbell S (1987) Ultrasonic assessment of complications during first trimester of pregnancy. Lancet ii: 1237–1240
Stabile I, Campbell S, Grudzinskas JG (1988a) Can ultrasound reliably diagnose ectopic pregnancy? Br J Obstet Gynaecol 95: 1247–1252
Stabile I, Westergaard JG, Grudzinskas JG (1988b) Ectopic pregnancy: diagnostic aspects. In: Chapman MG, Grudzinskas JG, Chard T (eds) Implantation. Springer-Verlag, London, pp 229–238
Stabile I, Warren R, Rodeck C, Grudzinskas JG (1988c) Measurements of placental, decidual and fetal proteins before and after chorionic villus sampling. Prenatal Diagn 8: 387–396
Stabile I, Olajide F, Chard T, Grudzinskas JG (1989) Maternal serum alphafetoprotein levels in anembryonic pregnancy. Hum Reprod 4: 204–205
Than GN, Tatra G, Szabo DG, Csaba K, Bohutt (1988) Beta-lactoglobulin homologue placental protein 14 (PP14) in serum of patients with trophoblastic disease and non-trophoblastic gynaecological malignancy. Arch Gynaecol 243: 131–137
Tsakok RTM, Koh M, Ratnam SS et al. (1983) Pregnancy associated proteins in trophoblastic disease. Br J Obstet Gynaecol 90: 483–486
Wald NG, Cuckle HS, Densem W et al. (1988) Maternal serum screening for Down's syndrome in early pregnancy. Br Med J ii: 883–887
Ward RHT, Grudzinskas JG, Bolton AE et al. (1985) Fetoplacental product as a prognostic guide following chorionic villus sampling. In: Fraccaro M, Simoni G, Brambati B (eds) First trimester diagnosis. Springer-Verlag, Berlin Heidelberg New York, pp 73–76
Westergaard JG, Chemnitz J, Teisner B et al. (1983) Pregnancy-associated plasma protein A – a possible marker in the classification and diagnosis of Cornelia de Lange syndrome. Prenatal Diagn 3: 2125–232
Westergaard JG, Teisner B, Sinosich MJ, Madsen LT, Grudzinskas JG (1985) Does ultrasound examination render biochemical tests obsolete in the prediction of early pregnancy failure? Br J Obstet Gynaecol 92: 77–83
Westergaard JG, Teisner B, Stabile I, Grudzinskas JG (1988) Ectopic pregnancy: diagnostic aspects. Protein and hormone measurements in ecoptic gestation. In: Tomoda S, Mizutani S, Narita O, Klopper A (eds) Endometrial and placental proteins: basic concepts and clinical applications. VSP International Science Publishers, The Netherlands, pp 615–622
Yovich JL, McColin JC, Willcox DL, Grudzinskas JG, Bolton AE (1986) The prognostic value of beta-hCG, PAPP-A, oestradiol and progesterone in early human pregnancies and the effect of medroxyprogesterone acetate. Aust NZ J Obstet and Gynaecol 26: 59–64

14. The Endocrinology of the Fetoplacental Unit in the Second Trimester of Pregnancy

T. Chard and J.G. Grudzinskas

The endocrinology of the human fetus and placenta presents a number of unique features when compared with the endocrinology of the normal adult. It is also a subject of great complexity, but certain generalizations are possible:

1. All glands and hormones characteristic of the adult are present in the fetus by the end of the first trimester. Control mechanisms (for example, pituitary-gonadal feedback) develop towards the end of the second trimester.
2. Fetal enodcrine systems are largely autonomous with respect to those in the mother so that the fetus has control over its own endocrine milieu from an early stage of pregnancy. Thus, normal children may be born to hypothyroid mothers. However, the fetus can respond to changes in maternal endocrine balance and the end-result of such a response may be pathological – for example, the excessive fetal growth associated with some cases of diabetes in the mother.
3. As a broad rule, protein and peptide hormones do not cross the placenta in significant quantities in either direction, while steroid hormones cross quite freely.
4. The fetal endocrine system has a number of unique "one-off" functions which are not repeated at any other stage of life. Examples include the differentiation of gonads and genitalia, and the initiation of parturition.

Table 14.1. Hormones of the human placenta

Human placental lactogen (hPL)
Human chorionic gonadotrophin (hCG)
Human placental growth hormone (hPGH)
Pro-opiomelanocortin (POMC) group (e.g. adrenocorticotrophin [ACTH])
Releasing hormones (e.g. gonadotrophin-releasing hormone [GnRH])
Progesterone
Oestrogens (principally oestriol)

5. Throughout pregnancy the placenta secretes large quantities of both proteins and steroid hormones (Table 14.1). From the end of the first trimester onwards, the function of these placental hormones is doubtful or non-existent.

Each of the main fetal endocrine systems will be reviewed in turn, followed by the endocrinology of the placenta.

Sex Hormones and Sexual Differentiation

The testis differentiates and becomes functional in the first trimester. However, development of the ovary only begins at a crown–rump (CR) length of about 115 mm (14 weeks) and ends at a CR of 190 mm (20 weeks). For this reason, the development of an XO female (Turner's syndrome) appears normal during the first trimester.

The most striking endocrine phenomenon of the early second trimester is the increase in serum testosterone levels in the male fetus which reach a peak at 10–15 weeks (Reyes et al. 1974; Tapanainen et al. 1981) After this, the levels of testosterone fall and approximate to those in the female fetus. It has been proposed that the testosterone secretion is directly stimulated by hCG. However, the number of hCG receptors in the testis only reaches a maximum at 15–18 weeks (Molsberry et al. 1982) and in vitro studies indicate that baseline testosterone secretion is *not* stimulated by hCG at 12–18weeks (Word et al. 1989). Pituitary gonadotrophins are not essential for gonadal/genital differentiation: the male anencephalic infant is born with normally differentiated (though hypoplastic) external genitalia. Male development depends on the production of hormones from the testis. In the absence of these the fetus develops as a female (Jost 1976).

The Sertoli cells secrete the anti-Müllerian hormone (AMH) which causes regression of the Müllerian ducts. The testosterone produced by the testis stimulates the development of prostatic buds in the urogenital sinus and the masculinization of the external genitalia. As in the adult, part of the action of testosterone is the result of conversion to dihydrotestosterone (DHT) in the target organ by the enzyme 5-alpha reductase. Testosterone itself stimulates Wolffian duct formation, while DHT is required for fusion of the labial-scrotal folds and the formation of the penile urethra and scrotum.

Growth

The genetic constitution of the fetus, together with constraints imposed by the size of the mother, are of greater importance in determining overall fetal size than is the action of hormones. Nevertheless, several fetal endocrine systems have a general involvement in the growth process (Chard 1989b).

Growth Hormone

Growth hormone (hGH) can be detected in the fetal circulation throughout the second trimester, reaching a peak at 20–24 weeks and thereafter falling rapidly until term (Kaplan et al. 1976); Suganuma et al. 1989). Surprisingly, since fetal hGH is identical to the adult form, it seems to have little or nothing to do with fetal growth. Despite the high concentration of serum GH, birth size is usually normal in children with congenital hypothalamic hypopituitarism or familial GH deficiency, as well as in anencephalic fetuses with only small amounts of circulating GH and dwarfs lacking receptors for GH (Laron dwarfs).

The structural similarities between human prolactin (hPRL) and human growth hormone (hGH) indicate that the two hormones might have a common evolutionary origin. A potential progenitor cell with the potential to secrete both hormones has been identified in human fetal pituitaries of 18–22 weeks' gestation, the so-called "somatomammotropes", in addition to the classical somatotropic and mammotropic cells.

Insulin

Diabetes in the mother, especially if uncontrolled, results in an overweight fetus. The high maternal blood glucose is reflected in the fetal circulation and stimulates the fetal pancreas to produce excess insulin. In turn, this may be responsible for the increase in fetal size. In fetal insulin deficiency, by contrast, it is common for the baby to be born underweight. Liggins (1976) suggested that "insulin is the most important growth hormone of the fetus".

Although the fetal pancreas responds to pathologically high levels of glucose, it probably does not operate as a glucostat. During normal gestation fetal blood glucose levels track those in the maternal circulation and are dependent less on fetal insulin than on the function of the maternal pancreas. The fetal pancreas responds sluggishly to changes in amino acid concentration.

Insulin-like Growth Factors

Insulin-like growth factors (IGFs) almost certainly play an important part in fetal growth (D'Ercole 1987; Chard 1989b). IGF-I (somatomedin-C) and IGF-II are part of a group of biologically active peptides which are structurally homologous with proinsulin. The IGFs in the circulation are associated with IGF-binding proteins. Thus circulating levels of free IGF are low, while tissue concentrations are high. Analysis of mRNA has shown that IGF-I mRNAs are detected in all human fetal tissues so far studied, except in cerebral cortex and hypothalamus; IGF-II mRNAs are consistently higher than IGF-I mRNAs in all tissues where IGF-II mRNAs were detectable (up to 650-fold in liver), suggesting that IGF-II is synthesized in greater quantities than IGF-I during early fetal life. The widespread distribution of these proteins also supports a local role for IGFs in human fetal development: the fact that the IGF-I gene is expressed in many tissues suggests that IGF-I induces growth by acting locally in its tissue of origin rather than reaching target cells via the bloodstream in an endocrine fashion. The action of IGF at the cellular level depends upon specific tissue receptors: type I receptors are similar to the insulin receptor whereas type II receptors bind IGFs but not insulin. Fetal tissues appear to have greater type I and type II IGF binding activity than the adult.

Pituitary–Thyroid Axis

The human fetal pituitary-thyroid axis is active from 10–12 weeks' gestation (Roti 1988). Fetal TSH peaks at 20–24 weeks. Placental transfer of TSH and the thyronines is minimal, if anything occurring from fetus to mother. Human fetal thyroid function is therefore virtually autonomous. However, thyroxine can be transferred from the mother as shown by cord blood thyroxine levels in neonates born with a complete inability to iodinate thyroid proteins and therefore to synthesize thyroxine (Vulsma et al. 1989). A mother suffering from hyperthyroidism can induce thyrotoxicosis in her child as a result of the transfer of immunoglobulin long-acting thyroid stimulator (LATS) or thyroid-stimulating immunoglobulins (TSIg).

The thyroid hormone, 3,3'5-triodothyronine (reverse T3, rT3) is found in considerably higher concentrations in the fetus than in the adult. During gestation the low serum levels of T3 are offset by the raised levels of rT3. The levels are very high at 15–30 weeks and decrease substantially thereafter.

Pituitary–Adrenal Axis

The human fetal pituitary secretes corticotrophin (ACTH) in response to corticotrophin-releasing hormone (CRH) as early as 14 weeks and shows normal adult responses throughout the rest of gestation. For example, the effect of CRH is inhibited by dexamethasone and enhanced by arginine vasopressin (Jaffe et al. 1988).

ACTH is derived from a large precursor molecule known as pro-opiomelanocortin (POMC). This is cleaved into several biologically active peptide hormones – endorphins, lipotrophins and melanocyte-stimulating hormones (MSH), as well as ACTH. In the human, the ACTH family of peptides is different in the fetus with relatively greater quantities of alpha-MSH and corticotrophin-like intermediate lobe peptide (CLIP) than ACTH. It has been proposed that alpha-MSH and CLIP may be factors in the control of fetal adrenal function. Low levels of alpha-MSH can stimulate the human fetal adrenal gland to produce dehydroepiandrosterone sulphate (DHEAS) without stimulating the formation of cortisol; alpha-MSH can also stimulate growth of the adrenal zona glomerulosa. In the human, alpha-MSH is deacetylated (Coates et al. 1988). This may reflect a particular form of post-translational processing of POMC. Different fragments of POMC can affect different aspects of adrenal function, e.g. the N-terminal fragments control adrenal mitogenesis and growth (Estivariz et al. 1988).

Both POMC and related peptides, including ACTH, are produced by the placenta. CRH is also produced in the human placenta and is believed to be a major source of CRH in the maternal and fetal plasma in late gestation and labour (Economides et al. 1987). The output is moderated by steroids, and changes with labour, suggesting that a regulatory system similar to that of the hypothalamic–pituitary axis might exist within the placenta (Jones et al. 1989).

The human fetal adrenal cortex has a distinct zone that lies under the thin rim of cells which will become the adult cortex. The "fetal zone" is the major part of the adrenal cortex throughout gestation and it is only at term, after involution of the fetal zone, that the adult or definitive cortex develops fully.

ACTH acts on the fetal adrenal to induce mRNAs for side chain cleaving enzymes (P-450 scc) and 17-hydroxylase (P-450c17) enzymes. Unlike the adult gland, repeated stimulation with ACTH does not desensitize the fetal gland (Jaffe et al. 1988).

Posterior Pituitary

The active hormones of the posterior pituitary (oxytocin and arginine vasopressin) are present from the first trimester onwards. Though both of these become functionally active near term (Chard 1989a), there is no evidence for any significant role in the midtrimester.

Placental Hormones

Human Placental Lactogen

Human placental lactogen (hPL) is closely related, both chemically and biologically, to pituitary prolactin and growth hormone (Chard 1979). It is secreted by the placental syncytiotrophoblast throughout pregnancy. The levels in maternal blood follow a sigmoid curve with the maximum rate of increase in the latter part of the second trimester and a plateau after 36 weeks.

The principal factors determining the levels of hPL in the circulation are the mass of functioning trophoblast and the rate of uteroplacental bloodflow. This explains why there is no systematic (as opposed to random) time-to-time variation in hPL levels (Houghton et al. 1982), and also why there is little or no change associated with standard physiological events (Pavlou et al. 1973). There have been numerous experimental studies on the release of hPL by placental tissues in culture. These have revealed a number of apparently significant phenomena. However, most of these experiments were performed in the presence of unphysiological concentrations of the stimulating material, and it seems unlikely that any of these factors play a significant role in the control of hPL levels.

Thus, in the case of hPL, there does not appear to be any of the feedback control which characterizes most endocrine systems.

The absence of classical feedback control mechanisms is accompanied by an apparent absence of biological function. The evidence for this rather nihilistic view has been reviewed in some detail (Chard 1990). However, there is a rare (1 in 3000) "experiment of nature" in which there is total deletion of the hPL gene and therefore no hPL in maternal blood (Simon et al. 1986). These pregnancies and the resulting neonates are entirely normal in every clinical respect; this virtually excludes hPL as an *essential* factor in a normal pregnancy.

At term there is a clear-cut relationship between hPL levels and the weight of both the fetus and placenta. There is also a possible relation to fetal sex, marginally higher levels being found in pregnancies with a female fetus. There is no comparable information available for the midtrimester.

Human Chorionic Gonadotrophin

Human chorionic gonadotrophin (hCG) is one of a family of glycoprotein hormones, the other members being luteinizing hormone (LH), follicle-stimulating hormone (FSH), and thyrotrophin-stimulating hormone (TSH). Each of these consists of two subunits: an alpha-subunit (92 amino acids) which is virtually identical in all four; and a beta-subunit which is characteristic of the individual hormone (Bahl et al. 1972; Morgan et al. 1975). The beta subunit of hCG is a single chain of 145 amino acids. The first 121 N-terminal amino-acids share 80% sequence homology with beta-LH; the C-terminus of beta-hCG has a 24 amino acid extension not present in beta-LH. Both subunits of the molecule are needed for biological activity but the beta subunit determines the specificity of the action (Strickland and Puett 1981). The alpha-subunit is coded by a single gene on chromosome 6 and the beta subunit by a family of seven genes on chromosome 19; only two of the latter genes appear to be active.

Chorionic gonadotrophin is produced by the syncytiotrophoblast (and possibly also by the cytotrophoblast) (Kurman et al. 1984). During most of pregnancy the alpha-subunit is synthesized in larger quantities than the beta-subunit (Boothby et al. 1983). Free alpha-subunit can be found in trophoblast cells and is released into culture medium in vitro, but the amount in the circulation is small relative to that of the intact molecule. Once the two subunits have dimerized the hormone is very rapidly released, virtually none being stored within the cell: unlike the pituitary gland, there is no evidence for calcium-dependent exocytosis of secreting granules (Hussa 1980).

Chorionic gonadotrophin is secreted by the blastocyst. It appears in maternal blood shortly after implantation and then rises rapidly until 8 weeks' gestation. Levels show little change at 8 to 12 weeks, then decline to 18 weeks and remain fairly constant until term (Braunstein et al. 1980; Kletzky et al. 1985).* There is some short-term variation in blood hCG levels but no circadian rhythm (Houghton et al. 1982). Release of hCG in vitro appears to be pulsatile (Barnea and Kaplan 1989). A small amount of free alpha-subunit also appears in maternal blood, but this shows a progressive increase in concentration to a plateau at 36 weeks (i.e. similar to other placental products such as hPL) (Benveniste and Scommegna 1981). The pattern of hCG in fetal blood is similar to that in the mother but at 2%–3% of the concentration (Clements et al. 1976). At term the levels in the female fetus are substantially higher than those in the male (Obiekwe and Chard 1983). The levels and pattern of hCG in amniotic fluid are similar to that in maternal blood (Kletzky et al. 1985). The half-life of the hormone shows multiple components, the initial faster phase being of 6 hours (Wehmann et al. 1984). In urine some hCG is in the form of intact hormone (20%–25%) while the remainder consists of free beta-subunit and, in particular, a fragment known as "beta-core" which is synthesized from hCG in the kidney.

The mechanisms which determine the levels of hCG in maternal blood are

* An almost identical pattern of early rise and fall is shown by the endometrial protein known as PP14 (Julkunen et al. 1985).

unknown. Unlike hPL and the steroid hormones, there is no relationship to the mass of the tissue of origin. A number of factors can influence release of hCG from placental tissues in vitro (Table 14.2). Much of the data concerns the possible role of GnRH, which undoubtedly is synthesized by the placenta (Gibbons et al. 1975; Khodr and Siler-Khodr 1978; Lee et al. 1981). However, although there appears to be extensive evidence for a role of GnRH in vitro, little or no effect has been shown with in vivo studies (Tamada et al. 1976; Perez-Lopez et al. 1984). Some of the studies shown in Table 14.2 have employed concentrations of materials which would generally be regarded as unphysiological. Finally, there does not appear to be any anatomical or physiological basis for suggesting that the type of feedback mechanisms which operate in the hypothalamic-pituitary gonadal axis should also apply to the placenta. It is difficult to escape from the conclusion that the trophoblast is, in effect, a free-running tissue, where the major factors determining levels over the short term (hours and days) are the mass of the trophoblast and uteroplacental bloodflow.

It has recently been shown that hCG synthesis in vitro can be stimulated by interferon-alpha (IFN-alpha) (Iles and Chard 1989). This is of particular interest in the light of the fact that the receptors for IFN-alpha are coded on chromosome 21, and that hCG levls are elevated in pregnancies with a trisomy 21 fetus (see below).

Table 14.2. Observations on various endogenous materials which affect the synthesis of hCG by the human placenta (trophoblast) in vitro

Material	Effect[a]	Authors
GnRH	S	Siler-Khodr et al. 1986; Khodr and Siler-Khodr 1978; Siler-Khodr and Khodr 1981 Haning et al. 1982; Barnea and Kaplan 1989; Belisle et al. 1989; Mathialagan and Rao 1989; Iwashita et al. 1989
GnRH antagonists	I	Siler-Khodr et al. 1983
Progesterone	I	Wilson and Jawad 1982; Wilson et al. 1984a; Barnea and Kaplan 1989; Iwashita et al. 1989
Progesterone	N	Zeitler et al. 1983; Belleville et al, 1978; Haning et al. 1982
Gonadal steroids (androgens and oestrogen)	N	Zeitler et al, 1983; Belleville et al. 1978 Wilson et al. 1980; Wilson et al. 1984; Haning et al. 1982
Oestradiol	S	Iwashita et al. 1989
Somatostatin	N	Macaron et al. 1978
Beta-adrenergics	S	Shu-Rong et al, 1982; Rabe et al. 1982
Glucocorticoids	S	Wilson et al. 1980; Wilson and Jawad 1982
Glucocorticoids	N	Morrish and Siy 1985
Epidermal growth factor (EGF)	S	Morrish and Siy 1985; Takemori et al. 1981
EGF	I	Huot et al. 1981
EGF	N	Wilson et al. 1984
Dibutyryl cyclic AMP and phosphodiesterase inhibitors	S	Zeitler et al. 1983; Morrish and Siy 1985; Handwerger et al. 1973; Winikoff and Braunstein 1985; Rabe et al. 1982; Haning et al. 1982; Hussa et al 1974, 1978; Hilf and Merz 1985

[a]S = stimulation; I = inhibition; N = nil.

In the first trimester hCG may be the major luteotrophic factor from the implanting embryo (Chapter 4). In the second trimester it has been postulated that hCG is the primary stimulus to testosterone synthesis by the fetal testis, but there is clear experimental evidence against this hypothesis (Word et al. 1989). It is also notable that there is no rise of testosterone coincident with the peak of fetal pituitary gonadotrophins at 20–22 weeks. Another fetal endocrine role proposed for hCG is an adrenocorticotrophic action. Again, however, the pattern of hCG secretion (assuming that this is the same in the fetus as in the mother) does not obviously correlate with the development of fetal adrenal function.

Oestriol

Oestriol is the third of the classical ovarian oestrogens (oestrone, oestradiol and oestriol); it has the characteristic aromatic A-ring of all oestrogens, together with hydroxyl groups at the 3, 15 and 16 positions.

The unique feature of oestriol is that it is produced by the syncytiotrophoblast from fetal precursors (Fig. 14.1) (Diczfalusy and Mancuso 1969; Ryan 1980; Chard and Klopper 1982). The fetal adrenal produces dehydroepiandrosterone (DHEA) and the fetal liver converts this to 16OH-DHEA. Both of these compounds circulate in the fetus as the sulphate conjugate. In the placenta the 16OH-DHEASO_4 is deconjugated by a sulphatase; the A-ring of the molecule is then acted upon by an aromatase to yield the form characteristic of oestrogens. Oestriol is then secreted into the maternal circulation. The pattern in maternal blood is a progressive rise throughout gestation.

The factors determining the levels of oestriol in the maternal circulation are the supply of fetal precursors, and the conversion of these to oestriol in the

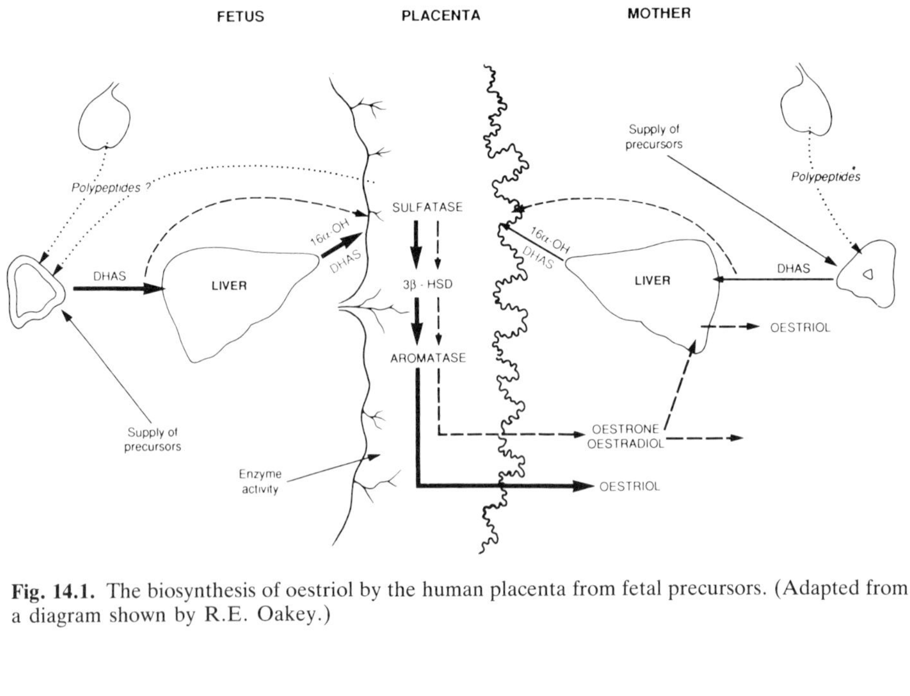

Fig. 14.1. The biosynthesis of oestriol by the human placenta from fetal precursors. (Adapted from a diagram shown by R.E. Oakey.)

placenta. Under normal circumstances it would appear that the latter is the rate-limiting step (Perry et al. 1986), and that the time-to-time control of oestriol secretion is the same as that of products such as hPL, namely, the mass of the trophoblast and the rate of uteroplacental bloodflow. Because of the unique synthetic pathway of oestriol, there are a number of unusual observations in experimental and pathological situations. These include:

1. Oestriol levels fall after administration of corticosteroids to the mother (Simmer et al. 1975; Elsner et al. 1979). These compounds cross the placenta, suppress the fetal pituitary-adrenal axis, and hence the production of DHEA.
2. Anencephaly (with an inactive fetal pituitary) and absence or hypoplasia of the fetal adrenal gland are associated with very low levels of oestriol.
3. Low levels of oestriol are associated with the rare condition of placental sulphatase deficiency in which the precursor (16OH-DHEASO_4) cannot be deconjugated and hence is not available for conversion in the placenta (Taylor 1982).

As with many placental products, there is no evidence for a specific physiological role of oestriol in pregnancy. Pregnancies in which oestriol is deficient (see above) appear to be normal in every other respect.

At term there is a relationship between maternal oestriol levels and fetal weight. There is no information on this relationship in midtrimester.

Progesterone

Progesterone is synthesized by the syncytiotrophoblast from maternal precursors. There is no evidence for feedback control mechanisms at any stage of pregnancy and the levels in the mother follow the sigmoid curve characteristic of the other trophoblast products. Progesterone is believed to play a key role in the maintenance of pregnancy, especially in ensuring quiescence of the endometrial/myometrial mechanisms, such as prostaglandin synthesis, which would otherwise lead to uterine contractions. Progesterone is also thought to be responsible for some of the main changes in maternal physiology such as relaxation of smooth muscle, hyperventilation, etc.

Maternal progesterone levels are related to the weight of the fetus and placenta at term.

Other Placental Hormones

In addition to the "classical" placental hormones described above, the human placenta secretes a number of other hormonal materials about which relatively little is known either from a biological or a clinical standpoint. These include placental growth hormone, releasing hormones, and various peptides related to the pro-opiomelanocortin family.

Placental growth hormone (hPGH) is a product of the so-called "V" gene which until recently was thought to be silent (Frankenne et al. 1988). It is closely related to both pituitary growth hormone and placental lactogen, but with greater somatotrophic activity than the latter. The pattern of secretion throughout pregnancy is similar to that of hPL. The description of a clinically normal

Table 14.3. Some specific non-hormonal protein products of the human fetus and placenta. It should be noted that the term "specific" is relative rather than absolute: all these materials occur in small amounts in some tissues in the non-pregnant state (especially seminal plasma and ovarian follicular fluid)

Product	Origin	Function	Control mechanism	Reference
Schwangerschaftsprotein (SP1)	Trophoblast	Unknown	Unknown	Bohn 1984
Placental protein 5 (PP5)	Trophoblast (+? decidua)	Anti-thrombin	Unknown	Salem and Chard 1982
Pregnancy-associated plasma protein A (PAPP-A)	Trophoblast	Anti-complementary Anti-elastase	Unknown	Stabile et al. 1988
Placental protein 12 (PP12)	Decidua	IGF-binding protein	Progesterone	Huhtala et al. 1988
Placental protein 14 (PP14)	Decidua	Beta-lactoglobulin	?Progesterone	Huhtala et al. 1988
Alpha-fetoprotein (AFP)	Fetal liver	Albumin analogue	Unknown	Alpert 1978

pregnancy with a total deficiency of hPGH (Simon et al. 1986) probably excludes an essential biological function.

The placenta appears to synthesize all the hypothalamic releasing hormones including gonadotrophin-releasing hormone (GnRH) (Lee et al. 1981) and corticotrophin-releasing hormone (CRH) (Sasaki et al. 1984; Economides et al. 1987). The sole exception is growth hormone-releasing hormone (GHRH) which appears to be almost totally absent from the placenta. There is much speculation and some experimental evidence to suggest that placental GnRH controls hCG synthesis; in addition, CRH relates to secretion of ACTH-like peptides and may itself be controlled by maternal-fetal corticosteroids. Since there is no evidence for significant time-to-time variation of the target hormones, it is unlikely that the releasing hormones play more than a permissive role under normal circumstances.

The full range of opioid peptides can be found in the human placenta, and this organ is likely to be the source of the elevated ACTH levels in the maternal circulation during pregnancy (Rees et al. 1975). It is not clear whether this plays any part in the increased circulating corticosteroid levels in pregnancy, which are largely the result of an increase in corticosteroid-binding globulin (CBG).

Other Placental Products

The human placenta secretes a number of "specific" non-hormonal proteins. Because these have some clinical implications similar to those of the placental hormones in midtrimester, they are listed in Table 14.3.

Alpha-fetoprotein

Though alpha-fetoprotein (AFP) is not itself a hormone, it is often measured in the same context as the other compounds discussed in this chapter and therefore merits brief review.

AFP is composed of a single polypeptide chain with a molecular weight of 69 kilodaltons. It consists of 590 amino acids and 39% of the amino acid sequence corresponds to that of albumin (Ruoslahti 1978; Morinaga et al 1983). Both AFP and albumin are coded on the long arm of chromosome 4. Unlike albumin it is a glycoprotein with 4% of carbohydrate residues. In amniotic fluid there are two types of AFP, differing in the structure of their carbohydrate chains and therefore in their ability to bind to concanavalin-A (Smith et al. 1979). Detection of different forms of AFP may be of value in the diagnosis of hepatocellular carcinoma (Aoyagi et al 1988).

There are low levels of AFP in normal subjects (2–25 ng/ml) (Kitau et al. 1988). In the fetus, AFP is synthesized by the liver, the gastrointestinal tract and the yolk-sac (Gitlin and Perricelli 1979; Belanger et al. 1982). The yolk-sac makes a major contribution in early gestation but later is largely replaced by hepatic synthesis. The concentration of AFP in fetal serum rises rapidly to reach a peak at 12–14 weeks' gestation at which time the levels are 2–3 g/l. Thereafter it falls until term with a sharp drop at 32–34 weeks (Gitlin 1975). The fall continues in the newborn with a half-life of 3–4 days during the first weeks of life, eventually reaching adult levels at 8 months (Wu et al. 1981). In amniotic fluid there is a steady fall in AFP levels from a peak in the first trimester; the source is complex and includes maternal blood, fetal urine and the yolk-sac. In the mother circulating AFP levels rise progressively to reach a peak at 32 weeks, then decrease towards term (Leek et a. 1985).

There is *no* information on mechanisms which may control the synthesis of AFP by the fetus and thus determine the concentrations in maternal and fetal fluids. Other than the relationship to gestational age (and certain pathological abnormalities) the only factor which influences AFP levels is fetal sex, the levels in umbilical blood at term being substantially higher if the child is a boy (Obiekwe et al. 1985).

The functions of AFP are also unknown. Probably the most convincing suggestion is that it serves an oncotic function similar to that of albumin (Alpert et al. 1971). Other possibilities include oestrogen binding (Uriel et al. 1972), though the activity of human AFP in this respect is far less than that of the more specific sex hormone-binding globulin (Swartz and Soloff 1974). It has also been suggested that AFP has immunosuppressive activity and thus plays a role in the maternal-fetal graft relationship. However, the experimental findings supporting this hypothesis (Murgita and Tomasi 1975) have not been confirmed by others (Littman et al. 1977).

Clinical Applications of Fetoplacental Hormone Determination in Midtrimester

Three main applications of fetoplacental hormone determinations have been described in midtrimester: prognosis of threatened abortion; prognosis of fetal risk in late pregnancy; and identification of congenital abnormalities.

Prognosis of Threatened Abortion

This topic has already been dealt with in more detail in Chapter 12. As a broad generalization, all fetoplacental products are reduced in association with the abortion process (Salem et al. 1984). This reduction is secondary to the destruction of the fetus and placenta: in other words, a reduction in fetoplacental products is not the primary cause of the abortion. The only exception to the fall in products is the very striking rise which may be observed in maternal AFP levels. This is the result of leakage of the very high levels of AFP from necrotic fetal tissues.

Prognosis of Fetal Risk in Late Pregnancy

A number of workers have proposed that measurement of fetoplacental products in midtrimester might be predictive of fetal complications in the third trimester, notably premature labour, growth retardation and placental abruption. In the case of AFP a clear association has been shown between elevated maternal levels and subsequent low birthweight; however, the association is not sufficiently strong to provide a useful clinical test (Chard et al. 1986). Descriptions of other possible associations, e.g. reduced SP1 and growth retardation, elevated PP5 and premature labour have not generally been confirmed in later studies (Rice et al. 1986).

Identification of Congenital Abnormalities Other than Down's Syndrome

The most widely applied test for any congenital abnormality is screening for neural tube defects (NTD) by measurement of maternal serum AFP. This will not be discussed here and is referred to simply because Down's syndrome detection (see below) has been a direct by-product of this screening process.

Other congenital abnormalities which can be identified by measurement of fetoplacental products include the group of disorders which lead to deficient oestriol production: anencephaly; absence or hypoplasia of the fetal adrenal; and placental sulphatase deficiency. The latter may be associated with ichthyosis in the infant. Another disorder, the Cornelia de Lange syndrome in the neonate, is associated with a deficiency of PAPP-A secretion (Westergaard et al. 1983). No specific abnormalities of the infant have been described in association with the known deficiencies of hPL or SP1.

Identification of Down's Syndrome

It is now quite clear that the presence of a Down's syndrome fetus is associated with a set of characteristic changes in the maternal levels of various fetoplacental products (Table 14.4) and that measurement of a group of these products provides a highly efficient screening test for the condition (Wald et al. 1988; see also Chapter 17). Here we will consider the possible mechanisms of these changes in the light of existing information on midtrimester fetal endocrinology.

It would be very attractive if alteration in a single product could be identified as the primary factor responsible for all the observed changes. For example, the oestriol deficiency in anencephaly can readily be explained on the basis of well-characterized physiology. There are, of course, numerous gaps in current knowledge of the control mechanisms of fetoplacental hormones. But even

Table 14.4. Changes in maternal levels of various fetoplacental products in midtrimester in a pregnancy with a Down's syndrome fetus

Authors	Product	Change
Merkatz et al. 1984	AFP	Reduced
Bogart et al. 1987	hCG	Increased
Canick et al. 1988	Oestriol	Reduced
Bartels and Lindemann 1988	SP1	Increased

allowing for this, there is no hypothesis, however speculative, which provides a simple explanation of the ensemble of changes listed in Table 14.4.

However, though precise mechanisms cannot be identified, it is possible to point to certain rather broader hypotheses which might account for the findings. The first such hypothesis was that a Down's syndrome fetus is generally immature, i.e. equivalent to a fetus of earlier gestational age. This was compatible with the known facts of the situation when these included only the elevated hCG and the reduced AFP and oestriol. But once it was recognized that SP1 was also elevated (Bartels and Lindeman 1988), this hypothesis was no longer tenable. Instead, it can now be postulated that Down's syndrome is associated with a relative elevation of trophoblast (i.e. placental) products (e.g. hCG, SP1) and a relative decrease of fetal products (AFP, oestriol). According to this hypothesis, other trophoblast products should prove to be elevated, e.g. hPL, progesterone and other fetal products to be reduced (e.g. DHEA). In addition, there is an important clinical implication. If there are two simple underlying processes (decreased fetal products and increased placental products), then the findings within any one group should be equivalent, i.e. if AFP is reduced, then E3 will be reduced pari passu. The practical implication is that most of the predictive value can be obtained using only one test from each group, a view supported by the actual findings in a large study (Wald et al. 1988).

If the general observation of raised trophoblast products and reduced fetal products is correct, it still begs the question of what underlies this phenomenon. There is no answer to this at the present time. We have recently evaluated the possibility that an inverse relationship between fetal and trophoblast products might obtain for all pregnancies, in which case Down's syndrome might simply represent one extreme of a normal spectrum. The findings of this study clearly show that the relationship, if any, is direct rather than inverse. Thus the changes observed in Down's syndrome are unique to that condition.

Conclusions

The hormonal events of midtrimester pregnancy are of great complexity, involving rapid development of all of the fetal endocrine systems and a major increase in the synthesis of hormones and other compounds by the placenta. The evolution of endocrine function in the midtrimester fetus has been characterized in some detail, and it is now possible to relate certain congenital abnormalities to specific events in the development of fetal endocrine glands. The pattern of secretion of materials by the placenta is also known in considerable detail, but the biological significance of many of these products remains enigmatic. Nevertheless, the pattern of changes in association with a chromosomally abnormal fetus (reduction in fetal products and increase in placental products), and the clinical importance of these changes in relation to screening for Down's syndrome, clearly indicates the need for further investigation of this important topic.

References

Alpert E (1978) Human alpha-fetoprotein (AFP) developmental and biological characteristics. In: Crandall BF (ed) Prevention of neural tube defects. Academic Press, New York, San Francisco, London, pp 19–26

Alpert E, Drysdale JW, Schur PH, Isselbacher KJ (1971) Human AFP: purification and physical properties. Fed Proc 30: 246

Aoyagi Y, Suzuki Y, Isemura M et al. (1988) The fucosylation index of alpha-fetoprotein and its usefulness in the early diagnosis of hepatocellular carcinoma. Cancer 61: 769–774

Bahl OP, Carlson RB, Bellisario R, Swaminathan N (1972) Human chorionic gonadotropin amino acid sequence of the alpha and beta subunits. Biochem Biophys Res Commun 48: 416–422

Barnea ER, Kaplan M (1989) Spontaneous gonadotropin-releasing hormone-induced and progesterone-inhibited pulsatile secretion of human chorionic gonadotropin in the first trimester placenta in vitro. J Clin Endocrinol Metab 69: 215–217

Bartels I, Lindemann A (1988) Maternal levels of pregnancy-specific beta-1-glycoprotein (SP-1) are elevated in pregnancies affected by Down's syndrome. Hum Genet 80: 46–48

Belanger L, Baril P, Guertin M et al. (1982) Oncodevelopmental and hormonal regulation of alpha-1-fetoprotein gene expression. Adv Enzyme Regul 21: 73–99

Belisle S, Petit A, Bellabarba D, Echer E, Lehoux JG, Gallo-Payet N (1989) Ca^{2+}, but not membrane lipid hydrolysis mediates human chorionic gonadotropin production by luteinizing hormone-releasing hormone in human term placenta. J Clin Endocrinol Metab 69: 117–121

Belleville F, Lasbennes A, Nabet P, Paysant P (1978) HCS-HCG regulation in cultured placenta. Acta Endocrinol (Copenh) 88: 169–181

Benveniste R, Scommegna A (1981) Human chorionic gonadotrophin alpha-subunit in pregnancy. Am J Obstet Gynecol 141: 952–961

Bogart MH, Pandian MR, Jones OW (1987) Abnormal maternal serum chorionic gonadotrophin levels in pregnancies with fetal chromosome abnormalities. Prenat Diagn 7: 623–630

Bohn H (1985) Biochemistry of placental proteins. In: Bischof P, Klopper A (eds) Proteins of the placenta. 5th Int Cong Placental Proteins, Karger, Basel, pp 1–25

Boothby M, Kukowska J, Boime I (1983) Imbalanced synthesis of human choriogonadotrophin alpha and beta subunits reflects the steady state level of the corresponding mRNAs. J Biol Chem 258: 9250–9253

Braunstein GD, Rasor J, Envgrall E, Wade ME (1980) Interrelationships of human chorionic gonadotrophin, human placental lactogen, and pregnancy-specific beta 1-glycoprotein throughout normal human gestation. Am J Obstet Gynecol 138: 1205–1213

Canick JA, Knight GJ, Palomaki GE, Haddow JE, Cuckle HS, Wald NJ (1988) Low second trimester maternal serum unconjugated oestriol in pregnancies with Down's syndrome. Br J Obstet Gynaecol 95: 330–333

Chard T (1979) Human placental lactogen. In: Gray CH, James VHT (eds) Hormones in blood. Academic Press, London, New York, San Francisco, pp 333–361

Chard T (1989a) Fetal and maternal oxytocin in human parturition. Am J Perinatol 6: 145–152

Chard T (1989b) Hormonal control of growth in the human fetus. J Endocrinol 123: 3–9

Chard T, Klopper A (1982) Placental function tests. Springer-Verlag, Berlin, Heidelberg, New York.

Chard T, Rice A, Kitau MJ, Hird JG, Grudzinskas JG, Nysenbaum AM (1986) Mid-trimester levels of alphafetoprotein in the screening of low birthweight Br J Obstet Gynaecol 93: 36–38

Clements JA, Reyes FI, Winter JSD, Faiman C (1976) Studies on human sexual development. III. Fetal pituitary and serum and amniotic fluid concentrations of LH, CG and FSH. J Clin Endocrinol Metab 42: 9–19

Coates PJ, Doniach I, Holly JPM, Rees LH (1989) Demonstration of desacetyl alpha-melanocyte-stimulating hormone in fetal and adult human anterior pituitary corticotrophs. J Endocrinol 120: 525–531

Diczfalusy E, Mancuso S (1969) Oestrogen metabolism in pregnancy. In: Klopper A, Diczfalusy E (eds) Foetus and placenta. Blackwell, Oxford, p 191

D'Ercole AJ (1987) Somatomedins/insulin-like growth factors and fetal growth. J Dev Physiol 9: 481–495

Economides D, Linton E, Nicolaides K, Rodeck CH, Lowry PJ, Chard T (1987) Relationship between maternal and fetal corticotrophin-releasing hormone-41 and ACTH levels in human mid-trimester pregnancy. J Endocrinol 114: 497–501

Elsner CE, Buster JE, Preston DL (1979) Interrelationships of circulating maternal steroid concentrations in third trimester pregnancies. III Effect of intravenous cortisol infusion on maternal concentrations of estriol, 16-alpha-hydroxyprogesterone, 17-alpha-dihydroprogesterone, Δ^5-pregnenolone, Δ^5-pregnenolone sulfate, dehydroepiandrosterone sulfate and cortisol. J Clin Endocrinol Metab 49: 30–36

Estivariz FE, Morano MI, Carino M, Jackson S, Lowry PJ (1988) Adrenal regeneration in the rat is mediated by mitogenic N-terminal pro-opiomelanocortin peptides generated by changes in precursor processing in the anterior pituitary. J Endocrinol 116: 207–215

Frankenne F, Closset J, Gomez F, Scippo ML, Smal J, Hennen G (1988) The physiology of growth hormones (GHs) in pregnant women and partial characterization of the placental GH variant. J Clin Endocrinol Metab 66: 1171–1180

Gibbons JM, Mitnick M, Chieffo V (1975) In vitro biosynthesis of TSH- and LH-releasing factors by the human placenta. Am J Obstet Gynecol 121: 127–131

Gitlin D (1975) Normal biology of AFP. Ann NY Acad Sci 259: 7–16

Gitlin D, Perricelli A (1970) Synthesis of serum albumin, prealbumin, alphafetoprotein, alpha-antitrypsin and transferrin by the human yolk sac. Nature 228: 995–997

Handwerger S, Barrett J, Tyrey L, Schomberg D (1973) Differential effect of cyclic adenosine monophosphate of the secretion of human placental lactogen and human chorionic gonadotrophin. J Clin Endocrinol Metab 36: 1268–1270

Haning RV, Choi L, Kigens AJ, Kuzman DL, Summerville JW (1982) Effects of dibutyryl adenosine 3′,5′-mono-phosphatase, luteinizing hormone-releasing hormone and aromatase inhibitor on simultaneous outputs of progesterone, 17 beta estradiol, and human chorionic gonadotropin by term placental explants. J Clin Endocrinol Metab 55: 213–218

Haning RV, Choi L, Kiggens AJ and Kuzma DL (1982) Effects of prostaglandins, dibutyryl cAMP, LHRH, estrogens, progesterone and potassium on output of prostaglandin F_2 alpha, HCG, estradiol and progesterone by placental minces. Prostaglandins 24: 495–506

Hilf G, Merz WE (1985) Influence of cyclic nucleotides on receptor binding, immunological activity, and microheterogeneity of human choriogonadotropin synthesized in placental tissue culture. Mol Cell Endocrinol 39: 151–159

Houghton DJ, Newnham JP, Lo K, Rice A, Chard T (1982) Circadian variation of circulating levels of four placental proteins. Br J Obstet Gynaecol 89: 831–835

Huhtala ML, Seppala M, Julkunen M, Koistinen R (1988) Characterisation, biological action and clinical studies of endometrial proteins. In: Chapman M, Grudzinskas G, Chard T (eds) Implantation. Springer-Verlag, London, pp 119–134

Huot RI, Foidart J-M, Nardone RM, Stromberg K (1981) Differential modulation of human chorionic gonadotropin secretion by epidermal growth factor in normal and malignant placental cells. J Clin Endocrinol Metab 53: 1059–1063

Hussa RO (1980) Biosynthesis of human chorionic gonadotropin. Endocrinol Rev 1: 268–294

Hussa RO, Story MT, Pattillo RA (1974) Cyclic adenosine monophosphate stimulates secretion of human chorionic gonadotropin and estrogens by human trophoblast in vitro. J Clin Endocrinol Metab 38: 338–340

Hussa RO, Pattillo RA, Rickert ACG, Scheuermann KW (1978) Effects of butyrate and dibutyryl cyclic AMP on hCG-secreting trophoblastic and non-trophoblastic cells. J Clin Endocrinol Metab 46: 69–76

Iles RK, Chard T (1989) Enhancement of ectopic ß-human chorionic gonadotrophin expression by interferon-alpha. J Endocrinol 123: 501–507.

Iwashita M, Watanabe M, Adachi T, et al. (1989) Effect of gonadal steroids on gonadotropin-releasing hormones stimulated human chorionic gonadotropin release by trophoblast cells. Placenta 10: 103–112

Jaffe RB, Mulcahey J, di Blasio AM, Martin MC, Blumenfeld Z, Dumesic DA (1988) Peptide regulation of pituitary and target tissue function and growth in the primate fetus. Rec Prog Horm

Res 44: 431–438

Jones A, Brooks AN, Challis JRG (1989) Steroids modulate corticotropin-releasing hormone production in human fetal membranes and placenta. J Clin Endocrinol Metab 68: 825–831

Jost A (1976) Sexual differentiation In: Beard RW, Nathanielsz PW (eds) Fetal physiology and medicine. WB Saunders, Philadelphia, pp 1–16

Julkunen R, Rutanen EM, Koskimies A, Ranta T, Bohn H, Seppala M (1985) Distribution of placental protein 14 in tissues and body fluids during pregnancy. Br J Obstet Gynaecol 92: 1145–1151

Kaplan SL, Grumbach MM, Aubert ML (1976) The ontogenesis of pituitary hormones and hypothalamic factors in the human fetus: maturation of central nervous system; regulation of anterior pituitary function. Rec Prog Horm Res 32: 161–193

Khodr G, Siler-Khodr TM (1978) The effect of luteinizing hormone-releasing factor on human chorionic gonadotropin secretion. Fertil Steril 30: 301–304

Kitau MJ, Grint PCA, Heath RB, Chard T (1988) Serum alphafetoprotein levels in subjects with hepatitis B virus. J Med Virol 26; 437–442

Kletzky OA, Rossman T, Bertolli SI, Platt LD, Mishell DR (1985) Dynamics of human chorionic gonadotropin, prolactin and growth hormone in serum and amniotic fluid throughout normal human pregnancy. Am J Obstet Gynecol 151: 878–884

Kurman RJ, Young RH, Norris HJ, Main CS, Lawrence WD, Scully RE (1984) Immunocytochemical localization of placental lactogen and chorionic gonadotropin in the normal placenta and trophoblastic tumours, with emphasis on intermediate trophoblast and the placental site trophoblastic tumor. Int J Gynecol Pathol 3: 101–121

Lee JN, Seppala M, Chard T (1981) Characterization of placental luteinizing hormone-releasing factor-like material. Acta Endocrinol (Copenh) 93: 394–397

Leek AE, Ruoss CF, Kitau MJ, Chard T (1975) Maternal plasma alphafetoprotein levels in the second half of normal pregnancy: relationship to fetal weight and maternal age and parity. Br J Obstet Gynaecol 82: 669–674

Liggins GC (1976) The drive to fetal growth. In: Beard RW, Nathanielsz PW (eds) Fetal physiology and medicine. WB Saunders, Philadelphia, pp 254–270

Littman BH, Alpert E, Rocklin RE (1977) The effect of purified alphafetoprotein on in vitro assays of cell mediated immunity. Cell Immunol 30: 35–42

Macaron C, Kynch M, Rutsky L, Halpern B, Brewer J (1978) Failure of somatostatin to affect human chorionic somatomammotropin and human chorionic gonadotropin secretion in vitro. J Clin Endocrinol Metab 47: 1141–1143

Mathialagan M, Rao AJ (1989) A role for calcium in gonadotrophin-releasing hormone (GnRH) stimulated secretion of chorionic gonadotrophin by first trimester human placental minces in vitro. Placenta 10: 61–70

Merkatz JR, Nitowsky HM, Macri JN, Johnson WE (1984) An association between low maternal serum alpha-fetoprotein and fetal chromosomal abnormalities. Am J Obstet Gynecol 148: 886–894

Molsberry RL, Carr BR, Mendelson CR, Simpson ER (1982) Human chorionic gonadotropin binding to human fetal testes as a function of gestational age. J Clin Endocrinol Metab 55: 791–794

Morgan FJ, Birken S, Canfield RE (1975) The amino acid sequence of human chorionic gonadotropin. The alpha subunit and beta subunit. J Biol Chem 250: 5247–5258

Morinaga T, Sakai M, Wegmann TG, Tamaoki T (1983) Primary structures of human alpha-fetoprotein and its mRNA (cDNA clones/the domain structures/molecular evolution). Proc Natl Acad Sci USA Biol Sci 80: 4604–4608

Morrish DW, Siy O (1985) Modulation of human chorionic gonadotrophin and placental lactogen secretion by epidermal growth factor in serum-free culture of normal human term placental cells. Clin Res 32: 28A

Murgita RA, Tomasi TB (1975) Suppression of the immune response by AFP. J Exp Med 141: 269–286

Obiekwe BC, Chard T (1983) Placental proteins in late pregnancy: relation to fetal sex. J Obstet Gynaecol 3: 163–164

Obiekwe BC, Malek N, Kitau MJ, Chard T (1985) Maternal and fetal alphafetoprotein (AFP) levels at term: relation to sex, weight and gestation of the infant. Acta Obstet Gynecol Scand 64: 251–253

Pavlou C, Chard T, Landon J, Letchworth AT (1973) Circulating levels of human placental lactogen in late pregnancy: the effect of glucose loading, smoking and exercise. Eur J Obstet Gynecol Reprod Biol 3: 45–49

Perez-Lopez FR, Robert J, Tejeiro J (1984) Prl, TSH, FSH, beta-hCG and oestriol reponses to repetitive (triple) LH/TRH administration in the third trimester of human pregnancy. Acta Endocrinol (Copenh) 106: 400–404

Perry L, Hickson R, Obiekwe BC, Chard T (1986) Maternal oestriol levels reflect placental function rather than fetal function. Acta Endocrinol (Copenh) 111: 563-566

Rabe T, Scheurer A, Muller A, Runnebaum B (1982) Pharmacologically induced changes in human beta-chorionic gonadotropin (beta-hCG) synthesis by human placenta in organ culture. Biol Res Pregnancy Perinatal 3: 139–147

Rees LH, Burke CW, Chard T, Evans SW, Letchworth AT (1975) Possible placental origin of ACTH in normal human pregnancy. Nature 354: 620–622

Reyes FI, Boroditsky RS, Winter JSD, Faiman C (1974) Studies on human sexual development II. Fetal and maternal serum gonadotropin and sex steroid concentrations. J Clin Endocrinol Metab 38: 612–617

Rice A, Chard T, Hird V, Grudzinskas JG, Nysenbaum AM (1986) Mid-trimester levels of placental protein 5 are not predictive of preterm labour. J Obstet Gynaecol 7: 18–19

Roti E (1988) Regulation of thyroid-stimulating hormones (TSH) secretion in the fetus and neonate. J Endocrinol Invest 11: 145–158

Ruoslahti E (1978) Isolation and biochemical properties of alpha-fetoprotein. In: Crandall BF, Brazier MB (eds) Prevention of neural tube defects. Academic Press, New York, pp 9–17

Ryan KJ (1980) Placental synthesis of steroid hormones. In: Tulchinsky D, Ryan KJ (eds) Maternal fetal endocrinology, WB Saunders, Philadelphia, p3

Salem HT, Chard T (1982) Clinical studies on placental protein 5 (PP5). In: Grudzinskas JG, Teisner B, Seppala M (eds) Pregnancy proteins. Biology, chemistry and clinical application. Academic Press, Sydney, pp 271–280

Salem HT, Ghaneimah SA, Shaaban MM (1984) Prognostic value of biochemical tests in the assessment of fetal outcome in threatened abortion. Br J Obstet Gynaecol 91: 382–385

Sasaki A, Liotta AS, Luckey MM, Margioria AN, Suda T, Krieger DT (1984) Immunoreactive corticotropin-releasing factor is present in human maternal plasma during the third trimester of pregnancy. J Clin Endocrinol Metab 59: 812–814

Shu-rong Z, Bremme K, Eneroth P, Nordberg A (1982) The regulation in vitro of placental release of human chorionic gonadotrophin, placental lactogen and prolactin. Effects of an adrenergic beta receptor agonist and antagonist. Am J Obstet Gynecol 143: 444–450

Siler-Khodr TM, Khodr GS (1981) Dose response analysis of GnRH stimulation of hCG release from human term placenta. Biol Reprod 25: 353–358

Siler-Khodr TM, Khodr GS, Valenzuela G, Rhode J (1986) Gonadotropin-releasing hormone effects on placental hormones during gestation I. alpha-human chorionic gonadotropin, human chorionic gonadotropin and human chorionic somatomammotropin. Biol Reprod 34: 345–354

Siler-Khodr TM, Khodr GS, Vickery BH, Nestor JJ (1983) Inhibition of hCG, alpha hCG and progesterone release from human placental tissue in vitro by GnRH antagonise. Life Sci 32: 2741–2745

Simmer HH, Frankland M, Greipel M (1975) On the regulation of fetal and maternal 16-alpha-hydroxydehydroepiandrosterone and its sulfate by cortisol and ACTH in human pregnancy at term. Am J Obstet Gynecol 121: 646–652

Simon P, DeCosta C, Brocas H, Schwers J, Vassart T (1986) Absence of human chorionic somatomammotropin during pregnancy associated with two types of gene deletion. Hum Genet 74: 235

Smith CJ, Kelleher PC, Belanger L, Dallaire L (1979) Reactivity of amniotic fluid AF with concanavalin A in the diagnosis off neural tube defects. Br Med J i: 920–921

Stabile I, Grudzinskas JG, Chard T (1988) Clinical applications of pregnancy protein estimations with particular reference to pregnancy-associated plasma protein A (PAPP-A). Obstet Gynecol Surv 43: 73–82

Strickland TW, Puett D (1981) Contribution of subunits to the function of luteinizing hormone/ human chorionic gonadotropin recombinants. Endocrinology 109: 1933–1942

Suganuma N, Seo H, Yamamoto N, Kikkawa F, Oguri H, Narita O, Tomoda Y, Matsui N (1989) The ontogeny of growth hormone in the human fetal pituitary. Am J Obstet Gynecol 160: 729–733

Swartz S, Soloff MS (1974) The lack of estrogen binding by human AFP. J Clin Endocrinol Metab 39: 589–591

Takemori M, Nishimura R, Ashitaka Y, Tojo S (1981) Release of human chorionic gonadotropin (hCG) and its alpha subunit (hCG-alpha) from perfused human placenta. Endocrinol Jpn 28: 757–768

Tamada T, Akabori A, Konuma S, Araki S (1976) Lack of release of human chorionic gonadotropin by gonadotropin-releasing hormone. Endocrinol Jpn 23: 531–533

Tapanainen J, Kellokumpu-Lehtinen P, Pelliniemi L, Huhtaniemi L (1981) Age-related changes in endogenous steroids of human fetal testis during early and midpregnancy. J Clin Endocrinol Metab 52: 98–102

Taylor NF (1982) Review: placental sulphatase deficiency. J Inher Metab Dis 5: 164–176
Uriel J, de Nechaud B, Dupiers M (1972) Estrogen binding properties of rat, mouse and man fetospecific serum proteins. Demonstrations by immunoautoradiographic methods. Biochem Biophys Res Commun 46: 1175–1180
Vulsma T, Gons MH, deVijlder JJM (1989) Maternal-fetal transfer of thyroxine in congenital hypothyroidism due to a total organification defect or thyroid agenesis. N Engl J Med 321: 13–16
Wald NH, Cuckle HS, Densem JW, et al. (1988) Maternal serum screening for Down's syndrome in early pregnancy. Br Med J 297: 883–887
Wehmann RE, Amr S, Rosa C, Nisula BC (1984) Metabolism, distribution and excretion of purified human chorionic gonadotropin and its subunits in man. Ann Endocrinol (Paris) 45: 291·295
Westergaard JG, Chemnitz J, Teisner B, et al. (1983) Pregnancy-associated plasma protein A: a possible marker in the classification and prenatal diagnosis of Cornelia de Lange syndrome. Prenatal Diagn 3: 225–232
Wilson EA, Jawad MJ (1982) Stimulation of human chorionic gonadotropin secretion by glucocorticoids. Am J Obstet Gynecol 142: 344–349
Wilson EA, Jawad MJ, Dickson LR (1980) Suppression of human chorionic gonadotropin by progestational steroids. Am J Obstet Gynecol 138: 708–713
Wilson EA, Jawad MJ, Powell DE (1984a) Effect of estradiol and progesterone on human chorionic gonadotropin secretion in vitro. Am J Obstet Gynecol 149: 143–148
Wilson EA, Jawad MJ, Vernon MW (1984b) Effect of epidermal growth factor on hormone secretion by term placenta in organ culture. Am J Obstet Gynecol 149: 579–580
Winikoff J, Braunstein GD (1985) In vitro secretory patterns of human chorionic gonadotrophin, placental lactogen and pregnancy-specific beta-1-glycoprotein. Placenta 6: 417–422
Word RA, George FW, Wilson JD, Carr BR (1989) Testosterone synthesis and adenylate cyclase activity in the early human fetal testis appear to be independent of human chorionic gonadotropin control. J Clin Endocrinol Metab 69: 204
Wu JT, Book L, Sudar K (1981) Serum alpha-fetoprotein levels in normal infants. Pediatr Res 15: 73–99
Zeitler P, Markoff E, Handwerger S (1983) Characterization of the synthesis and release of human placental lactogen and human chorionic gonadotropin by an enriched population of dispersed placental cells. J Clin Endocrinol Metab 37: 812–818

15. Endometrial Proteins

R. Koistinen, M. Julkunen, L. Riittinen, A. M. Suikkari and M. Seppälä

Introduction

Research on endometrial function and implantation has usually dealt with morphological changes in response to endocrine stimuli during the menstrual cycle, pregnancy, menopause and cancer. Biochemical events related to morphological changes have been studied during the past 10 years. Like all tissues, the endometrium contains a great number of proteins, many of which are more or less ubiquitous. Our studies have concentrated on placental and endometrial protein secretion and on the local actions of these proteins in the endometrium and elsewhere in the body. This review summarizes our studies on two proteins, namely insulin-like growth factor-binding protein (IGFBP-1) and endometrial protein PP14 (placental protein 14).

Insulin-Like Growth Factor-Binding Protein (IGFBP-1)

Insulin-like growth factor-binding proteins are a heterogeneous group of proteins with molecular weights from 24 kDa to 160 kDa (Furlanetto 1980). One of these proteins has been isolated from placenta and named placental protein 12 (PP12) (Bohn and Kraus 1980). Povoa and his coworkers (1984) have isolated a small molecular weight IGF-binding protein and determined its N-terminal amino acid sequence. Our studies have shown that PP12 has the same N-terminal amino acid sequence as the amniotic fluid binding protein (Koistinen et al. 1986). It has been proposed that this protein be named IGFBP-1 (Vancouver meeting on IGF-binding proteins, 1989). Our studies have shown that IGFBP-1 is synthesized by secretory and decidualized endometrium, not by the placenta (Rutanen et al. 1985; 1986).

Bell and coworkers have isolated a protein from human pregnancy endometrium and named it $alpha_1$-pregnancy associated endometrial globulin (alpha$_1$-PEG) (Bell et al. 1985). This protein has been found to be immunologically similar to PP12 (Bell and Bohn 1986), and its N-terminal amino acid sequence is also similar to that of amniotic fluid IGFBP (Bell and Keyte 1988). During 1988, five groups independently reported results of molecular cloning of IGFBP-1 (Brewer et al. 1988; Brinkman et al. 1988; Grundmann et al. 1988, Julkunen et al. 1988a; Lee et al. 1988). All except one group (Brewer et al. 1988) have reported essentially the same primary structure for this protein.

Cellular Origin of IGFBP-1

Immunohistochemical studies have localized alpha$_1$-PEG in endometrial stromal cells (Waites et al. 1988). Early studies using polyclonal anti-PP12 antiserum have demonstrated staining in both the stroma and in the glands (Wahlström and Seppälä 1984). This difference may be due to specificity of the antisera or to the amount of IGFBP-1 present in these cells. Positive immunohistochemical staining is no proof of synthesis, and also the receptor-bound proteins can give a positive result (Wahlström et al. 1983).

We have found that cultured endometrial stromal cells secrete IGFBP-1 (Bützow, unpublished observation). The final evidence of synthesis derives from studies on incorporation of labelled ^{35}S-methionine into IGFBP-1 in tissue or cell culture, and by the demonstration of specific messenger ribonucleic acid (mRNA) in the tissue or cells. We have shown that secretory/decidualized endometrium and ovarian granulosa cells can incorporate labelled methionine into immunodetectable IGFBP-1 (Rutanen et al. 1985; 1986; Suikkari et al. 1989a), and IGFBP-1 mRNA has been detected in the same tissues and also in the liver (see later). Using in situ hybridization Julkunen and her coworkers (to be published) have found IGFBP-1 mRNA in secretory endometrial stroma.

Purification and Characterization

Human mid-trimester amniotic fluid is an abundant source of IGFBP-1 for purification. Koistinen and coworkers (1987a) used gel filtration, hydrophobic interaction high performance liquid chromatography and anion-exchange chromatography to obtain highly purified IGFBP-1 at milligram quantities. This protein retained its IGF-binding capacity. The hydrophobic interaction chromatography step is particularly efficient. IGFBP-1 is effectively retained with equilibrating buffer, whereas most other proteins are not. After this step the major immunoreactive fraction migrates as one band at 34 kD in sodium dodecylsulphate polyacrylamide gel electrophoresis (SDS-PAGE).

A human decidual cDNA library was constructed by Julkunen and coworkers (1988a), and polyclonal antisera against IGFBP-1 were used to identify positive IGFBP-1 cDNA clones. The authenticity of the cDNA was verified by in vitro transcription/translation experiments and by the identity of the 10 N-terminal amino acids deduced for the mature peptide. IGFBP-1 consists of 259 amino acids including a 25-residue putative signal peptide. The molecular mass of mature IGFBP-1 deduced from the cDNA is 25.3 kDa (Julkunen et al. 1988a).

Our results on the deduced sequences are quite similar to those reported by Brinkman et al. (1988) and Lee et al. (1988). They differ only in one amino acid near the C-terminus, at position Met/Ile-228 (nucleotides ATG/ATA). The protein contains 18 cysteine residues, which are conserved in the growth hormone-dependent IGFBP-3 (Wood et al. 1988).

A hydrophobic domain covering the residues 30–50 is particularly rich in cysteine. Perhaps these Cys residues explain why the mobility in SDS-PAGE changes so much after reduction. IGFBP-1 consists of one -Arg-Gly-Asp-sequence near the C-terminus, known to represent the cell attachment site (Ruoslahti and Pierschbacher 1986). Busby and coworkers (1988) have found two types of IGFBP, one of which attaches to the cell surface and the other which does not. In their preliminary studies the attachment could be prevented by the tripeptide Arg-Gly-Asp (Brewer et al. 1988). However, the primary structure of their IGFBP differs from that of the other IGFBP-1 sequences between residues 30 and 46.

Southern blot analysis of genomic DNA suggested that there is a single IGFBP-1 gene within the human genome (Julkunen et al. 1988a). In situ hybridization studies with a cDNA encompassing the entire protein coding region of IGFBP-1 localized the gene to bands p12–p13 on chromosome 7 (Alitalo et al. 1989). Southern blot analysis revealed a polymorphic site with the enzyme Bgl II, which splits the gene near the Ile coding sequence. This is, however, different from the Ile^{228} coding sequence.

Expression of the IGFBP-1 Gene

RNAs from a number of human tissues were analysed for the presence of IGFBP-1 mRNA sequences by RNA blot hybridization. RNA was isolated by the LiCl-urea method (Auffray and Rougeon 1980) from the following human tissues: liver, kidney, adrenal, endometrium, myometrium, placenta and decidua, as well as from a human hepatoma cell line (HepG2), and enriched for poly(A)-RNA by oligo/dT-cellulose chromatography (Aviv and Leder 1972). Poly(A)-RNA samples were fractionated by electrophoresis on agarose gels containing 2.2 M formaldehyde (Rave et al. 1979) and transferred to nitrocellulose filters. The filters were hybridized with ^{32}P-labelled IGFBP-1 cDNA (Julkunen et al. 1988a). The IGFBP-1 gene encodes a single 1.6kb mRNA species expressed most abundantly in term decidua. IGFBP-1 mRNA was also found in secretory endometrium, early decidua, liver and HepG2 cells, but not in term placenta, kidney, adrenal (Julkunen et al. 1988a) or myometrium (Koistinen, unpublished observation). In the fetus, IGFBP-1 mRNA is expressed in the liver only (Brinkman et al. 1988). There are reports indicating that IGFBP-1 gene is expressed in Wilm's tumour (Lee et al. 1988), in some breast cancer cells (Yee et al. 1989), and in granulosa cells and borderline malignant ovarian cystadenoma (Koistinen et al. submitted).

Radioimmunoassay (RIA)

Polyclonal antibody to IGFBP-1 was generated by immunizing a rabbit with the main protein peak from hydrophobic interaction chromatography. For RIA,

IGFBP-1 was iodinated with $Na^{125}I$ using the lactoperoxidase method (Seppälä et al. 1987b). Otherwise the assay was performed as described elsewhere (Rutanen et al. 1982). No other proteins (FSH, hCG, PRL, PP14, PP10, SP_1, alpha subunit of LH, IGF-I) cross-reacted in this RIA. The sensitivity of the assay is 2.3 µg/l.

Immunofluorometric Assay (IFMA)

This method uses a two-step solid phase technique (Koistinen et al. 1987b). The antibody was purified using affinity chromatography on an IGFBP-1 Sepharose column, which was prepared by coupling purified IGFBP-1 to CNBr-activated Sepharose. Affinity-purified antibody was immobilized by adsorbing it onto polystyrene microtitre wells, incubated with the sample and, after washing, the labelled antibody was added. Antibody against IGFBP-1 was labelled with isothiosyanatophenyl-EDTA-europium(III) derivative (Hemmilä et al. 1984), and the fluorescence in each well was measured. The measuring range of the IFMA was 0.25–250 μug/l.

Clinical Studies

Our studies have demonstrated that serum IGFBP-1 level is insulin-dependent (Suikkari et al. 1988; 1989c). The circulating IGFBP-1 levels are inversely correlated with serum insulin concentrations and independent of the glucose level. This has also been found by another group (Holly et al. 1988). There is diurnal variation in serum IGFBP-1 levels both during pregnancy (Rutanen et al. 1984b) and in the non-pregnant state (Drop et al. 1984; Baxter and Cowell 1987; Holly et al. 1988). These changes are likely to reflect changes in liver-derived IGFBP-1 secretion in response to insulin. Insulin and IGF-1 have been found to decrease the release of IGFBP-1 from HepG2 liver cancer cells (Singh et al., to be published).

Subnormal serum IGFBP-1 levels have been found (Suikkari et al. 1989d) in patients with polycystic ovarian disease (PCOD). This is seen in about one-third of cases. These women are characterized by a higher degree of obesity and a tendency to be more hirsute. They also have a higher serum insulin concentration and testosterone to sex hormone binding globulin (SHBG) ratio. Their SHBG level is often subnormal. Recent studies by Kiddy et al. (1990) have shown that diet-induced weight loss is accompanied by a significant decrease in serum insulin and IGF-1 levels, as well as in serum free testosterone levels, whereas the levels of SHBG and IGFBP-1 rise. Hyperinsulinaemia and insulin resistance are characteristics of obese women with PCOD, and high insulin and IGF-1 levels appear to stimulate androgen production in the ovary (Barbieri and Hornstein 1988). It can be speculated on the basis of these results that the effect of weight loss on endocrine status is likely to start from decreasing insulin and IGF-1 concentrations, followed by increased SHBG and IGFBP-1 secretion from the liver and decreased androgen production in the ovary. At the same time the bioavailability of testosterone and IGF-1 may decrease.

Patients with insulinoma and hyperinsulinaemia have very low serum IGFBP-1 levels, which normalize after removal of the tumour (Suikkari et al. 1988).

In patients with type 1 diabetes the serum IGFBP-1 is elevated depending on the level of insulin deficiency. The acute effect of insulin on serum IGFBP-1 concentration has been studied after induction of normoglycaemic hyperinsulinaemic conditions by the insulin clamp technique (Suikkari et al. 1989c) Hyperinsulinaemia has been found to reduce serum IGFBP-1 levels by 40%–70% in patients with type 1 and type 2 diabetes or insulinoma, and also in healthy subjects (Brismar et al. 1988; Suikkari et al. 1988; 1989c).

Patients with advanced ovarian cancer (Iino et al. 1986a) or primary liver cancer (Rutanen et al. 1984a) often have elevated serum IGFBP-1 levels. Obviously malignant hepatocytes produce IGFBP-1, which has also been found in hyperplastic nodules of cirrhosis.

Seppälä and Than (1987) have found elevated levels of IGFBP-1 in benign cystadenoma fluids of the ovary, and also in luteinized granulosa cells of the ovary and in follicular fluid after ovarian hyperstimulation (Seppälä et al. 1984). During ovarian hyperstimulation the circulating IGFBP-1 level increases, and this increase is more pronounced in those women who have more developing follicles (Seppälä et al. 1988a). This increased IGFBP-1 may derive from the ovary, because no simultaneous change takes place in serum insulin levels (Suikkari et al. 1989b).

In view of the multiple sites of IGFBP-1 synthesis, as substantiated by detection of both the protein and its mRNA, the endometrium probably contributes little to the changes in circulating levels in non-pregnant patients with diabetes, liver disorders, PCOD or ovarian hyperstimulation. This is corroborated by findings of no systematic variation in serum IGFBP-1 levels during the menstrual cycle (Suikkari et al. 1987). However, the situation is different during pregnancy (see below).

Pregnancy and Pregnancy-Related Disorders

Serum IGFBP-1 concentration increases during pregnancy (Bognar et al. 1981; Rutanen et al. 1982) The highest levels are seen after 22 weeks' pregnancy. In preeclampsia the IGFBP-1 concentration is abnormally high (Iino et al. 1986b), and the same is true in intrauterine growth retardation (Howell et al. 1985). There is an inverse correlation between serum IGFBP-1 level and birthweight in women with type I or gestational diabetes and in their infants (Hall et al. 1986). It can be speculated that elevated IGFBP-1 is associated with decreased bioavailability of a growth factor (IGF-1) in fetal growth retardation.

In gestational trophoblastic disease the serum IGFBP-1 level may be elevated, but the changes are not so dramatic as those of hCG (Rutanen et al. 1982). Whereas the measurement of serum IGFBP-1 concentration may not add to the clinical management of gestational trophoblastic disease, the biological action of IGFBP-1 in respect to choriocarcinoma is intriguing in the light of studies by Ritvos and coworkers (1988). They have demonstrated that IGFBP-1 of decidual origin inhibits the binding of IGF-I to its receptors in choriocarcinoma cells. IGFBP-1 also inhibits uptake of aminoisobutyric acid by cultured choriocarcinoma cells. Pekonen and coworkers (1988) have found that decidual cytosols containing high IGFBP-1 concentrations can inhibit the binding of IGF-1 to its placental receptors. These results suggest a role for decidual IGFBP-1 in the control of placental growth.

Placental Protein 14

Background

Placental protein 14 (PP14) was originally isolated from the placenta (Bohn et al. 1982). Our studies have demonstrated that PP14 is synthesized by secretory/decidualized endometrium, not the placenta (Julkunen et al. 1986b, 1988b). This protein appears in the literature under several names: alpha$_2$-pregnancy associated endometrial globulin, or alpha$_2$-PEG, (Bell and Bohn 1986), alpha-uterine protein, AUP (Sutcliffe et al. 1982), human chorionic alpha$_2$-globulin (Petrunin et al. 1976), and progestogen-associated endometrial protein, PEP (Joshi et al. 1982).

Purification

We have purified PP14 from mid-trimester amniotic fluid using two different methods (Riittinen et al. 1989b). The first employs gel filtration, anion exchange chromatography and reversed-phase high performance liquid chromatogrphy. In the second method, instead of reversed-phase high performance liquid chromatography (HPLC), octyl-Sepharose CL-4B has been used. This is done to avoid any possible denaturating effect of acetonitrile. Purified PP14 migrates as a 28kDa band in SDS-PAGE. In Western blot analysis this band reacts with anti-PP14 antiserum.

The use of amniotic fluid for the purification of PP14 offers several advantages over placenta as the starting material. First, the concentration of PP14 is high as compared to that of other proteins. Second, the concentration of hCG is low. Special attention has been paid to removing the remaining traces of hCG in the purified PP14 preparation so as to obtain material for studies on its biological actions. The second method includes an anti-hCG absorption step. Before the adsorption PP14 contains 0.00013% hCG and after the adsorption the amount is 0.00003%. This contamination is miniscule and unlikely to interfere in biossays using ovarian granulosa cells. Purification of PP14 from amniotic fluid makes it possible to purify milligrams of this protein for biological studies.

Primary Structure

The N-terminal amino acid sequence of PP14 was the first to be described among this group of similar proteins (Huhtala et al. 1987). Significant homology was detected between PP14 and ß-lactoglobulins from various species. Thereafter it was not surprising that alpha$_2$-PEG was also found to have a N-terminal sequence similar to PP14 (Bell et al. 1987). Westwood et al. (1988) have reported a slightly different N-terminal sequence for PP14. In addition to ß-lactoglobulins, other proteins, notably those belonging to the retinol-binding protein family, have significant homology to PP14 (Seppälä et al. 1988b; Westwood et al. 1988). However, our studies have failed to demonstrate that PP14 is a retinol-binding protein.

Julkunen et al. (1988b) have isolated the cDNA encoding PP14 from a human decidual cDNA library. They have sequenced the cDNA and deduced the entire primary structure of PP14. PP14 consists of 180 amino acids, of which 18 correspond to a putative signal peptide. The predicted molecular weight of pre-PP14 is 20 555 and that of the mature protein is 18 787. The N-terminal sequence of amniotic fluid PP14 (Riittinen et al. 1989b) and that of PP14 purified from placenta (Huhtala et al. 1987) are identical to the deduced amino acid sequence from the cDNA. Sequencing of PP14 cDNA has confirmed its kinship to ß-lactoglobulins for the entire sequence. The amino acid homology to horse ß-lactoglobulin is 53.4%, and these two proteins contain the same number of amino acids. The folding of PP14 and ß-lactoglobulins may be similar, because all four cysteinyl residues, which form the disulphide bridges, are conserved in the sequence of PP14. The nucleotide sequence includes three potential glycosylation sites compatible with the glycosylated nature of secreted PP14 (Julkunen et al. 1988b) containing 17.5% carbohydrate (Bohn et al. 1982).

Expression of the PP14 Gene

RNA from various tissues was isolated using the LiCl/urea method. RNAs were enriched for poly(A)-containing RNA by oligo(dT)-cellulose chromatography and fractionated on 1% agarose/2.2 M formaldehyde gel electrophoresis and transferred to a nitrocellulose filter. The filter was hybridized with ^{32}P-labelled cRNA probe. PP14 mRNA is expressed in early pregnancy decidua and secretory endometrium, but not in placenta, liver, kidney or adrenals. It is interesting to note that human milk contains PP14, but the levels decline rapidly during the first postpartum days. MCF-7 cells, a human breast cancer cell line that expresses the ß-lactoglobulin gene, do not contain PP14 mRNA (Julkunen et al. 1988b). Southern blot analysis of human DNA suggests that either the PP14 gene is very large, consisting of about 20 kilobase pairs, or there are several PP14-related gene sequences in the human genome.

Immunoassays

We have developed assays based on both RIA (Julkunen et al. 1985; Seppälä et al. 1987b) and IFMA techniques (Riittinen et al. 1989a), the latter being more sensitive. It is a sandwich-type solid phase method which utilizes affinity-purified polyclonal antibodies. The antibodies, raised in rabbits, were purified using Sepharose-bound purified PP14. These antibodies were used in a solid phase in polystyrene microtitre wells and also as a tracer, labelled with europium (III) chelate. The samples were incubated in microtitre wells, washed and the europium-labelled antibodies were added. After thorough washing the enhancement solution was added and the fluorescence was measured. The measuring range of IFMA is 0.6–1000 µg/l. We have also generated monoclonal antibodies to PP14 and developed an RIA with a sensitivity of 10 µg/l (Riittinen et al., to be published).

Clinical Studies

In women with normal ovulatory cycles the serum PP14 levels become elevated during the last week of luteal phase (Julkunen et al. 1986a). This PP14 is probably endometrium-derived, because secretory endometrium produces significant amounts of PP14 at that time, and PP14 has not been found in other tissues (Julkunen et al. 1986b). The levels are lowest at midcycle and highest at the onset of the next period, when the progesterone level has already declined (Julkunen et al. 1986a). No similar increase is seen in anovulatory women. These findings may be of clinical relevance in the assessment of endometrial function in infertile women. It seems possible to identify, at the onset of menstrual bleeding, whether the previous cycle had been ovulatory or anovulatory, and whether the endometrium had responded to the ovulatory levels of progesterone or not.

Studies by Seppälä and coworkers (1987b) have shown that, in ovulatory women with unexplained infertility, it is possible to increase their circulating PP14 concentration by giving them micronized oral progesterone. This finding may become important in view of another finding of low serum PEP levels in patients with inadequate luteal phase (Joshi et al. 1986). It is not known whether primary endometrial dysfunction would exist as a cause of infertility. Studies on endometrial protein secretion are underway to elucidate this question.

In our studies on postmenopausal endometrium we have not found PP14 in atrophic endometrium, and the circulating levels are low in postmenopausal women (Seppälä et al. 1987a). Sustained cyclical oestrogen-progestogen replacement treatment is followed by elevated serum PP14 levels in the end of that cycle. We have found considerable individual variation in the PP14 responses to the same treatment regime indicating individual differences in endometrial responsiveness. We have also found some differences in serum PP14 responses to various progestogens after similar oestrogen priming. These preliminary results must be confirmed by studying larger numbers of women in each treatment group.

Hysterectomized women exhibit a much smaller increase (7%) of serum P14 concentration in response to hormone replacement than those with an intact uterus (a 48% increase) (Seppälä et al. 1988b). Current techniques of hysterectomy, when it does not include ovariectomy, usually leave distal parts of the fallopian tubes unremoved. The remaining parts of the tubes may account for this slight elevation of serum PP14 level in hysterectomized women, as PP14 has been detected in the fallopian tubes (Julkunen et al. 1986d).

Serum progesterone levels may not be the only factor influencing serum PP14 concentration. Careful studies on infertile women have demonstrated that serum oestradiol level on day 9 of the cycle has a significant correlation with the subsequent serum PP14 level on days 22–23. (Seppälä et al. 1989). This finding emphasizes the importance of endometrial priming in the follicular phase to its subsequent maturation and secretory capacity in the luteal phase.

After a conception cycle the serum PP14 levels continue to rise until weeks 8–10 of pregnancy, and then decline (Julkunen et al. 1985; Seppälä et al. 1988a). The profile of PP14 levels resembles that of hCG. However, PP14 and hCG are totally unrelated, both structurally and immunologically.

Endometriosis tissue contains PP14. In patients with endometriosis the serum PP14 levels follow similar cyclical variation as in apparently healthy women. When the low midcycle levels were analysed with respect to clinical stage of disease in endometriosis patients, those with stage III endometriosis had significantly higher levels than those with stage I disease, or those with no disease at all (Telimaa et al. 1989). The levels decline after radical surgery or during sustained treatment with danazol (Than et al. 1987), or with medroxyprogesterone acetate (Telimaa et al. 1989).

Overlap of PP14 values between healthy women and patients with endometriosis is considerable and invalidates the use of serum PP14 measurement as a guide to detect active disease. Perhaps this is due to the coexisting secretion of PP14 by the normal endometrium.

The role of PP14 in fertility regulation is unknown. Studies using purified PP14 and decidual extract have indicated immunosuppressive effects in mixed lymphocyte cultures (Bolton et al. 1987). This effect could be reduced by treatment with immunoabsorption with anti-PP14 antibodies. Riittinen and coworkers (unpublished) have studied the effect of purified PP14 on phytohaemagglutinin-stimulated T cell proliferation, and have found no inhibition.

Summary

A review is presented on purification, molecular cloning and sequencing of the cDNA, localization of the mRNA, and clinical studies of two human endometrial proteins present in midtrimester amniotic fluid. One of them, IGFBP-1, is synthesized by endometrial stromal cells, ovarian granulosa cells and the liver, whereas the other protein, PP14, appears to be mainly a product of endometrial glands. Clinical situations in which the circulating levels of IGFBP-1 are changed include pregnancy, preeclampsia, fetal growth retardation, diabetes, insulinona, polycystic ovarian disease and certain clinical treatment regimens such as ovarian hyperstimulation. Serum PP14 becomes elevated in the last week of the luteal phase, and the levels continue to rise if pregnancy ensues. Serum PP14 levels may give information on endometrial responsivencss to endocrine and paracrine stimuli.

Acknowledgements. This work was supported by grants from the Finnish Social Insurance Institution, the Academy of Finland and the Sigrid Jusélius Foundation.

References

Alitalo T, Kontula K, Koistinen R et al. (1989) The gene encoding the human low-molecular weight insulin-like growth factor binding protein (IGF-BP25): regional localization to 7p12-p13 and description of a DNA polymorphism Hum Genet 83: 335–338

Auffray C, Rougeon F (1980) Purification of mouse immunoglobulin heavy-chain messenger RNAs from total myeloma tumor RNA. Eur J Biochem 107: 303–341

Aviv H, Leder P (1972) Purification of biologically active globin messenger RNA by chromatography on oligothymidylic acid cellulose. Proc Natl Acad Sci USA 69: 1408–1412

Barbieri RL, Hornstein MD (1988) Hyperinsulinemia and ovarian hyperandrogenism. Cause and effect. Endocrinol Metab Clin North America 17: 685–703

Baxter RC, Cowell CT (1987) Diurnal rhythm of growth hormone-independent binding protein for insulin-like growth factors in human plasma. J Clin Endocrinol Metab 65: 432–440

Bell SC, Bohn H (1986) Immunochemical and biochemical relationship between human pregnancy-associated secreted endometrial alpha$_1$- and alpha$_2$-globulins (alpha$_1$- and alpha$_2$-PEG) and the soluble placental proteins 12 and 14 (PP12 and PP14). Placenta 7: 283–294

Bell SC, Keyte JW (1988) N-terminal amino acid sequence of human pregnancy-associated endometrial alpha$_1$-globulin, an endometrial insulin-like growth factor (IGF) binding protein – evidence for two small molecular weight IGF-binding proteins. Endocrinology 123: 1202–1204

Bell SC, Patel S, Hales HW, Kirwan PH, Drife JO (1985) Immunochemical detection and characterization of pregnancy-associated endometrial alpha$_1$- and alpha$_2$-globulins secreted by human endometrium and decidua. J Reprod Fertil 74: 261–270

Bell SC, Keyte JW and Waites GT (1987) Pregnancy-associated endometrial alpha$_2$-globulin, the major secretory protein of the luteal phase and first trimester pregnancy endometrium, is not glycocylated prolactin but related to ß-lactoglobulins. J Clin Endocrinol Metab 65: 1067–1071

Bognar ZJ, Than GN, Csaba IF, Szabo D (1981) Placental protein 12 levels of maternal and fetal sera and amniotic fluid at delivery. IRCS Med Sci 9: 1088

Bohn H, Kraus W (1980) Isolierung und Charakterisierung eines neuen plazentaspezifichen protein (PP12). Arch Gynecol 229: 279–291

Bohn H, Kraus W, Winckler W (1982) New soluble placental tissue proteins: their isolation, characterization, localization and quantification. In: Klopper A (ed) Immunology of human placental proteins. Praeger Publ. Placenta S4: 67–81

Bolton AE Pockley AG, Clough KJ, et al. (1987) Identification of placental protein 14 as an immunosuppressive factor in human reproduction. Lancet i: 593–595

Brewer MT, Stetler GL, Squires CH, Thompson RC, Busby WH, Clemmons DR (1988) Cloning, characterization, and expression of a human insulin-like growth factor binding protein. Biochem Biophys Res Commun 152: 1289–1297

Brinkman A, Groffen C, Kortleve DJ, van Kessel AG, Drop SLS (1988) Isolation and characterization of a cDNA encoding the low molecular weight insulin-like growth factor binding protein (IBP-1). EMBO J 7: 2417–2423

Brismar K, Gutniak M, Povoa G, Werner S, Hall K (1988) Insulin regulates the 35 kDa IGF binding protein in patients with diabetes mellitus. J Endocrinol Invest 11: 599–602

Busby WH Jr, Klapper DG, Clemmons DR (1988) Purification of a 31 000-dalton insulin-like growth factor binding protein from human amniotic fluid. Isolation of two forms with different biologic actions. J Biol Chem 263: 14203–14210

Drop SLS, Kortleve DJ, Guyda HJ (1984) Immunoassay of a somatomedin-binding protein from human amniotic fluid: levels in fetal, neonatal and adult sera. J Clin Endocrinol Metab 59: 908–915

Furlanetto RW (1980) The somatomedin C binding protein: evidence for a heterologous subunit structure. J Clin Endocrinol Metab 51: 12–19

Grundmann U, Nelich C, Bohn H, Rein T (1988) Cloning of cDNA encoding human placental protein 12 (PP12): binding protein for IGF-I and somatomedin. Nucl Acids Res 16: 8711

Hall K, Hansson U, Lundin G, et al. (1986) Serum levels of somatomedins and somatomedin-binding protein in pregnant women with type I or gestational diabetes and their infants. J Clin Endocrinol Metab 63: 1300–1306

Holly JMP, Biddlecombe RA, Dunger DB, et al. (1988) Circadian variation of GH-independent IGF-binding protein in diabetes mellitus and its relationship to insulin. A new role for insulin? Clin Endocrinol 29: 667–675

Hemmilä I, Dakubu S, Mukkala V-M, Siitari H, Lövgren T (1984) Europium as a label in time-resolved immunofluorometric assay. Anal Biochem 137: 335–343

Howell RJS, Perry LA, Choglay NS, Bohn H, Chard T (1985) Placental protein 12 (PP12): a new test for the prediction fo the small-for-gestional-age infant. Br J Obstet Gynaecol 92: 1141–1144

Huhtala M-L, Seppälä M, Närvänen A, Palomäki P, Julkunen M, Bohn H, (1987) Amino acid sequence homology between human placental protein 14 and ß-lactoglobulins from various species. Endocrinology 120: 2620–2622

Iino K, Seppälä M, Heinonen PK, Sipponen P, Rutanen E-M (1986a) Elevated levels of a somatomedin-binding protein PP12 in patients with ovarian cancer. Cancer 58: 2294–2297

Iino K, Sjöberg J, Seppälä M (1986b) Elevated circulating levels of decidual protein, placental protein 12, in preeclampsia. Obstet Gynecol 68: 58–60

Joshi SG, Bank JF, Henriques ES, Makarachi A, Matties G (1982) Serum levels of a progestagen-associated endometrial protein during the menstrual cycle and pregnancy. J Clin Endocrinol Metab

55: 642–648
Joshi SG, Rao R, Henriques EE, Raikar RS, Gordon M (1986) Luteal phase concentrations of a progestagen-associated endometrial protein (PEP) in the serum of cycling women with adequate or inadequate endometrium. J Clin Endocrinol Metab 63: 1247–1249
Julkunen M (1986) Human decidua synthesizes placental protein 14 (PP14) in vitro. Acta Endocrinol 112: 271–277
Julkunen M, Rutanen E-M, Koskimies AI, Ranta T, Bohn H, Seppälä M (1985) Distribution of placental protein 14 in tissues and body fluids during pregnancy. Br J Obstet Gynaecol 92: 1145–1151
Julkunen M, Apter D, Seppälä M, Stenman U-H, Bohn H (1986a) Serum levels of placental protein 14 reflect ovulation in nonconceptual menstrual cycles. Fertil Steril 45: 47–50
Julkunen M, Koistinen R, Sjöberg J, Rutanen E-M, Wahlströn T, Seppälä M (1986b) Secretory endometrium synthesizes placental protein 14. Endocrinology 118: 1782–1786
Julkunen M, Raikar RS, Joshi SG, Bohn H, Seppälä M (1986c) Placental protein 14 and progestogen-dependent endometrial protein are immunologically indistiguishable. Hum Reprod 1: 7–8
Julkunen M, Wahlström T, Seppälä M (1986d) Human fallopian tube contains placental protein 14. Am J Obstet Gynecol 154: 1076–1079
Julkunen M, Koistinen R, Aalto-Setälä K, Seppälä M, Jänne OA, Kontula K (1988a) Primary structure of human insulin-like growth factor-binding protein/placental protein 12 and tissue-specific expression of its mRNA. FEBS Lett 236: 295–301
Julkunen M, Seppälä M, Jänne OA (1988b) Complete amino acid sequence of human placental protein 14. A progesterone-regulated uterine protein homologous to ß-lactoglobulin. Proc Natl Acad Sci USA 85: 8845–8849
Kiddy DS, Hamilton-Fairley D, Seppälä M, et al. (1990) Diet-induced changes in sex hormone-binding globulin and free testosterone in women with normal or polycystic ovaries: correlation with serum insulin and insulin-like grwoth factor I. Clin Endocrinol (in press)
Koistinen R, Kalkkinen N, Huhtala M-L, Seppälä M, Bohn H, Rutanen E-M (1986) Placental protein 12 is a decidual protein that binds somatomedin and has an identical N-terminal amino acid sequence with somatomedin-binding protein from human amniotic fluid. Endocrinology 118: 1375–1378
Koistinen R, Huhtala M-L, Stenman U-H, Seppälä M (1987a) Purification of placental protein PP12 from human amniotic fluid and its comparison with PP12 from placenta by immunological, physiochemical and somatomedin-binding properties. Clin Chim Acta 164: 293–303
Koistinen R, Stenman U-H, Alfthan H, Seppälä M (1987b) Time-resolved immunofluorometric assay of 34-kDa somatomedin-binding protein. Clin Chem 33: 1126–1128
Lee Y-L, Hintz RL, James PM, Lee PDK, Shively JE, Powell DR (1988) Insulin-like growth factor (IGF) binding protein complementary deoxyribonucleic acid from human HEPG2 hepatoma cells: predicted protein sequence suggests an IGF binding domain different from those of the IGF-I and IGF-II receptors. Mol Endocrinol 2: 404-411
Pekonen F, Suikkari A-M, Mäkinen T, Rutanen E-M (1988) Different insulin like growth factor binding species in human placenta and decidua. J Clin Endocrinol Metab 67: 1250–1257
Petrunin DD, Gryaznova IM, Petrunina YA, Tatarinov YS (1976) Immunochemical identification of organ-specific human placental alpha$_2$-globulin and its content in the amniotic fluid (in Russian). Byull Eksp Biol Med 82: 803–804
Povoa G, Enberg G, Jörnvall H, Hall K (1984) Isolation and characterization of a somatomedin-binding protein from mid-term human amniotic fluid. Eur J Biochem 144: 199–204
Rave N, Crkvenjakov R, Boedtker H (1979) Identification of procollagen mRNAs transferred to diazobenzyloxymethyl paper from formaldehyde agarose gels. Nucl Acids Res 6: 3559–3567
Riittinen L, Stenman U-H, Alfthan H, Suikkari A-M, Bohn H, Seppälä M (1989a) Time-resolved immunofluorometric assay for placental protein 14. Clin Chim Acta 183: 115–124
Riittinen L, Julkunen M, Seppälä M, Koistinen R, Huhtala M-L (1989b) Purification and characterization of endometrial protein PP14 from midtrimester amniotic fluid. Clin Chim Acta 184: 19–30
Ritvos O, Ranta T, Jalkanen J et al. (1988) Insulin-like growth factor (IGF) binding protein from human decidua inhibits the binding and biological action of IGF-1 in cultured choriocarcinoma cells. Endocrinology 122: 2150–2157
Ruoslahti E, Pierschbacher MD (1986) Arg-Gly-Asp a versatile cell recognition signal. Cell 44: 517–518
Rutanen E-M, Bohn H, Seppälä M (1982) Radioimmunoassay of placental protein 12: levels in amniotic fluid, cord blood, and serum of healthy adults, pregnant women, and patients with trophoblastic disease. Am J Obstet Gynecol 144: 460–463
Rutanen E-M, Wahlström T, Koistinen R, Sipponen P, Jalanko H, Seppälä M (1984a) Placental

protein 12 (PP12) in primary liver cancer and cirrhosis. Tumor Biol 5: 95–102

Rutanen E-M, Koistinen R, Wahlström T, Bohn H, Ranta T, Seppälä M (1985) Synthesis of placental protein 12 by human decidua. Endocrinology 116: 1304–1309

Rutanen E-M, Seppälä M, Pietilä R, Bohn H (1984b) Placental protein 12 (PP12): factors affecting levels in late pregnancy. Placenta 5: 243–248

Rutanen E-M, Koistinen R, Sjöberg J, et al. (1986) Synthesis of placental protein 12 by human endometrium. Endocrinology 118: 1067–1071

Seppälä M, Wahlström T, Koskimies AI, et al. (1984) Human preovulatory follicular fluid, luteinized cells of hyperstimulated preovulatory follicles, and corpus luteum contain placental protein 12: J Clin Endocrinol Metab 58: 505–510

Seppälä M, Alfthan H, Vartiainen E, Stenman U-H (1987a) The postmenopausal uterus: the effect of hormone replacement therapy on the serum levels of secretory endometrial protein PP14/ß-lactoglobulin homologue. Hum Reprod 2: 741–743

Seppälä M, Rönnberg L, Karonen S-L, Kauppila A (1987b) Micronized oral progesterone increases the circulating level of endometrial secretory PP14/ß-lactoglobulin homologue. Hum Reprod 2: 453–455

Seppälä M, Than G (1987c) Insulin-like growth factor-binding protein PP12 in ovarian cyst fluid. Arch Gynecol Obstet 241: 33–35

Seppälä M, Julkunen M, Koskimies A, Laatikainen T, Stenman U-H, Huhtala M-L (1988a) Proteins of the human endometrium: basic and clinical studies toward a blood test for endometrial function. Ann NY Acad Sci 541: 432–444

Seppälä M, Riittinen L, Julkunen M, et al. (1988b) Structural studies, localization in tissue and clinical aspects of human endometrial proteins. J Reprod Fertil S 36: 127–141

Seppälä M, Martikainen H, Rönnberg L, Riittinen L, Kauppila A (1989) Suppression of prolactin secretion during ovarian hyperstimulation is followed by elevated serum levels of endometrial protein protein PP14 in the late luteal phase. Hum Reprod 4: 389–391

Suikkari A–M, Rutanen E-M, Seppälä M (1987) Circulating levels of immunoreactive insulin-like growth factor-binding protein in non-pregnant women. Hum Reprod 2: 297–300

Suikkari A-M Koivisto VA, Rutanen E-M, Yki-Järvinen H, Karonen S-L, Seppälä M (1988) Insulin regulates the serum levels of low molecular weight insulin-like growth factor-binding protein. J Clin Endocrinol Metab 66: 266–272

Suikkari A-M, Jalkanen J, Koistinen R, et al. (1989a) Human granulosa cells synthesize low molecular weight insulin-like growth factor-binding protein. Endocrinology 124: 1088–1090

Suikkari A-M, Koistinen R, Yki-Järvinen H, Koivisto VA, Koskimies A, Seppälä M (1989b) Association of insulin-like growth factor-binding protein (IGF–BP25) with serum insulin and reproductive functions. Proc Vancouver Meeting on IGF-binding proteins. Hintz RL (ed), Vancouver

Suikkari A-M, Koivisto VA, Koistinen R, Seppälä M, Yki-Järvinen H (1989c) Dose-response characteristics for suppression of low molecular weight plasma insulin-like growth factor-binding protein by insulin. J Clin Endocrinol Metab 68: 135–140

Suikkari A-M, Ruutiainen K, Erkkola R, Seppälä M (1989d) Low levels of low molecular weight insulin-like growth factor-binding protein in patients with polycystic ovarian disease. Hum Reprod 4: 136–139

Sutcliffe RG, Joshi SG, Paterson WF, Bank JF (1982) Serological identity between human uterine protein and human progestagen-dependent endometrial protein. J Reprod Fertil 65: 207–209

Than G, Seppälä M, Julkunen M, et al. (1987) The effect of danazol on the circulating levels of 34K insulin-like growth factor-binding protein (PP12) and endometrial secretory protein PP14. Hum Reprod 2: 549–551

Telimaa S, Kauppila A, Rönnberg L, Seppälä M (1989) Elevated serum levels of endometrial secretory protein PP14 in patients with advanced endometriosis: suppression by treatment with danazol and high dose medroxyprogesterone acetate. Am J Obstet Gynecol 161: 866–871

Wahlström T, Seppälä M (1984) Placental protein 12 (PP12) is induced in the endometrium by progesterone. Fertil Steril 41: 781–784

Wahlström T, Huhtaniemi I, Hovatta O, Seppälä M (1983) Localization of luteinizing hormone, follicle-stimulating hormone, prolactin and their receptors in the human and rat testis using immunohistochemistry and radioreceptor assay. J Clin Endocrinol Metab 57: 825–830

Waites GT, James RFL, Bell SC (1988) Immunohistological localization of the human endometrial secretory protein pregnancy-associated endometrial alpha$_1$-globulin, an insulin-like growth factor-binding protein, during the menstrual cycle. J Clin Endocrinol Metab 67: 1100–1104

Westwood OMR, Chapman MG, Totty N, Philip R, Bolton AE, Lazarus NR (1988) N-terminal sequence analysis of human placental protein 14, purified in high yield from decidual cytosol. J Reprod Fertil 82: 493–500

Wood WI, Cachianes G, Henzel WJ, et al. (1988) Cloning and expression of the growth hormone-dependent insulin-like growth factor-binding protein. Mol Endocrinol 2: 1176–1185

Yee D, Favoni RE, Lupu R, et al. (1989) The insulin-like growth factor binding protein BP-25 is expressed by human breast cancer cells. Biochem Biophys Res Commun 158: 38–44

16. Maternal Serum AFP Screening for Fetal Malformations and Down's Syndrome

B. Nørgaard-Pedersen

Introduction

The aim of antenatal screening for fetal malformations, especially neural-tube defects (NTD) and Down's syndrome, is to identify women with a sufficiently high risk of having an affected fetus to justify carrying out special diagnostic procedures such as a detailed ultrasound screening and amniocentesis including laboratory analyses of amniotic fluid for alpha-fetoprotein (AFP), acetylcholinesterase (AChE), and chromosomes.

Since Brock and Sutcliffe (1972) demonstrated elevated levels of AFP in amniotic fluid samples from pregnancies with neural-tube defects, development has taken place rapidly (for review see Wald and Cuckle, 1984). First the UK-collaborative studies have shown that amniotic fluid AFP (A-AFP) is an almost specific diagnostic test for NTD; that maternal serum APF (S-AFP) can be used as a screening test for NTD; and that amniotic fluid AChE (A-AChE) is an important confirmatory test for NTD. Furthermore, ultrasound scanning is becoming increasingly efficient in the detection for severe malformations; indeed, it has been claimed that it is as effective as S-AFP in screening for severe malformations, but no randomized studies have been carried out.

Merkatz et al (1984) showed that S-AFP is low in Down's syndrome pregnancies and this observation has been confirmed in several studies. Other markers such as oestriol (E_3) and human chorionic gonadotrophin (hCG) have now been added (Bogard et al. 1987; Canick et al. 1988 Wald et al. 1988a; 1988b Nørgaard-Pedersen et al. 1990). The addition of these markers for Down's syndrome has increased the need for risk reporting of laboratory analyses. The increase in the AFP database for spina bifida, anencephaly, abdominal wall defects, twins, etc. makes this possible not only for Down's syndrome, but also for malformations. Risk reporting is also important since a randomized study by Tabor et al. (1986) showed an amniocentesis-related abortion risk of about 1%. The risk of abnormality should always be weighed against the risk of amniocentesis. Finally, the introduction of chorionic villus sampling (CVS), in place of amniocentesis, has increased the need for S-AFP and/or US-screening, since malformations are not detected by CVS. A revised prenatal diagnostic policy is therefore essential though the details are not yet certain.

AFP Screening for Fetal Malformations

The first prenatal diagnosis of NTD in Denmark was carried out in 1974; both A-AFP and S-AFP were elevated. Since then, all amniotic fluid samples taken for prenatal diagnostic purposes have been screened for AFP leakage disorders by AFP estimation. Maternal S-AFP screening was not started until 1980 mainly because Denmark is a low incidence area for NTD, and also because S-AFP methods were not reliable until then (Nørgard-Pedersen et al. 1985). Furthermore, the confirmatory laboratory tests for amniotic fluid i.e. AChE testing and concanavalin A reactivity of AFP were not available. Finally, the US scanning facilities for follow-up and amniocentesis were not optimal. As shown in Table 16.1 nearly 100 000 pregnancies have been screened at two university departments (Hvidovre and Rigshospitalet) and two country hospitals (Kolding and Sønderborg). As seen in Table 16.1 about 14 000 pregnancies are now screened every year, i.e. about a quarter of the total pregnant population in Denmark.

In Denmark the total number of births per year is about 55 000. A nationwide S-AFP screening programme should detect about 110 malformations. The flow scheme below shows the predicted outcome of a nationwide screening programme for high S-AFP.

During the first two years of the pilot screening programme a detailed analysis of all 11 198 screened pregnancies was carried out (Tables 16.2 and 16.3). This was done in order to ensure that the numbers of high and low AFP values were

Table 16.1. Prenatal diagnosis of severe fetal malformation in Denmark

Year	No. of amniotic fluids	No. of malformations				No. of serum samples
		Total		By screening only		
		NTD	Other	NTD	Other	
1980	2790	5	3	(2)	(0)	
1981	3274	22	7	(13)	(5)	
1982	3852	25	18	(12)	(12)	25 969
1983	4554	18	16	(8)	(14)	
1984	4143	19	12	(14)	(5)	11 359
1985	3448	14	11	(10)	(8)	11 745
1986	4457	14	17	(5)	(9)	13 017
1987	4043	14	19	(9)	(9)	14 446
1988	4299	20	12	(8)	(6)	14 927
Total	34 860	151	115	(81)	(68)	91 463

The numbers in brackets are malformations detected by S-AFP screening only. NTD: neural-tube defects. Other: other malformations especially gastrointestinal defects.

55 000 pregnancies
60 000 S-AFP
3.7% S-AFP elevated
3.7% US-scan (2000)
0.9% amniocenteses (500)
0.2% malformations (110)

Increased S-AFP
Detected: 110
34 anencephaly
30 spina bifida
20 abdominal wall defects
26 other abnormalities

Normal S-AFP
Not detected: 6
3 spina bifida
3 encephalocele
(skin-covered)

acceptable and that the number of amniocenteses was about 1.0%. Since these claims were fulfilled it was decided to monitor detected and undetected malformations only.

Table 16.2. Results of S-AFP analyses of 11 198 screening pregnancies at the four centres (a two-year study)

Centre	Hvidovre	Kilding	RH	Sdr.borg	Total (%)
Number of patients	3679	1451	2498	3570	11 198 (100)
1st S-AFP high	157	52	94	112	415 (3.7)
2nd S-AFP normal	19	13	16	39	87 (0.8)
2nd S-AFP not taken[a]	93	16	45	16	170 (1.5)
1st and 2nd S-AFP high	45	23	33	57	158 (1.4)
Number of amniocenteses	40	25	26	36	118 (1.1)
NTD detected	5	4	2	4	15 (0.13)
Other abnormalities detected	4	0	1	0	5 (0.044)
NTD not detected	1	0	1	0	2 (0.018)
1st S-AFP low	47	28	94	98	267 (2.4)

[a]Missed, spontaneous or threatened abortion, twins, correction of gestational age by ultrasonography, etc.

Table 16.3. AFP screening – detailed follow-up of 11 198 patients

	Total number	1st S-AFP elevated
Total number	11 198	415 (37.%)
Normal pregnancy	9 401	251 (2.7%)
Missed abortion	51	15 (29.4%)
Imminent abortion	384	25 (6.5%)
Vaginal bleeding	167	17 (10.2%)
Placental insufficiency	403	20 (5.0%)
Placental abruption	35	3 (8.6%)
Preeclampsia/hypertension	358	10 (2.8%)
Hydramnios	27	3 (11.1%)
Oligohydramnios	9	4 (44.4%)
Cystitis/cystopyelitis	88	5 (5.7%)
Hydatidiform mole[a]	7	2 (28.6%)
Twin pregnancy	107	47 (43.9%)

[a]Two partial moles, both with high S-AFP, five classic moles, all with non-pregnant levels of S-AFP.

Table 16.4. Incidence of neural-tube defects (NTD) and abdominal wall defects (AWD) per 10 000 pregnancies for the AFP screening population and per 10 000 total births (live and stillborn) from Fyns county for 1979, 1980 and 1981

	Screening population	Fyns county
NTD total	*15.7*	*10.8*
Anencephaly	8.3	4.1
Spina bifida	6.2	6.7[a]
Encephalocele	1.2	–
AWD total	*5.4*	*6.7*
Omphalocele	2.9	4.0
Gastroschisis	2.5	2.7

[a]Spina bifida and encephalocele.

After the first 24 023 screened pregnancies, a comparison was made between the incidence of NTD and abdominal wall defects (AWD) in the screened population and among 10 000 total births (Table 16.4) (Nørgaard-Pedersen et al. 1984) As can be seen, there is good agreement between the two populations except for anencephaly. This may be due to late spontaneous abortion in some cases of anencephaly.

Our detection rates have been similar to the UK-Collaborative Study for spina bifida and anencephaly. During the eight-year screening period we have also obtained laboratory data for spina bifida, anencephaly, abdominal wall defects and twins, which are similar to those found in the UK-Collaborative Study. Based on these distributions and the incidence of the different abnormalities it is possible to carry out risk calculations (Nørgaard-Pedersen et al. 1985).

AFP Screening for Down's Syndrome

Since Merkatz et al. (1984) observed that pregnancies associated with fetal Down's syndrome had reduced levels of S-AFP, several studies have examined the possibility of using S-AFP as a screening test for Down's syndrome. We have

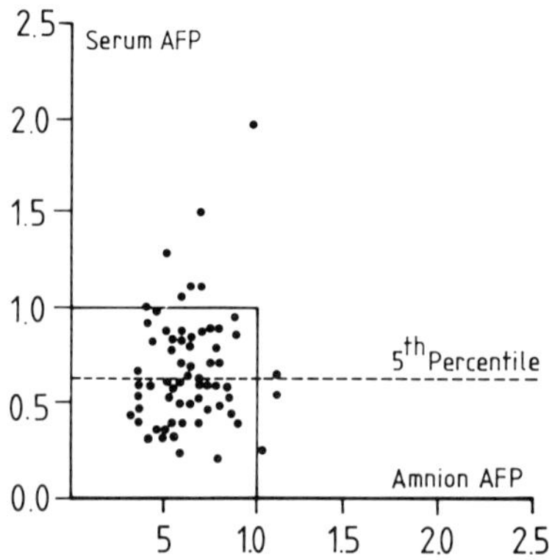

Fig. 16.1. Levels of AFP in serum and amniotic fluid in MoM from 65 pregnant women with fetal Down's syndrome.

confirmed this observation in the Danish population. Our data for 86 cases of Down's syndrome showed a median of 0.64 (Tabor et al. 1986).

AFP is low in both serum and amniotic fluid from pregnancies with fetal Down's syndrome, but there is no correlation between the two parameters (see Fig.16.1). It is, however, noteworthy that none of the 65 cases in Fig. 16.1 had S-AFP and A-AFP greater than 1.0 MoM (Multiple of the Median) simultaneously. This information may be used to determine whether chromosome analysis should be carried out.

It is possible to calculate the risk for Down's syndrome by combining age and S-AFP. Based upon S-AFP distribution among 86 cases of Down's syndrome and the age-related risk for Down's syndrome, we have been able to construct so-called iso-risk curves (Tabor et al. 1987). In Fig. 16.2 we have chosen a probability of 1 : 400 since this corresponds to the lower limit of referral for amniocentesis for the youngest women (35 years of age) in Denmark. Our calculations were applied to the Danish birth distribution by maternal age for 1983. The total number of births was 51 086 in that year and the expected number of infants with Down's syndrome was 62.3. The maternal S-AFP levels and age are shown as an iso-risk curve in (1 : 400) Fig. 16.2. The 95% reference intervals

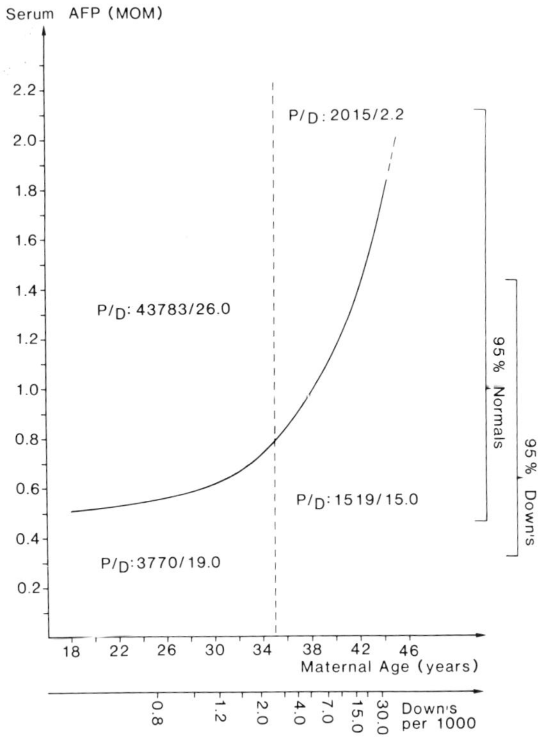

Fig. 16.2. Iso-risk curve (1 : 400) for Down's syndrome based upon maternal age and serum AFP (expressed in MoM). The 95% reference intervals for normals (n=2018) and Down's syndrome (n=86) are shown. The median serum AFP in Down's syndrome pregnancies was 0.64 MoM. The lowest abscissa (Down's per 1000) shows the risk of having a Down's syndrome infant based on age alone. P=number of pregnancies; D=number of Down's syndrome cases. Number of births in Denmark 1983=51 087 (Tabor et al. 1987).

for normal pregnancies (n= 2018) and Down's syndrome (n=86) are shown. The median for Down's syndrome was 0.64 MoM.

The outcome of different screening strategies is shown in Table 16.5. Based upon maternal age at or above 35 years, amniocentesis in 6.9% of all pregnant women in Denmark would detect 27.7% of Down's syndrome fetuses. Based upon the iso-risk curve (1 : 400) 9.4% amniocenteses would detect 53.0% of Down's syndrome fetuses.

In a prospective screening study for fetal chromosone abnormalities using maternal S-AFP, 14 272 women were screened by S-AFP and ultrasound. In 571 women (4.2%) S-AFP was below the 5th percentile (corresponding approximately to 0.55 MoM). Amniocentesis was offered to 226 women because of low S-AFP alone; 188 (83.2%) accepted amniocentesis and 3 cases of fetal trisomy were found i.e. a yield of 1 fetal trisomy per 63 amniocenteses. This study was started 1 January 1985 and about 50 000 pregnancies have now been screened. Although detailed information has not yet been collected, the number of amniocenteses per trisomy is about the same.

Recently, however, it has been shown that serum oestriol (E3) is also low in pregnancies with Down's syndrome, and human chorionic gonadotrophin (hCG) is high. These markers can therefore be used together with AFP and maternal age to calculate the risk for Down's syndrome (see Table 16.5 and Fig 16.3) (Nørgaard-Petersen et al. 1990).

In a new population of 42 Down's syndrome pregnancies the median values were 0.70 MoM for AFP, 0.74 for E3, and 1.57 MoM for hCG (Table 16.6).

Using a discriminatory analysis the linear function that best distinguished normal sera and Down's syndrome sera was found to be D = E3 + 1.072 AFP − 0.572 hCG. From Fig. 16.3 it can be seen how many amniocenteses would be necessary to obtain a certain detection rate of Down's syndrome using different

Table 16.5. Screening for Down's syndrome

Criteria	Age						No. of amniocenteses per Down's
	34 and below		35 and above		Total		
	All	Down's	All	Down's	All	Down's	
Age	0	0	100.0	100.0	61	27.7	204
Age+AFP	61	40.4	43.3	86.0	9.4	53.0	146
Age+E3+AFP	4.7	41.5	38.0	80.7	7.0	52.4	110
Age+E3+AFP+hCG	5.3	48.0	34.8	83.1	7.3	57.6	105
Age+hCG+AFP	5.6	44.0	38.2	83.1	7.8	54.7	117

Table 16.6 Average and standard deviation (SD) of log MoM values in normal and Down's syndrome pregnancies for AFP, oestrio and hCG

	Down's syndrome sera n = 42		Normal sera n = 291	
	average	SD	average	SD
AFP	−0.154	0.198	0.010	0.152
Oestriol	−0.129	0.202	0.003	0.118
hCG	0.195	0.317	0.009	0.248
Discrimination function D	−0.4051	0.386	0.008	0.272

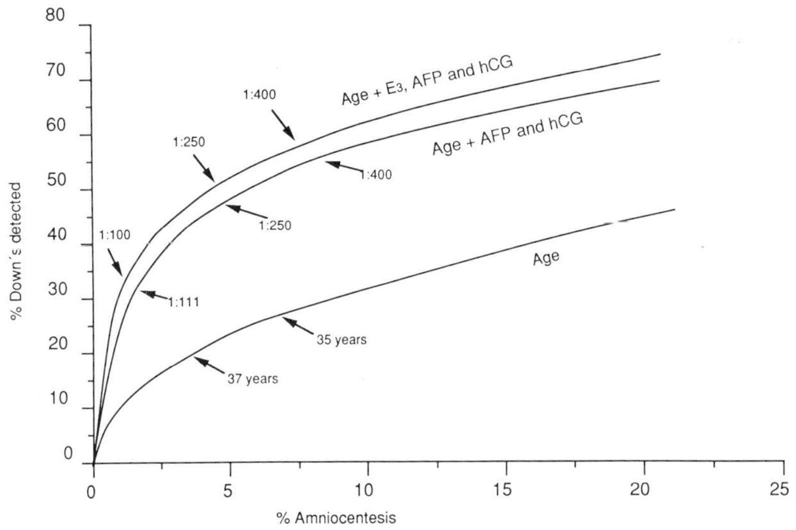

Fig. 16.3. Percentage of amniocenteses required to detect a certain proportion of Down's syndrome pregnancies, using three different screening strategies: either maternal age alone, a combination of maternal age, AFP and hCG, or a combination of maternal age, AFP, hCG and oestriol. Different cut-offs are marked on the two curves combining age and biochemical markers, so that all women to the left of a cut-off have a risk exceeding the cut-off (Nørgaard-Pedersen et al. 1989).

screening strategies. A function based on AFP and hCG (D = AFP– 0.448 hGC) gives discrimination which is nearly as good as the one based upon E3, AFP and hCG. If a risk cut-off level of 1 : 400 is used, AFP and hCG combined with maternal age would give a detection rate of 54.7% with a false positive rate (amniocentesis) of 7.8% and an average risk of being affected for those referred to amniocentesis of 1 : 117. We have found a weak, but significant correlation between Log MoM values for AFP and E3 for the 42 Down's pregnancies and for the normal pregnancies. There was no significant correlation beween any of these markers and hCG. Therefore, the combination of AFP and hCG should be chosen because hCG is easier to determine than E3 (Nørgaard-Pedersen et al. 1990).

Cost Benefit of S-AFP and/or Ultrasound Scanning in Denmark

In 1988 a working group reported on: "Analyses of the economic consequences of S-AFP screening and ultrasound screening in antenatal care". This report was based upon the following facts and presumptions:

1. S-AFP and US-screening are assumed to be equally effective in detection of the different malformations.
2. About 50% of the malformations are already detected by the present indications for amniocentesis in Denmark.
3. About 70% of US-screening capacity is already present in Denmark according to an US-scanning report from the Danish National Health Board, which does not recommend US-screening but only scanning on indication.
4. Cost savings were calculated for spina bifida only, not including anencephaly, abdominal defect, etc.

The advantages and disadvantages of introducing prenatal screening are shown in Table 16.7.

The savings in costs are a minimum estimate because it has only been possible to calculate the costs for the first 7 years of the child's life. In addition, for each of the two screening methods a number of other fetal abnormalities will be detected; these have not been included in the calculations.

If both S-AFP screening and ultrasound are introduced, the annual costs – on the basis of the assumptions built into the analysis – lie between 13.2 million kr and 14.7 million kr. The working group also made calculations about screening

Table 16.7. Advantages and disadvantages of introducing prenatal screening

Disadvantages	*Advantages*
Direct costs	Cost savings
S-AFP screening approx. 3.6 million kr Ultrasound 11.4–12.9 million kr	10.1–16.4 million kr
Carrying out 59 induced abortions	Avoidance for 59 families of a stillbirth or a severely handicapped child.
Provoking 2 or 3 unwanted miscarriages each year (as a result of the increased risk of miscarriage following amniocentesis)	Better treatment possibilities and better survival for children with abdominal wall defects.
Unnecessary anxiety in the middle of pregnancy for women with normal fetuses who have additional investigations following screening	Increased peace of mind for women with normal fetuses
Greater disappointment for whose women who despite the test have a handicapped child	

Table 16.8. Direct costs and cost savings for different risk groups in screening for Down's syndrome by a combination of maternal age and S-AFP

Risk for Down's syndrome	No. of amniotic fluid analyses/ abortions	Direct costs (mill. kr)	Cost savings (mill. kr)
0.006	1402/20.3	4.535	14.718
0.004	2536/25.9	8.134	18.778
0.003	3775/30.1	11.982	21.823
0.0025	4806/33.0	15.206	23.925
0.002	6380/36.5	20.117	26.463
The present age indication (35 years and above)	3500/17	11.008	12.325

for Down's syndrome based upon S-AFP and maternal age. Table 16.8 shows the direct costs and cost savings for different risk groups.

For all the different risk groups, the cost savings for the first 7 years of the child's life exceed the direct cost of screening. Since there are also cost savings after the 7th year of life the difference will be considerably greater than that shown in Table 16.8.

Future of Antenatal Screening in Denmark

Nationwide screening is now under consideration by the Danish National Health Board. A randomized study on S-AFP and US-screening will be important for deciding whether S-AFP and/or US-screening should be recommended. Patient acceptance should also be evaluated. A positive screening result causes anxiety, but this should be weighed against the number of fetal abnormalities detected per number of amniocenteses, since the abortion risk after amniocentesis is about 1%. The key issue is providing information to all pregnant women so that each woman can make her own decision.

References

Bogart MH, Pandian MR, Jones OW (1987) Abnormal maternal serum chorionic gonadotropin levels in pregnancies with fetal chromosome abnormalities. Prenat Diagn 7: 623-630

Brock DJH, Sutcliff RG (1972) Alphafetoprotein in the antenatal diagnosis of anencephaly and spina bifida. Lancet ii: 197–199

Canick JA, Knight GJ, Palomaki GE, Haddow JE, Cuckle HS, Wald NJ (1988) Low second trimester maternal serum unconjugated oestriol in pregnancies with Down's syndrome. Br J Obstet Gynaecol 95: 330–333

Merkatz IR, Nitowsky HM, Johnson WE (1984) An association between low maternal serum alpha-fetoprotein and fetal chromosomal abnormalities. Am J Obstet Gynecol 148: 886–894

Nørgaard-Pedersen B, Bagger PV, Bang J et al. (1984) Screening for serum alphafetoprotein for detection of congenital deformities in the 16th–18th weeks of pregnancy. Results of 24 023 investigations. Ugeskr Læg 146: 3253–3259

Nørgaard-Pedersen B, Bagger P, Bang J et al. (1985) Maternal serum alpha-fetoprotein screening for fetal malformations in 28 062 pregnancies. A four-year experience from a low-risk area. Acta Obstet Gynecol Scand 64: 511–514

Nørgaard-Pederson B, Olesen Larsen S, Arends J, Svenstrup B, Tabor A (1990) Maternal serum markers in the screening for Down's syndrome. Clin Genet 37: 35–43

Tabor A, Philip J, Madsen M, et al. (1986) Randomized controlled trial of genetic amniocentesis in 4606 low-risk women. Lancet i: 1287–1293

Tabor A, Larsen SO, Nielsen J et al. (1987) Screening for Down's syndrome using an iso-risk curve based on maternal age and serum alpha-fetoprotein level. Br J Obstet Gynaecol 94: 636-642

Wald NJ, Cuckle HS (1984) Open neural-tube defects. In: Wald NJ (ed) Antenatal and neonatal screening. Oxford University Press, Oxford, New York, Tokyo, pp 25–73

Wald NJ, Cuckle HS, Densem JW, et al. (1988a) Maternal serum unconjugated oestriol as an antenatal screening test for Down's syndrome. Br J Obstet Gynaecol 95: 334–341

Wald NJ, Cuckle HS, Densem JW, et al. (1988b) Maternal serum screening for Down's syndrome in early pregnancy. Br Med J 297: 883–887

17. Biochemical Screening for Down's Syndrome

N. Wald and H. Cuckle

Background

Until the early 1980s the only effective method of identifying women with a risk of having a fetus with Down's syndrome sufficient to justify a diagnostic amniocentesis was to use maternal age; older women, say 40 years of age or more, were offered an amniocentesis whilst younger women were not. Unfortunately, there is considerable overlap in the distribution of maternal age in pregnancies with and without Down's syndrome and most affected pregnancies occur in young women. Using an age cut-off level of 40 years, about 1% of women are eligible for an amniocentesis and this would lead to the detection of about 15% of pregnancies associated with Down's syndrome. By lowering the cut-off to 35 the detection rate is increased to about 35% but with an increase in the amniocentesis rate to about 7%. Offering amniocentesis to younger women who have had a previous Down's syndrome pregnancy is accepted practice, but it has only a negligible effect on the overall detection rate; about 1% of affected pregnancies will arise in such women. In practice, few screening programmes based on maternal age and previous family history have achieved a reduction in the birth prevalence of Down's syndrome of more than 15%.

Serum Screening

The value of maternal serum alpha-fetoprotein (AFP) measurement at 16–18 weeks of gestation, in conjunction with an ultrasound biparietal diameter (BPD) measurement, is well established as a method of screening for open neural tube defects. The same specimen of blood can also be used to screen for Down's syndrome by performing two additional biochemical tests, namely the measurement of unconjugated oestriol (uE3) and human chorionic gonadotropin (hCG) and using these together with AFP and maternal age to estimate the risk to the individual of having an affected pregancy (Wald et al. 1988; Norgaard-

Table 17.1. A basic serum screening programme for open neural tube defects and Down's syndrome

1. A maternal serum AFP, uE3 and hCG test is carried out at 16–18 weeks of gestation based on dates and an ultrasound BPD measurement is made. (Anencephaly should be identified at this stage). The values are expressed in MoM's, using the gestational age estimate based on BPD. If a scan has already been done the AFP tests should be carried out at 16 weeks based on BPD.
2. The result is regarded as positive if (a) the AFP level is raised, say ≥2.5 MoM, or (b) the risk of Down's syndrome, calculated from the serum levels and age, is high, say ≥1 : 250.
3. If the result is positive an amniocentesis and a detailed ultrasound scan is performed. An amniotic fluid AFP test is carried out on women with raised serum AFP levels; a karyotype is carried out on women with a high risk of Down's syndrome. (An AFP and a karyotype determination are often performed on all amniotic fluid samples although this will have a negligible effect on the detection of neural tube defects and Down's syndrome.)
4. An amniotic fluid AFP result is regarded as positive if it is equal to or greater than a cut-off level of 2.0 MoM using the estimate of gestational age based on the BPD, but if this estimate is 1–34 days earlier than the dates estimate, the dates estimate is used.
5. If the amniotic fluid AFP result is positive a gel AChE test is done.
6. A termination of pregnancy is offered if the AChE result is also positive, or if the karyotype is positive.

AChE = Acetylcholinesterase; AFP = alpha-fetoprotein; BPD = biparietal diameter; hCG = human chorionic gonadotropin; MoM = multiple of normal median; uE3 = unconjugated oestriol.

Pedersen et al. 1990). Table 17.1. shows the steps involved in such a screening programme for neural tube defects and Down's syndrome, and Table 17.2 shows the expected outcome of screening all pregnancies in England and Wales. The estimates of performance are likely to be better than those shown for three reasons:

1. Ultrasound examination will visualize some of the spina bifida lesions (particularly in women with raised maternal serum AFP levels).
2. Women with positive or ambiguous amniotic fluid results will have a repeat amniocentesis.
3. Ultrasound gestational dating will usually be performed in women with positive Down's syndrome screening tests.

Sufficient data are not at present available to quantify these effects.

Table 17.3 shows the detection rate and the false positive rate associated with different risk cut-off levels. At a risk cut-off level of 1 : 250, the detection rate for Down's syndrome is 61% and the false positive rate is 5%.

The main advantage of the use of the new biochemical markers for Down's syndrome is that, for a given amniocentesis rate, a much greater proportion of Down's syndrome pregnancies can be identified than if maternal age is used alone. At an amniocentesis rate of 5% the detection rate is about 60% using the new markers and maternal age compared with about 30% using age alone. To achieve this extra detection, some women thought to be at high risk on account of their age alone will, as a result of their biochemical results, be classified as being at low risk. They can be counselled accordingly and may choose to avoid an amniocentesis. Other women, thought to be at low risk on account of their relatively young age, may be classified as being at high risk on account of their biochemical results and can be offered an amniocentesis. This more accurate

Table 17.2. Expected outcome of screening for open neural tube defects and Down's syndrome at 16–18 weeks of gestation in all pregnancies in England and Wales (say 600 000 births per year) using the scheme given in Table 17.1 (figures are also given for anterior abdominal wall defects)

	Anencephaly	Open spina bifida	Anterior abdominal wall defect	Down's syndrome	Unaffected
Total	1080	960	150	780	597 030
Positive screening test	1080	864	110	476	46 568
Amniotic fluid AFP ⩾ 2 MoM and positive AChE	ND	838	75	ND	67[a]
Positive karyrotype	ND	ND	ND	476	0
Offer of termination of pregnancy	1080	838	75	476	67[a]

From Wald and Cuckle (1989), modified to take account of the results of the Second Report of Collaborative AChE Study: Wald, Cuckle and Nanchahal (1989).
ND = Not done; MoM = multiple of normal median.
[a]Excludes miscarriages and other serious abnormalities.

Notes

1. Birth prevalences per 1000 births are as follows: 1.8 anencephaly, 1.6 open spina bifida, 0.25 anterior abdominal wall defects and 1.3 Down's syndrome.
2. Open spina bifida screening detection rate is 90% and the false positive rate is 2.8%. The biparietal diameter determination can be expected to detect all cases of anencephaly.
3. Down's syndrome screening detection rate is 61% and the false positive rate is 5.0%. Nearly all the false positive will be additional to those for neural tube defect screening.
4. Anterior abdominal wall defect screening detection rate is 73%, and amniotic fluid AFP and AChE detection rate is 75%.
5. Open spina bifida amniotic fluid AFP and AChE detection and false positive rates are 97% and 0.40%, respectively, in women with raised serum AFP levels.

Table 17.3. Combined maternal age and serum AFP, uE3 and hCG screening for Down's syndrome at 14–20 weeks of gestation: detection rate, false positive rate and odds of a Down's syndrome birth according to risk cut-off level[a]

Risk cut-off level	Detection rate (%)	False rate (%)	Average Down's syndrome risk in positives
1 : 100	44	1.7	1 : 29
1 : 150	52	2.8	1 : 42
1 : 200	57	3.9	1 : 54
1 : 250	61	5.0	1 : 65
1 : 300	64	6.1	1 : 75
1 : 350	67	7.2	1 : 85

Adapted from Wald et al. (1988).
[a]A woman has a positive screening result for Down's syndrome if the risk is equal to or greater than the risk cut-off.

reassignment of women into high- and low-risk categories substantially improves the effectiveness of screening.

Table 17.4 shows the risk of having a pregnancy associated with Down's syndrome for women of different ages according to the various levels of the three serum markers. The biochemical markers have a striking effect on the risk; for example, in a 35-year-old woman the risk varies from 1 : 16 if the AFP, uE3 and hCG values are 0.4, 0.4 and 2.0 MoM, respectively, to 1 : 52 000 if the values were, respectively, 2.5, 1.4 and 0.5 MoM.

Table 17.4. Risk of having a Down's syndrome term pregnancy according to selected maternal serum AFP, uE3 and hCG levels

Maternal serum			Maternal age (completed years)				
AFP	uE3	hCG	20	25	30	35	40
0.4	0.4	2.0	1 : 65	1 : 60	1 : 40	1 : 16	1 : 6
1.0	0.4	2.0	1 : 280	1 : 240	1 : 170	1 : 69	1 : 20
1.0	1.0	2.0	1 : 1400	1 : 1300	1 : 860	1 : 360	1 : 110
1.0	1.0	1.0	1 : 5700	1 : 500	1 : 3400	1 : 1400	1 : 420
2.5	1.4	1.0	1 : 68 000	1 : 60 000	1 : 41 000	1 : 17 000	1 : 5000
2.5	1.4	0.5	1 : 210 000	1 : 180 000	1 : 120 000	1 : 52 000	1 : 15 000
NK	NK	NK	1 : 1500	1 : 1400	1 : 910	1 : 380	1 : 110

NK = not known; MoM = multiple of normal median.

Disadvantages of Restricting Serum Screening to "Younger" Women

In spite of the benefits of serum screening using the new markers on all pregnant women regardless of their age, some screening centres still use maternal age as an initial screening test, offering women who are, say, aged 35 years or more, an amniocentesis immediately, and restricting serum screening to younger women. The risk cut-off level often adopted among these younger women is equivalent to the risk of a 35-year-old women having a pregnancy associated with Down's syndrome. This two-step policy has serious disadvantages, both as a public health measure and for the individual woman.

The policy, if applied to the population of England and Wales, would yield a detection rate of 72%, but 13% of women would need an amniocentesis. Since the same detection rate can be achieved with an amniocentesis rate of 10% if all women were screened, 3% of all women would have an amniocentesis unnecessarily (including 69% of those aged 35 years or more). Conversely, if this level of amniocentesis were thought acceptable, a detection rate of 77% could be achieved with the same amniocentesis rate (13%) if all women were screened; the two-step policy means a 5% reduction in the detection rate.

The case for rejecting the two-step policy is as compelling at the individual level as it is at the population level. While women aged under 35 years would be treated fairly in the sense that all women above a specified risk cut-off level would be offered an amniocentesis, those women aged 35 or more would not; those older women who would be routinely offered an amniocentesis include a large proportion who could be identified as being at low risk if they had the serum screening test; many would be found to have a risk of Down's syndrome that was lower than of a 20-year-old woman and would welcome the opportunity of accepting the small risk in return for avoiding the hazards of amniocentesis. This can be seen from Table 17.4. If the AFP, uE3 and hCG levels were 0.4, 0.4 and 2.0 MoM respectivley, the risk of Down's syndrome is so high that an amniocentesis would be indicated *regardless of the woman's age:* if they were 2.5, 1.4 or 0.5 respectively, the risk would be so low that there would be no need to offer any of the women an amniocentesis. With both of these extreme sets of biochemical results maternal age is irrelevant in judging whether a diagnostic amniocentesis is needed. This is not to say that age should be ignored; there are less extreme sets of biochemical results, such as those shown in the third row of Table 17.4, for which age would influence the decision to have an amniocentesis. Table 17.4 illustrates that age should not be used as an initial method of separating those who should have serum screening and those who should not.

Computer-Assisted Test Interpretation

As we have described, serum screening for Down's syndrome relies on the use of four variables simultaneously (maternal age, serum AFP, uE3 and hCG) to determine the risk of Down's syndrome in each woman. Women are screen-positive if their risk lies above a specified cut-off level or screen-negative if it falls below it. Such risk estimation can be performed by computer-assisted test interpretation (CATI). Indeed it would be difficult to accomplish the necessary

The Medical College of St Bartholomew's Hospital
Department of Environmental and Preventive Medicine Tel: 982 6143

NEURAL TUBE DEFECT AND DOWN'S SYNDROME SCREENING Report dated 14-FEB-89

Surname : SCOTT
Forename(s) : Barbara
ID Code : 142930
Date of Birth : 11-01-49
IMP : 02-10-88
Date of Sample : 09-02-89
Doctor : Dr A Jones
Report Address : 75 Harley Street
London W1

CLINICAL DETAILS AND TEST RESULTS
Previous NTD : None
Previous Down's : None
Maternal Age at EDD : 40 years
Scan Measure : BPD
Gestation at Date of Sample : 18 weeks 4 days (by dates)
: 18 weeks 4 days (by scan)
Weight : Not known
MS-AFP Level : 56 iu/mL; 1.27 MoM
MS-uE3 Level : 7.3 nmol/L; 1.65 MoM
MS-hCG Level : 8.2 iu/mL; 0.43 MoM

INTERPRETATION
Screening Result : Screen Negative
Risk of Down's : 1 in 5900 (at Term)
Comment : Although a greater risk of Down's would be expected from the maternal age alone (1 in 110) the risk is, in fact, lower on account of the level of AFP, uE3 and hCG

Fig. 17.1. Example of a report for a woman aged 40 years found to be at low risk of having a pregnancy associated with Down's syndrome. The names of the patient and her doctor have been changed and are fictitious.

The Medical College of St Bartholomew's Hospital
Department of Environmental and Preventive Medicine Tel: 982 6143

NEURAL TUBE DEFECT AND DOWN'S SYNDROME SCREENING Report dated 14-MAR-89

Surname	: HOLLIS
Forename(s)	: Mary
ID Code	: 104698
Date of Birth	: 01-01-69
IMP	: 14-11-88
Date of Sample	: 06-03-89
Doctor	: Dr H Smith
Report Address	: Southborough General Hospital

CLINICAL DETAILS AND TEST RESULTS

Previous NTD	: None	
Previous Down's	: None	
Maternal Age at EDD	: 20 years	
Scan Measure	: CRL	
Gestation at Date of Sample	: 16 weeks 0 days (by dates)	
	: 16 weeks 1 days (by scan)	
Weight	: 60.5 Kgs	
MS-AFP Level	: 12 iu/mL;	0.38 MoM
MS-uE3 Level	: 2.5 nmol/L;	0.58 MoM
MS-hCG Level	: 55.8 iu/mL;	1.81 MoM

INTERPRETATION

Screening Result	: ★★★Screen Positive★★★
Reason	: Increased risk of Down's syndrome
Risk of Down's	: 1 in 100 (at Term)
Comment	: The risk of Down's is greater than that expected from the maternal age alone (1 in 1500)

Fig. 17.2. Example of a report for a woman aged 20 years found to be at high risk of having a pregnancy associated with Down's syndrome. The names of the patient and her doctor have been changed and are fictitious.

risk estimation without this aid and the approach permits the risk estimate to take account of other factors such as maternal weight, ultrasound measures of gestational age, ethnic origin, diabetic status and multiple pregnancy which can affect the interpretation of the test. Fig. 17.1 shows an example of a CATI report from a 40-year-old woman found to have a high risk of having Down's syndrome pregnancy and 17.2 shows an example from a 20-year-old woman found to have a high risk.

Conclusion

Down's syndrome is the commonest cause of severe mental retardation. To be able to avoid the birth of 60% or more of affected pregnancies is a significant advance in antenatal screening. Undoubtedly antenatal screening and selective abortion is a second-best option, but in the absence of any method of primary prevention (for example, of a method to avoid the non-dysjunction of chromosome 21) screening is the only available preventive measure. It was more than 10 years before AFP screening for open neural tube defects was routinely offered and even now there are districts where the service is not offered. The challenge now is not more research in screening (although this will certainly take place); it is in the application of the technique so that it is provided for all women who want it with efficiency, economy and compassion.

References

Nørgaard-Pedersen B, Olsen Larsen S, Arends J, Svenstrup B, Tabor A (1990) Maternal serum markers in screening for Down's syndrome. Clin Genet 37: 35–43

Wald NJ, Cuckle HS (1989) Biochemical detection of neural tube defects and Down's syndrome. In: Turnbull Sir Alec, Chamberlain G (eds) Obstetrics. Churchill Livingstone, Edinburgh London Melbourne New York, pp269–289

Wald NJ, Cuckle HS, Densem JW, et al. (1988) Maternal serum screening for Down's syndrome in early pregnancy. Br Med J 297: 883–887

Wald NJ, Cuckle H, Nanchahal K (1989) Amniotic fluid acetylcholinesterase measurement in the prenatal diagnosis of open neural tube defects. Second report of the collaborative acetylcholinesterase study. Prenatal Diag 9: 813–829

Subject Index